Anaesthesia, Analgesia and Intensive Care

Anaesthesia, Analgesia and Intensive Care

Edited by

Anthony P Adams

Professor of Anaesthetics,
University of London,
United Medical and Dental Schools of Guy's
and St. Thomas's Hospitals;
Hon. Consultant Anaesthetist,
Guy's Hospital, London

and

Jeremy N Cashman

Consultant Anaesthetist,
St. George's Hospital, London

Edward Arnold

A division of Hodder & Stoughton
LONDON   MELBOURNE   AUCKLAND

© 1991 Anthony P Adams and Jeremy N Cashman

First published in Great Britain 1991

British Library Cataloguing in Publication Data

Adams, Tony
  Anaesthesia, analgesia and intensive care.
  I. Title II. Cashman, Jerry
  617.9

  ISBN 0 340 54927 0

Typeset in 10/11pt Palatino by Hewer Text Composition Services, Edinburgh.
Printed in Great Britain for Edward Arnold, a division of
Hodder and Stoughton Limited, Mill Road, Dunton Green,
Sevenoaks, Kent TN13 2YA by St Edmundsbury Press Ltd,
Bury St Edmunds, Suffolk, and bound by Hartnolls Ltd, Bodmin, Cornwall.

Preface

Anaesthesia is arguably the most useful subject taught in the undergraduate curriculum. The practical aspects encompassed by the specialty are taught in the clinical part of the course but rely much on basic scientific knowledge gained in the preclinical period. Clinical physiology and applied pharmacology instantly come to life as part of anaesthesia.

Anaesthesia is the largest single hospital specialty in Britain. Moreover, anaesthetists are gregarious and friendly people who are in the habit of keeping up-to-date by various means, including attending scientific meetings. On one such occasion the editors and their friends decided that the medical student was not comprehensively served by the existing range of textbooks and so decided to produce their own version. London University is responsible for the training of over 30 per cent of medical students in Great Britain and contains many of the most famous medical schools in the world. The contributors to this book thus represent practically every teaching centre in London.

This concept is a clear and simplified account of what anaesthesia entails. The basis of sound practice is a thorough understanding of the principles of anatomy, physiology, pharmacology and medicine in the care of patients. This is supported by accounts of how patients are prepared for operation, monitoring of vital signs, practical skills (such as vascular access, control of the airway), oxygen therapy, fluid therapy, electrolyte and acid-base balance, and common complications in surgical patients. Anaesthesia is not just about what happens in the operating theatre, therefore this book also covers intensive care, the provision of pain relief after operation, analgesia for women in labour, and the problems of patients with chronic pain. A whole chapter is devoted to the very important subject of cardiopulmonary resuscitation; in many centres now a student will not be 'signed up' unless he or she can demonstrate theoretical and practical proficiency in this field.

A solid undergraduate training in anaesthesia will equip the student with a far-ranging variety of practical skills, together with knowledge applicable to the wider practice of medicine, particularly as applied to the unconscious patient, trauma, life-threatening situations and the basic care of the critically ill.

The medical student needs to know how simple apparatus works so it can be applied safely in an emergency. He or she also needs to know about the advantages, disadvantages and problems concerning the use of local anaesthetics. Children present special problems. There is not enough time in the curriculum to learn all there is to know. However, this book aims to provide abundant information so that the student will be able to achieve the best use of his clinical attachment to the anaesthetist in the operating theatre. In due course he or she will find these skills, learnt through the discipline of 'anaesthesia', of enormous benefit in a wide variety of ways after graduation.

APA

London, 1991

JNC

The motto of the Association of Anaesthetists of Great Britain and Ireland is 'In Somno Securitas' or safety in sleep, while that of the American Society of Anesthesiologists is 'Vigilance'. The motto of the European Academy of Anaesthesiology is 'Dormitas Protego' or protection in sleep. The shield of the heraldic emblem of the new College of Anaesthetists (previously the Faculty of Anaesthetists of the Royal College of Surgeons of England) has the motto 'Divinum Sedare Dolorem' which may be translated as 'It is praiseworthy to relieve pain'; the supporters on the coat of arms are John Snow and Joseph Clover, the first two physician anaesthetists in the UK. Dr John Snow, the most important figure in the establishment of anaesthesia, gave anaesthesia in his private practice and in the leading London teaching hospitals of his time. Joseph Clover, a surgeon by training, inherited this mantle on Snow's death.

Contents

Contributors

A P Adams MB, BS, PhD, FCAnaes, FFARCS
Professor of Anaesthetics in the University of London, United Medical and Dental Schools of Guy's and St. Thomas's Hospitals; Hon. Consultant Anaesthetist, Guy's Hospital, London

R F Armstrong FFARCS
Consultant Anaesthetist, University College Hospital, London

B A Astley FFARCS
Consultant Anaesthetist, University College Hospital, London

W Aveling MA, MB, B Chir, FFARCS
Consultant Anaesthetist, The Middlesex Hospital, London

P K Barnes MB, BS, FFARCS, DA
Consultant Anaesthetist, Magill Department of Anaesthetics, Westminster Hospital, London

D R G Browne MBBS, MSc, FFARCS
Consultant Anaesthetist in charge of Intensive Care, The Royal Free Hospital, London

I Calder MB, ChB, DOGst RCOG, FFARCS
Consultant Anaesthetist, The National Hospital for Neurology and Neurosurgery and the Royal Free Hospital, London

J N Cashman BSc, MB, BS, FFARCS
Consultant Anaesthetist, St. George's Hospital, London

R H Ellis MB, BS, DRCOG, FCAnaes, FFARCS
Consultant Anaesthetist, St. Bartholomew's Hospital, London

J A Gil-Rodriguez MD, FFARCS, DA
Consultant Anaesthetist, St. Mary's Hospital, London

T H Howells MB, ChB, FCAnaes, DA
Emeritus Consultant Anaesthetist, The Royal Free Hospital, London

D M Justins MBBS, FCAnaes
Consultant Anaesthetist and Director, Pain Management Centre, St.
Thomas's Hospital, London

B Morgan MB, ChB, FCAnaes
Consultant Anaesthetist, Queen Charlotte's and Chelsea Hospital,
London

A P Rubin FFARCS
Consultant Anaesthetist, Charing Cross Hospital, London

K J Wark MBBS, FFARCS
Consultant Anaesthetist, Guy's Hospital, London

P M Tate MB, BS, FFARCS
Consultant Anaesthetist, The Royal London Hospital, London

D A Zideman BSc, MB, BS, FcAnaes
Consultant Anaesthetist, The Hammersmith Hospital, London

1

Anaesthesia and analgesia
A.P. Adams

- What is anaesthesia?
- Anaesthesia and the student
    scope, aims and objectives
- The beginnings of inhalation anaesthesia

What is anaesthesia?

Anaesthesia is the art or science of removing sensation of, and reaction to, a surgical procedure. Anaesthesia means loss of all modalities of sensation whether it be the sense of pain, touch, temperature or position sense. Analgesia means absence of the sensation of pain alone although other modalities may be preserved. General anaesthesia thus implies the loss of all forms of sensation throughout the whole body and is associated with unconsciousness. General analgesia doesn't exist because attempts to produce such a state inevitably end up producing general anaesthesia. Regional blocks are very popular because a region of the body such as a limb or limbs can be made either pain-free (regional analgesia) or free of all forms of sensation (regional anaesthesia). The term 'local' in the context of 'local anaesthesia' or 'local analgesia' is too loose and is best avoided.

Modern general anaesthesia comprises the triad of unconsciousness, muscle relaxation and analgesia. These effects are commonly produced by administering different drugs, each for its own specific desired action, rather than use of a single agent. At the conclusion of surgery the patient usually awakens spontaneously when the inhalational anaesthetic agents producing unconsciousness are discontinued. Specific antagonists may be given to 'reverse' the effects of certain drugs such as the non-depolarizing muscle relaxants (Chapter 3).

Sedation as used in dentistry must never be so deep that general anaesthesia is produced by accident. During i.v. sedation for dental procedures the operator must always be in verbal contact with the patient, i.e. the patient *must* always be awake. The same safeguard should apply to sedative techniques used in other areas of medicine where investigative or diagnostic procedures are carried out (e.g. gastroscopy, and radiological procedures). All these procedures require proper monitoring of the patient's vital functions (Chapter 5).

Anaesthesia is often described as a 'sharp-end' specialty. This means it is a specialty where correct decisions have to be made very quickly indeed, in a minute or two if not in seconds. Anaesthesia is thus an exciting speciality in which to practise. It is the largest hospital specialty in the National Health Service in the UK; there are about 2400 consultant anaesthetists. Nowadays about 50 per cent of graduates in medicine are women and the proportion of women in the UK at consultant anaesthetist grade is about 20 per cent. Anyone aspiring to a career in anaesthesia is best advised to complete at least 1 year in a subject such as general (internal) medicine, chest medicine or surgery, or cardiology. Anaesthesia has become a demand specialty both in the USA and in the UK. In the UK there are schemes whereby married women can elect to continue their training on a part-time basis in order to cope with domestic commitments. Although similar opportunities exist in other specialties competition for such posts in anaesthesia is strong; there are too few posts for the numbers wishing to take advantage of them.

The personality of the anaesthetist is an interesting one. He or she must have a good grasp of acute medicine and be good at practical procedures. The nature of anaesthetists is such that they tend to be interested in gadgets and to be innovative. The anaesthetist functions very much as a member of a team and indeed is often called upon to be a leader. He has often been termed the surgeon's physician because of his knowledge of medicine. Many an anaesthetist has the tale of a patient referred to the physicians for an opinion as to fitness for surgery. The physician says 'OK for anaesthesia but give him plenty of oxygen'! The anaesthetist is trained to be a careful observer and this skill alone should enable him to cope with over 75 per cent of problems which present with his patients during anaesthesia. The anaesthetist also has the ability to recognize problems instantly and thus react immediately to a crisis. It is not like other aspects of medicine where everybody goes away to cogitate and come up with a solution later. Some forms of anaesthesia have been likened to long periods when nothing much seems to be happening punctuated by short periods of acute activity of a crisis nature; this is the astronaut analogy. The psychologist Lisl Klein reported on the role of the anaesthetist in 1980. She remarked on the fact that the greatest pleasure was in seeing a patient, having undergone a potentially life-threatening situation, awaken and recover.

There is perhaps nothing more tragic than the death of an otherwise fit and healthy patient during a surgical operation, or during an anaesthetic for dentistry. The tragedy of the situation often reflects the triviality of the surgical procedure. Indeed, the first anaesthetic death recorded occurred in County Durham and concerned a 15-year-old girl Hannah Greener who, in January 1848 during an operation for the removal of an ingrowing toenail, died under the influence of chloroform.

However, there is a situation where continued existence can, arguably, be worse than if death had occurred. When things go wrong during anaesthesia and surgery, cerebral damage due to hypoxia is likely. Consider the situation where the patient is turned into a 'vegetable' — the vegetative state. The human misery involved is enormous and the damages awarded, depending on the expectation of life, occupation and responsibilities of the patient, prospective cost of nursing care and so on, can nowadays amount to over a million pounds.

Anaesthesia and the student

What does the medical student learn during his or her time attached to the anaesthetic firm? Clinical teaching in anaesthesia is arranged very much on a one to one basis so the student has — at last — the chance to be taught on a highly personal level. It is difficult, if not impossible, for more than one person at a time to be performing a practical procedure, whether it be setting up an i.v. infusion ('drip'), holding on a facemask and oxygenating an unconscious patient, using a laryngoscope and intubating the trachea with an endotracheal tube or a host of other 'hands on' practical procedures. All these procedures will stand the newly qualified doctor in very good stead from the very first day he or she starts as a houseman right up to the end of a professional career in medicine, irrespective of chosen specialty, in hospital or general practice. Every doctor must be able to practise skills learnt during the anaesthetic attachment with confidence: skills needed for effective cardiopulmonary resuscitation, management of the unconscious patient and so on.

Scope, aims and objectives
The aim of a period of attachment to an anaesthetic department is to produce a good doctor who is able to cope with a variety of critical and emergency situations. Most of these require intelligent application of expertise with practical procedures. He, or she, will also be trained to be able to sustain life in acute crisis situations until senior help can be summoned. It is a mistake to believe that the student is going to administer anaesthetics from the day he or she obtains a medical qualification just as it is unlikely that a qualified doctor will immediately go out and operate for acute appendicitis, but it may be argued that the skills taught in the anaesthetics part of the undergraduate curriculum are of more value to the newly qualified doctor than many other subjects.

A large amount of pharmacology, cardiopulmonary physiology and of the principles of clinical measurement can be learnt from the drugs and techniques used by anaesthetists. The expertise gained by the student from the anaesthetics attachment includes:
- Proficiency in the care of the unconscious patient; whether unconscious due to trauma, drugs or disease.
- Experience in the recognition and treatment of both airway obstruction and underventilation of the lungs.
- Awareness of the hypoxaemia that occurs without upper airway obstruction or with frank underventilation, and thoroughly understanding the principles of oxygen therapy.
- Becoming thoroughly experienced in the assessment of a patient's cardiovascular system, its current performance and any sudden changes.

- Becoming skilled in vascular access, i.e. venepuncture in general and setting up i.v. infusions ('drips') in particular; arterial puncture; measurement of central venous pressure. This necessitates applying the knowledge learnt in anatomy about the course of the veins in the body and appreciating the dangers of traumatizing related anatomical structures. A thorough knowledge of the requirements and range of equipment used (sizes and varieties of venous cannulae, i.v. infusion sets, connectors, fluid filters).
- Proficiency in the performance of cardio-pulmonary-cerebral resuscitation.
- Appreciation of the special problems of children.
- To practise observing the acute effects of drugs given intravenously.

The student has a marvellous opportunity to see the responses of his patient to several classes of drug.
- The effects of i.v. anaesthetic induction agents (p. 34).
- The effects of the neuromuscular-blocking drugs (muscle relaxants) (p. 38). Such agents vary in onset and duration and may produce important side-effects and interactions. The student also gets an opportunity to observe how the effects of such drugs are antagonized by antidotes.
- The use of potent analgesics in the relief of acute and chronic pain. How pain may be assessed and the various methods for the treatment of pain after surgical operations. The side-effects and complications of the opioid drugs (Chapter 18).
- The institution and maintenance of artificial ventilation (controlled mechanical ventilation of the lungs).
- An appreciation of the preoperative and postoperative needs of the surgical patient; anxiolysis, oxygenation, provision of analgesia, fluid requirements and acid-base balance (Chapter 6).
- An appreciation of critical care medicine (intensive care). In the intensive care (or therapy) unit (ICU/ITU) a host of clinical problems are encountered; respiratory and cardiovascular support in critically-ill patients suffering from a wide variety of medical and surgical conditions; total parenteral nutrition (Chapter 19).

The beginnings of inhalation anaesthesia

Substances which could make some surgical operations tolerable were known to the ancient civilizations of Greece and Assyria. In the thirteenth century mandrake was used as an anaesthetic, and analgesic 'potions' have been mentioned extensively in literature. The unreliability of many of these preparations helped in the success of that well-loved anaesthetic agent — alcohol. In the mid-sixteenth century Andreas Vesalius showed that animals could be kept alive by the rhythmic inflation of their lungs with air pumped through an opening in the windpipe with bellows. Robert Hooke, Robert Boyle's assistant, conducted experiments in 1667 on animals in which he was able to maintain life by blowing through their lungs with bellows. The possibility that some diseases could benefit from the inhalation of gases or vapours generated interest in the study of oxygen and the nature of respiration. Nitrous oxide was discovered by Joseph Priestley in 1772. He also discovered carbon dioxide and oxygen (1771). The analgesic properties of nitrous oxide were discovered by Humphry Davy who came within an ace of discovering its property as a general anaesthetic agent. Davy's research on nitrous oxide was published in 1800. Another Englishman, Henry Hill Hickman (1800–1830), explored the potential of carbon dioxide as an anaesthetic and found that temporary loss of consciousness in animals would result without interference with respiration. Hickman therefore deserves credit as having been the first to prove that the pain of a surgical operation can be abolished by the inhalation of a gas. However, he was unable to persuade surgeons at home or abroad to allow him to try the gas on their patients.

William Thomas Green Morton, a dentist, experimented with sulphuric ether and painlessly extracted a tooth from Eben Frost on 30 September 1846. However, anaesthesia really began on 16 October 1846 when Morton gave the first successful public demonstration of general anaesthesia. This took place at the Massachusetts General Hospital, and the operating theatre, now a lecture theatre, is called the 'Ether Dome'. The surgeon was Dr John C Warren who, having painlessly removed a tumour from the neck of a young man named Gilbert Abbott who was under the effects of Morton's ether, is said to have exclaimed to the assembled onlookers 'gentlemen this is no humbug!'. Thus began the era of painless surgery but no name had yet been coined for the discovery.

Morton called it 'The Letheon', a name derived from the river Lethe of Greek mythology. Mythological belief was that a draught of the water of Lethe could erase all painful memories. However, Oliver Wendell Holmes wrote to Morton at the latter's request on 21 November 1846:

Dear Sir, Everybody wants to have a hand in a great discovery. All I do is to give you a hint or two, as to names, or the name, to be applied to the state produced by the agent. The state should, I think, be called 'Anaesthesia', the adjective will be 'Anaesthetic'. Thus we might say 'the state of anaesthesia', or 'the anaesthetic state'. The means employed would properly be called the anti-aesthetic agent. Perhaps it might be allowable to say anaesthetic agent, but this admits of question. I would have a name pretty soon, and consult some accomplished scholar, such as President Everett or Bigelow, Snr. before fixing upon the terms which will be repeated by the tongues of every civilized race of mankind. Respectfully yours, Oliver Wendell Holmes.

On 28 November 1846 Dr Jacob Bigelow wrote to his friend and colleague Dr Francis Boott, an American expatriate living in London, to tell him of the events surrounding the introduction of 'a new anodyne process' (ether anaesthesia) that day in Boston. Boott arranged with a friend of his, James Robinson, a leading London dentist, to carry out some experiments. The result was that on Saturday 19 December 1846, James Robinson gave ether to a young woman, Miss Lonsdale, and then removed a diseased molar tooth in the presence of Dr Boott and his family. The surgeon Robert Liston and William Squire, then a medical student, had both seen Robinson at work, and 2 days later they performed the first major operation under ether (administered by Squire). This was the amputation of the leg of a butler,

William Churchill, at University College Hospital, London. It was some-thing of a paradox that the first textbook of anaesthesia *A Treatise on the Inhalation of the Vapour of Ether* should have been published in Britain, by Robinson, rather than in America.

Others, however, had experimented with sulphuric ether and nitrous oxide before Morton's classic demonstration. William Crawford Long in Georgia, USA, had used ether 6 years before Morton but possibly because of the religious intolerance of the day he never published his findings until December 1849, 3 years after Morton's discovery had been reported in the *Boston Medical and Surgical Journal* in 1846 by both Bigelow and Warren.

Horace Wells, a dentist in Hartford, Connecticut, and Gardner Quincy Colton, another dentist, discovered the analgesic effects of nitrous oxide or 'laughing gas'. Wells noticed that a student, who badly bruised his leg whilst indulging in a laughing gas frolic organized in Hartford in December 1844 by Colton, felt no pain. Wells obtained permission from Dr Warren to speak to a surgical class at Harvard Medical School and concluded by administering nitrous oxide to a boy for the extraction of a tooth. Unfortunately for Wells the boy cried out and the audience pronounced the discovery to be a hoax, although later the boy admitted that he hadn't felt any pain. If Wells' demonstration had been deemed successful he would have been credited as the discoverer of surgical anaesthesia. He used the gas successfully in his own dental practice in Hartford in 1845. Wells then, is credited with conceiving the idea of anaesthesia and publicizing the possibility of its use.

James Young Simpson, an Edinburgh obstetrician, introduced chloroform as an alternative to ether for the relief of pain in childbirth. He got the idea from David Waldie, a Liverpool chemist. Simpson and his assistants tried chloroform on themselves and, satisfied as to its properties, intro-duced it immediately into his practice. There were strong religious objec-tions to the use of chloroform in childbirth but Simpson waged a successful campaign. The use of chloroform in obstetrics was assured when Queen Victoria accepted its use during the birth of Prince Leopold, her eighth child, on 7 April 1853; John Snow administered the chloroform intermittently on a handkerchief to produce analgesia (the so-called *chloroform à la reine*).

Further reading

Academic departments of anaesthesia in undergraduate education: an undervalued resource.
    London: The College of Anaesthetists.
Adams A P, Hewitt P B, Rogers M C, (eds). *Emergency Anaesthesia.* London: Edward
    Arnold, 1986.
Career guide to anaesthetics. London: Association of Anaesthetists of Great Britain &
    Ireland.
Edmonds-Seal J, Eaton J W, McNeilly R H. Part-time training for doctors with
    domestic commitments (DDC). *Anaesthesia* 1980; **35**: 1027.
Edmonds-Seal J, Mitchell J V. The Oxford training scheme in anaesthesia and other
    matters. *Anaesthesia* 1979; **34**: 776–83.

Ellis R H. *James Robinson on the inhalation of the vapour of ether*. (Facsimile edition of *A treatise on the inhalation of the vapour of ether for the prevention of pain in surgical operations* by James Robinson originally published in London by Webster & Company, 1847.) London: Ballière Tindall, 1983.

Gordon R. *The sleep of life*. Harmondsworth: Penguin Books, 1976.

Keys T E. *The history of surgical anesthesia*. New York: Dover Publications, 1945.

Klein L, 1980. *The role of the anaesthetist. An exploratory study*. London: Association of Anaesthetists of Great Britain & Ireland.

Royal College of Physicians of London. *Resuscitation from Cardiopulmonary Arrest. Training and Organisation*, 1987.

Sykes W S. *Essays on the first hundred years of anaesthesia*. London: Livingstone, 1961: Vols I & II.

Sykes W S. In: Ellis R H, ed. *Essays on the first five hundred years of anaesthesia*. London: Churchill Livingstone, 1982: Vol III.

Theatre Safeguards. The Medical Defence Union, 1988.

Zorab, J S M. Applying for a post in anaesthesia. *Anaesthesia* 1980; **35**: 601–607.

2

Anaesthetic physiology
J.N. Cashman

- Cardiovascular physiology
    - factors influencing cardiac output
    - factors influencing peripheral resistance
    - factors influencing blood pressure
    - cardiovascular effects of anaesthetic agents
    - physiological responses to hypovolaemia
    - special circulations
- Respiratory physiology
    - the mechanics of respiration
    - pulmonary gas exchange
    - gas transport to the periphery
    - control of respiration
- Neurophysiology
    - sensory mechanisms
    - motor mechanisms
    - autonomic nervous system
- Haematological system
    - blood components
    - haemostasis
    - blood groups
    - blood transfusion
- Renal physiology
- Gastrointestinal physiology

Cardiovascular physiology

The main purpose of the circulatory system is to deliver oxygen and nutrients to the body and to remove the waste products of metabolism. It has other subsidiary functions including a role in thermoregulation.

The circulatory system is comprised of the heart, a four-chambered pump which pumps blood into the arterial system. Also the arteries which are distensible and serve to convert the pulsatile ejection of the heart into the steady flow which is presented to the arterioles (the site of greatest vascular resistance) and then to the capillary bed. Finally blood returns to the heart via the veins which act as capacitance vessels, with 60–70 per cent of the circulating blood volume present in the venous system.

The heart receives a sympathetic and a parasympathetic innervation. The former from the superior, middle and inferior cardiac ganglia of the sympathetic chain (T_{1-5}) and the latter via the vagi (cranial nerve X). Sympathetic stimulation increases not only heart rate by increasing the rhythmicity of the sino-atrial (sa) node (chronotropy), but it also increases the speed and force of contraction of myocardial muscle (inotropy). Vagal stimulation profoundly reduces the rate of impulse generation by the sa node but there is no vagal innervation of the ventricles. The vascular tree, with the exception of the special circulations (see below), is overwhelmingly under sympathetic control.

Factors influencing cardiac output

The average adult has a blood volume of 5–6 litres and a resting cardiac output of 5.5 litres per minute. Cardiac output is the product of heart rate and stroke volume.

stroke volume → cardiac output ← heart

Stroke volume

Stroke volume is dependent on the size of the heart, the contractility of the myocardium and on the venous return.

The size of the heart is dependent on blood volume and vascular capacity. In normal circumstances blood volume is constant (but see Physiological responses to hypovolaemia), with the result that it is changes in vascular capacity which mainly influence the size of the heart. Venous 'pooling' is

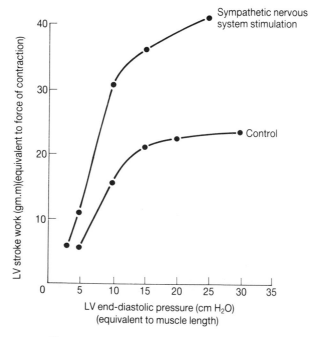

Fig. 2.1   Ventricular function curves.

associated with accommodation of a larger volume of blood in the veins with less available for return to the heart; this reduction in venous return results in a fall in cardiac output.

The contractility of the myocardium can be strikingly influenced either by increasing the initial length of the cardiac muscle fibres (Starling's Law) or by increasing the power of contraction of fibres at any given length, usually as a result of sympathetic nervous system stimulation. According to Starling's Law the initial diastolic length of ventricular muscle fibres determines their force of contraction, thus contraction is increased with increasing ventricular filling (Fig. 2.1). The normal heart never expels the whole of the end-diastolic content when it beats, there being a small residual volume. The amount of blood ejected in systole expressed as a percentage of the end-diastolic volume is called the 'ejection fraction' and is commonly reduced in heart failure.

Sympathetic nervous system stimulation also increases the contractile power of cardiac muscle at any particular load (i.e. muscle length) by increasing its velocity of contraction (Fig. 2.2). Primary and secondary

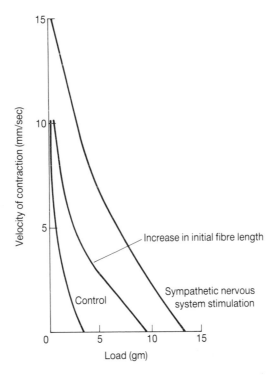

An increase in the initial fibre length results in the development of a greater isometric force (P_o) but no increase in maximum velocity of contraction (V_{max}).

An increase in sympathetic nervous system activity is associated with an increase in both P_o and V_{max}.

Fig. 2.2 Ventricular force-velocity curves.

sympathetic stimulation, circulating catecholamines and certain drugs including digitalis glycosides, dopamine and beta-sympathomimetic agents, will increase myocardial contractility, whilst trauma, hypoxia, acidosis and most anaesthetic drugs will decrease myocardial contractility (see below).

Venous return is influenced by a number of factors including gravity, muscle and respiratory pumps, arteriolar and venous tone and blood volume.

Heart rate

The normal heart rate of 60–80 beats per minute is generated by the sa node, however, heart rate is influenced by a number of factors.

Autonomic tone

The balance between the sympathetic and parasympathetic nervous systems. At rest the heart beats at a rate influenced by vagal tone with little tonic influence by cardiac sympathetic nerves. Abolition of vagal tone (e.g. by administration of atropine) results in a dramatic rise in heart rate. During acute haemorrhage increased sympathetic discharge will speed up heart rate. Input from higher centres, such as occurs in response to anxiety and pain, will also influence heart rate.

Baroreceptors

High-pressure stretch receptors exist in the first part of the carotid arteries (carotid sinus), the aortic arch and the ventricles of the heart, whilst low-pressure stretch receptors exist in the atria and pulmonary trunk. All of these baroreceptors, with the exception of the carotid sinus (cranial IX), are vagally innervated and provide a negative-feedback mechanism for cardiovascular control. Falls in systemic arterial pressure are associated with a decrease in firing rate of the carotid sinus nerve resulting in reflex increases in heart rate and vice versa. The low-pressure stretch receptors are mainly involved in blood volume regulation but rises in venous return cause a reflex rise in heart rate (Bainbridge reflex).

Chemoreceptors

Heart rate is also influenced by hypoxia and hypercarbia. Stimulation of the carotid-body chemoreceptors causes vasoconstriction, reflex hypertension and bradycardia. In spontaneously breathing subjects, secondary reflexes arising from lung afferents override the chemoreceptor reflex and cause a tachycardia. The chemoreceptors exert little effect in normal circumstances but in conditions of lack of oxygen (see Physiological responses to hypovolaemia) their powerful discharge helps to maintain systolic blood pressure.

Miscellaneous

Circulating hormones such as thyroxine and catecholamines will also influence heart rate.

Factors influencing peripheral resistance

Peripheral resistance depends on two variables: blood viscosity and size of blood vessels.

viscosity → peripheral resistance ← size of blood vessel

Viscosity

The relative viscosity of blood increases with cooling and also as haematocrit rises above its normal value of 45 per cent (Fig. 2.3). Plasma proteins which are necessary for axial streaming in the smaller blood vessels reduce viscosity.

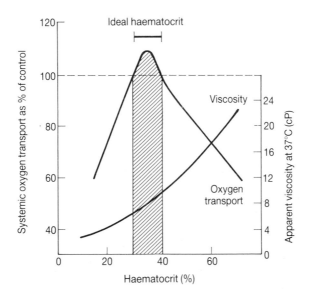

Fig. 2.3   Whole blood viscosity and oxygen transport as functions of haematocrit.

Blood vessel size

The site of greatest peripheral resistance is the arterioles, and arteriolar tone is maintained by sympathetic activity. The blood vessels respond to circulating catecholamines and also receive a sympathetic innervation from the vasomotor centre. The vasomotor centre receives input from baroreceptors, chemoreceptors, higher centres, sensory nerves, the respiratory centre and also directly in response to hypoxia and hypercarbia. Increased sympathetic activity results in vasoconstriction and decreased activity results in vasodilatation. Vasodilator nerves occur only in the blush areas and are of no significance in blood pressure control. Axon reflex from stimulation of sensory (pain) fibres, tissue injury and hypersensitivity produces cutaneous vasodilatation and release of histamine (triple response), which in turn produces marked dilatation of arterioles and capillaries.

Increased activity of secretomotor nerves leads to production of vaso-dilator substances such as bradykinin. Metabolites will also produce vasodilatation, especially if allowed to accumulate as occurs with increased metabolism (exercise) or decreased flow (tourniquet, cross clamping).

Vasoconstriction will occur in response to serotonin which is released from platelets at the site of tissue injury and in response to renin–angiotensin–aldosterone release. Hypoxia and hypercarbia have an indirect vasoconstrictor action via the chemoreceptors and vasomotor centre, but a local vasodilator effect on blood vessels. Cutaneous vasoconstriction occurs in response to cold.

Factors influencing blood pressure

The amount of blood ejected by the heart (cardiac output) balanced against the resistance to flow offered by the peripheral circulation (peripheral resistance) determines the pressure generated in the great vessels.

$$\text{stroke volume} \rightarrow \text{cardiac output} \leftarrow \text{heart rate}$$
$$\downarrow$$
$$\text{blood pressure}$$
$$\uparrow$$
$$\text{viscosity} \rightarrow \text{peripheral resistance} \leftarrow \text{size of blood vessel}$$

Cardiovascular effects of anaesthetic agents

Inhalational agents

All inhalational agents are direct depressants of myocardial cells to a greater or lesser extent and all cause vasodilatation due to a direct effect on vascular smooth muscle. These effects are dose dependent. Halothane and enflurane produce a reduction in blood pressure mainly as a result of decreases in cardiac output secondary to myocardial depression, whereas the reduction in blood pressure associated with isoflurane is mainly due to a decrease in peripheral resistance.

The three agents differ in their effects on heart rate. Halothane tends to cause a decrease and isoflurane an increase in heart rate whereas enflurane has little overall effect. Ventricular dysrhythmias occur only very rarely with enflurane and isoflurane but may occur with halothane, especially in the presence of hypoxia and respiratory acidosis. Nodal rhythm is also commonly associated with halothane.

All inhalational agents depress the baroreceptor reflex, with halothane and enflurane being the most potent and isoflurane the least. The result is an impaired ability to increase heart rate in response to falls in blood pressure.

Intravenous agents

Most intravenous agents (except ketamine) produce different degrees of reduction in myocardial contractility and of vasodilatation, and they reduce sympathetic discharge. Thus cardiac output is reduced due to decreased myocardial contractility (thiopentone>propofol>etomidate), heart rate slows due to decreased sympathetic tone and venous return is reduced due to vasodilatation. However, the baroreceptor reflex remains largely intact and there is a reflex increase in heart rate in response to hypotension in order to maintain cardiac output.

Physiological responses to hypovolaemia

Hypovolaemia results in an inadequate flow of blood perfusing the capillaries of various tissues and organs with subsequent damage to those tissues and organs. Causes of hypovolaemic shock include haemorrhage, fluid seepage from wounds or burn sites, severe electrolyte disturbances (with removal of water from the intravascular compartment) and tissue dehydration, as occurs in cholera.

Compensatory mechanisms mean that the sudden loss of up to 30 per cent of the circulating blood volume, and also chronic losses of larger volumes, can be tolerated. Acute blood loss results in a decrease in blood pressure with baroreceptor-mediated reflex vasoconstriction in resistance and capacitance vessels which increases peripheral resistance. The reduced blood volume is associated with decreased cardiac filling which in turn results in a decline in cardiac output. However, the increased sympathetic discharge will result not only in an increase in heart rate but also in force of contraction which tends to maintain cardiac output. Decreased capillary filling favours the net movement of fluid into the vascular compartment. This mechanism can restore 10–15 per cent of the blood volume within 5 minutes but is associated with haemodilution. Vasoconstriction is associated with a fall in glomerular filtration with concomitant fluid retention and release of renin. Formation of angiotensin and aldosterone cause further vasoconstriction and water retention. The reduced blood volume and decreased tissue blood

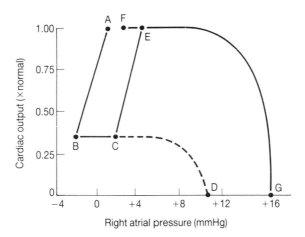

A – B : Effect of acute blood loss
B – A : Effect of prompt volume replacement
B – C (– D) : Effect of prolonged hypovolaemia with decreased myocardial contractility
C – E : Effect of delayed volume replacement to control cardiac output
E – F : Effect of recovery of myocardial function
E – G : Irreversible 'shock'

Fig. 2.4 Relationship between cardiac output and right atrial pressure during the course of haemorrhagic shock.

flow lead to a decrease in oxygen content of mixed venous blood. Chemoreceptor stimulation results in increased respiration and in cardio-vascular stimulation. Increased levels of circulating catecholamines cause hyperglycaemia and increased lipid mobilization, whilst increased levels of cortisol cause protein catabolism and glycogenolysis.

All of these compensatory mechanisms will maintain blood pressure and cardiac output to the vital organs. However, if hypovolaemia is progressive or prolonged the compensatory mechanisms begin to fail. This is because cellular hypoxia and the build-up of lactate and other metabolites, with resultant acidosis, cause a deterioration in cellular function. Prolonged myocardial hypoxia is associated with a deterioration in cardiac function and a failing Starling relationship, with progressive impairment of myocardial contractility (Fig. 2.4). In the peripheral circulation anaerobisis and acidosis cause vascular relaxation; with vasodilatation there is release of toxins from the ischaemic capillary beds. This endotoxaemia further depresses myocardial function. Eventually these changes become irreversible.

Special circulations

Coronary circulation

About 80 per cent of the total coronary flow occurs in diastole. Increases in heart rate reduce coronary flow due to a reduction in the diastolic period. During systole, flow in the subendocardial region is limited by the heart's contraction hence this layer's greater sensitivity to ischaemia.

Hypoxia is one of the most potent factors controlling coronary flow. The Arterio-venous (A–V) oxygen difference is very large so that increases in oxygen demand can only be met by increases in flow rather than increases in extraction. Thus coronary flow is directly related to coronary oxygen consumption. Hypercarbia and acidosis have only a slight dilator effect.

Adrenaline and noradrenaline increase coronary flow secondary to an increase in contractile force and metabolism. Sympathetic nervous system stimulation increases flow and the resultant hyperaemia outlasts the period of stimulation.

Cerebral circulation

The cerebral circulation exhibits very marked autoregulation, having a constant blood flow over a wide range of perfusion pressures. The cerebral circulation is unaffected by the sympathetic vasoconstrictor nerves. Local chemical changes are the most important determinants of cerebral vascular resistance and of these hypercarbia is the main factor affecting cerebral blood vessels. Increases in carbon dioxide cause dilatation but hypoxia also has a mild vasodilator effect. Inhalational anaesthetic agents all have a vasodilator effect (halothane>enflurane>isoflurane).

Pulmonary circulation

The pulmonary circulation is a low-pressure system, with only a limited capacity to alter vascular resistance. Passive changes in pulmonary vascular resistance occur as a result of changes in cardiac output, gravity (posture), and respiration (spontaneous or controlled). Active changes in pulmonary vascular resistance occur in response to alterations in blood gases. Hypoxia is a potent vasoconstrictor and localized hypoxia plays an important part in the distribution of pulmonary blood flow. Chronic hypoxia results in increases in pulmonary artery pressure and right ventricular hypertrophy. Hyperoxia can cause vasodilatation whilst hypercarbia and acidosis cause mild vasoconstriction. The autonomic innervation of the pulmonary vessels plays little part in the control of vessel size.

Renal circulation

Autoregulation involving the renin–angiotensin system maintains flow over a blood pressure range of 50–180 mmHg. Hypoxia causes vasoconstriction and hypercarbia causes vasodilatation. Sympathetic stimulation causes vasoconstriction. Most anaesthetic agents reduce blood flow.

Respiratory physiology

The major function of the respiratory system is to ensure effective gas exchange whereby oxygen necessary for cellular metabolism enters the bloodstream and carbon dioxide is removed from it.

The mechanics of respiration

Respiration

Quiet breathing is characterized by the rhythmic expansion and relaxation of the thorax and lungs. The diaphragm, innervated by the phrenic nerves (cervical roots 3, 4 and 5), is the most important muscle of ventilation. The external intercostal muscles, innervated by the intercostal nerves, are less important and paralysis of the intercostal muscles alone, as may occur with excessive spread of local anaesthetic from an epidural, does not seriously impair breathing. The accessory muscles of inspiration, which include pectoralis major, the scalene muscles and the sternomastoids, are not used during quiet breathing. Expiration is a passive process resulting from the elastic recoil of the lungs. Active expiration, as occurs during exercise and in hyperventilation states, primarily involves the muscles of the anterior abdominal wall, assisted by the internal intercostal muscles. Anaesthesia results in decreased intercostal activity and impairment of diaphragmatic activity.

Lung volumes

Measurement of the amount of air contained in the lungs throughout the respiratory cycle is an important assessment of lung function. The size of the thorax and lungs determines the lung capacities, whilst lung volumes are determined by inspiratory and expiratory effort. There are four volumes and four capacities (Fig. 2.5).

Tidal volume (V_T) is the volume of gas inhaled during a normal inspiration. *Residual volume* (RV) is the volume of gas remaining in the lungs at the end of a maximal expiratory effort. It normally comprises 20–25 per cent of the total lung capacity, but this value increases with age and with any decrease in

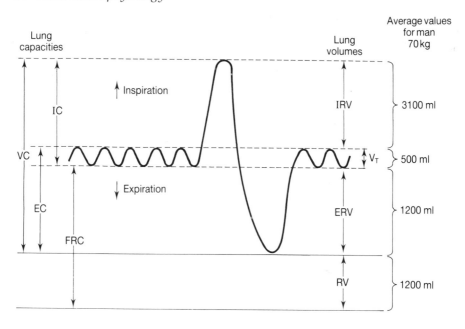

Fig. 2.5   Lung spirometry.

elastic recoil of the lungs. *Vital capacity* (VC) is the volume of gas entering the lungs following a maximal inspiratory effort from the RV. *Functional residual capacity* (FRC) is the volume of gas remaining in the lung at the end of a normal expiration. FRC is the most important of all the lung volumes because it represents gas remaining in the lung which continues to take part in gas exchange; it is therefore a measure of oxygen reserve. Anaesthesia and surgery (particularly abdominal and thoracic) are associated with reductions in FRC and VC. After abdominal surgery FRC can fall to 70 per cent of its preoperative level and remain depressed for up to 7 days. Causes of a fall in FRC include

- increased elastic recoil of the lungs
- changes in inspiratory and expiratory muscle activity
- small airways closure and subsequent trapping of gas
- cephalad displacement of the diaphragm

Static and dynamic properties of the lungs

During inspiration the respiratory muscles must work to overcome the elastic recoil forces of the lungs and thoracic wall (static lung properties) and also the non-elastic resistive forces including resistance to the flow of gas through the airways, surface active agents, shearing forces and tissue resistance (dynamic lung forces). To overcome the non-elastic components requires approximately 30 per cent of the energy expenditure of breathing, and resistance to gas flow constitutes nearly 80 per cent of this energy waste. Work done to combat resistance forces is maximal in mid-inspiration.

Static compliance is a measure of elasticity and is defined as the relation between lung volume and the pressure required to generate that volume. It is comprised of lung compliance and chest wall compliance, both of which affect FRC. Overall compliance decreases under anaesthesia. Chest wall compliance is also reduced in obese patients.

There are 23 generations of airways, with the 23rd generation airways having a total cross-sectional airway diameter greatly in excess of that of the trachea. The major site of airways resistance to gas flow is at the level of the 3rd and 4th generation airways; 60–70 per cent of the total airways resistance to breathing occurs in these large generation airways (with 20 per cent from airways less than 2 mm in diameter and 10 per cent from the trachea and upper airways; Fig. 2.6). In addition, airways resistance increases with decreasing lung volume.

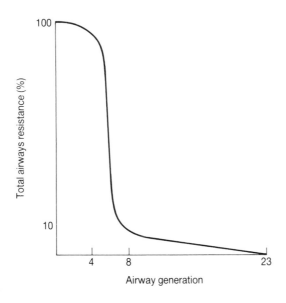

Fig. 2.6 Influence of airway generation on resistance to gas flow.

Some alveoli close off from the rest of the respiratory tract, especially at very low lung volumes. The closing volume is that volume of gas remaining in the lungs at which the airways collapse and trapping of gas occurs. Closing volume increases with age and may even move into the V_T range.

Pulmonary gas exchange

Alveolar ventilation

Alveolar ventilation refers to the volume of gas entering the alveoli per minute and taking part in gas exchange and can be considered as the product of tidal minus dead-space volume and respiratory rate.

The *dead space* is that portion of the airways not available for gas exchange. The ratio of physiological dead space to V_T (normally less than 30 per cent in young adults) represents wasted ventilation and is increased under general anaesthesia. Physiological dead space is made up of anatomical and alveolar dead space. Alveolar dead space is the portion of lung which has the potential for gas exchange and which although remaining ventilated is not perfused. Alveolar dead space increases with age, reduction in cardiac output, pulmonary embolism, hypothermia, general anaesthesia and induced hypotension. Anatomical dead space is made up of that portion of the lungs and conducting airways which do not have the capacity for gas exchange. Anaesthetic circuits and equipment will increase anatomical dead space.

Hypoventilation will result in hypoxia and can occur following the administration of CNS depressant drugs (e.g. narcotics and general anaesthetic agents). Other causes of hypoventilation include:

- decreased central drive, as occurs with trauma and drugs
- spinal cord lesions (above C3–5), also poliomyelitis
- nerve lesions — peripheral neuropathy and Guillain-Barré syndrome
- neuromuscular junction defects e.g. myasthenia gravis
- muscle defects/weakness e.g. myopathies
- rib cage deformities e.g. flail chest and kyphoscoliosis
- airways obstruction e.g. asthma

Gas diffusion across alveolar membrane

Gas exchange occurs at the level of the alveolar-capillary membrane, where only 2–3 cells separate alveolar gas from the bloodstream. Oxygen and carbon dioxide cross the alveolar membrane by diffusion. The rate of diffusion depends upon the concentration gradient across the alveolar membrane (alveolar P_{O_2} = 13.3 kPa or 100 mmHg, capillary P_{O_2} = 5.3 kPa or 40 mmHg, hence driving pressure = 8 kPa or 60 mmHg), the area available for diffusion (enormous since the total surface area of the lungs equals 50–100 m^2) and the rate of removal of oxygen and carbon dioxide. In the case of oxygen, removal is by capillary blood with equilibrium taking place within one third of the transmit time for blood in an alveolar capillary. In addition, the rate of transfer of oxygen also depends on its rate of chemical combination with haemoglobin (which in its turn depends on the shape and position of the oxygen dissociation curve). Impaired diffusion of oxygen will result from any pathological process which increases the thickness of the alveolar-capillary membrane (e.g. lung fibrosis) or which results in a reduced pulmonary blood flow. The rate of diffusion of carbon dioxide from capillary into alveolus is 20 times more rapid than that of oxygen in the reverse direction. Pulmonary gas exchange has been shown to be impaired under general anaesthesia and this may be the result in part of changes in Ventilation/perfusion $\dot{V}/\dot{Q}$ distribution and also falls in FRC.

$\dot{V}/\dot{Q}$ matching

Ventilation (V) must be matched with perfusion (Q) for optimal gas exchange. In the upright subject at normal lung volumes, alveoli at the apex are well inflated and larger than those at the base. Therefore for a given volume of gas inhaled there is a proportionately greater change in the basal as opposed to apical alveoli. The bottom of the lung expands more than the apex in response to a given pressure; disease states exaggerate these differences enormously. Thus ventilation at the top of the lung is less than at the bottom. Alveoli at the base of the lungs may be compressed and collapse, especially with splinting of the diaphragm as occurs in obesity, abdominal distension and postoperative abdominal pain.

These changes in regional ventilation are matched by a similar but more marked pattern of variation in regional blood flow, with the bases much better perfused than the apices. This distribution is mainly the result of hydrostatic forces, but at low lung volumes, blood flow to the apices may exceed basal blood flow. Pulmonary artery pressure may not be sufficient to keep capillaries at the apex of the lung open all the time (<hydrostatic pressure), capillaries therefore flip open during systole only.

Regional variations in perfusion may occur as a result of hypoxic pulmonary vasoconstriction (a reduced volume of blood flow through underventilated regions). The hypoxic segment is associated with vascular constriction and therefore a decrease in flow. Matching of ventilation to perfusion is obviously crucial to efficient gas exchange. Anaesthesia can markedly impair this matching. The distribution of ventilation has been shown to be shifted towards the non-dependent regions of the lungs due to changes in chest-wall shape and motion, and to airways closure in the dependent parts of the lung. Hypoxic pulmonary vasoconstriction is inhibited by all anaesthetic vapours with the result that unventilated regions may remain perfused thus significantly increasing the shunt.

Gas transport to the periphery

The major proportion of oxygen is transported in combination with haemo-globin with only a very small proportion transported dissolved in plasma.

The amount of oxygen dissolved in blood is proportional to its partial pressure. In the lungs, normal arterialized blood with an O_2 tension of 13.3 kPa (100 mmHg) contains 0.3 ml of oxygen per 100 ml blood.

Normal adult haemoglobin consists of 4 protein chains (2 α and 2 β) with a haem group attached to a histidine residue. Iron in haemoglobin is in the ferrous form but may be oxidized to the ferric form by a number of drugs, resulting in methaemoglobin. The bonding between chains determines the shape of the haemoglobin molecule which in turn influences the affinity of the haemoglobin molecule for oxygen. The affinity of haemoglobin for oxygen is further influenced by temperature, pH, erythrocyte levels of 2–3 DPG and even the number of oxygen atoms attached (Fig. 2.7).

Oxygen combines loosely and reversibly with haemoglobin. Each mole-cule of haemoglobin can combine with four atoms of oxygen, but the association of each atom of oxygen alters the affinity of the haemoglobin molecule to associate with subsequent atoms of oxygen, resulting in the characteristic sigmoid shape of the oxygen-dissociation curve. This sigmoid shape has many physiological advantages. Thus minor changes in alveolar Po_2 have little effect on the flat upper part of the curve whereas the steep middle part of the curve means that large amounts of oxygen are released to the tissues with relatively small falls in Po_2, thus maintaining oxygenation of the tissues. The oxygen dissociation curve may be shifted to the right or left. A shift to the left is associated with an increased tendency for oxygen to be released to the tissues. A fall in pH, a rise in CO_2, a rise in temperature

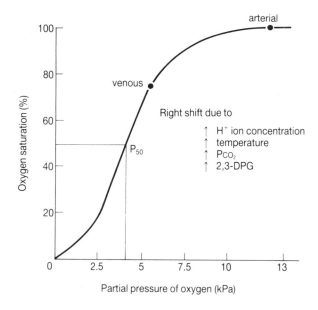

Fig. 2.7   Oxygen haemoglobin dissociation curve.

and increases in 2–3 DPG levels all favour a right shift and hence greater unloading of oxygen to the tissues.

Carbon dioxide is carried in the blood in one of three ways: in solution, in the form of bicarbonate and attached to protein as carbamino compounds. Carbon dioxide is twenty times more soluble than oxygen and carriage of CO_2 in solution plays a significant role.

Most of the CO_2 carried in the blood is present in the form of bicarbonate. Bicarbonate is formed as a result of hydration of carbon dioxide by the action of carbonic anhydrase, present in the red blood cell, to form carbonic acid. Carbonic acid in turn ionizes to form a hydrogen ion and a bicarbonate ion.

$$H_2O + CO_2 \rightleftharpoons H_2CO_3 \rightleftharpoons H^+ + HCO_3^-$$

The haemoglobin within the red cell combines with H^+ in order to prevent a change of pH and the bicarbonate ion diffuses out of the cell in exchange for a chloride ion which moves into the cell (the chloride shift). Buffering of H^+ utilizes oxyhaemoglobin resulting in the formation of reduced haemoglobin and the release of oxygen to the tissues. This process is reversed in the alveolar capillary. The fact that the deoxygenation of blood increases its ability to carry carbon dioxide is known as the Haldane effect.

Control of respiration

Respiration is an automatic process under the control of a central respiratory centre located in the medulla of the brain stem. The respiratory centre receives inputs from central and peripheral chemoreceptors, irritant and mechanoreceptors in the lungs and from higher centres in the central nervous system.

Chemical control of breathing

Peripheral chemoreceptors are located in the carotid body and also in the aortic arch (although the latter probably predominantly subserve circulatory responses). They have a very high blood flow in relation to their size and hence only a very small arterio-venous oxygen difference exists. The peripheral chemoreceptors rapidly respond to falls in the partial pressure of oxygen but will also respond to rises in H^+ concentration and in the partial pressure of carbon dioxide. The peripheral chemoreceptors are thought to respond to the oscillations in partial pressure of carbon dioxide that occur during the normal respiratory cycle.

At rest at least 60 per cent of the respiratory drive is derived from the central chemoreceptors. The central chemoreceptors are located on the ventro-lateral aspect of the medulla and respond to changes in CSF H^+ concentration. The CSF pH is controlled within very narrow limits, however carbon dioxide freely crosses the blood–brain barrier with the result that the partial pressure of carbon dioxide in the blood ECF is identical to the partial pressure in the CSF. A rise in the partial pressure of carbon dioxide in the CSF results in a rise in CSF H^+ concentration. However, because CSF is poorly buffered a small change in H^+ concentration will result in a rapid respiratory response. Carbon dioxide–ventilatory response curves can be constructed by measuring the minute ventilation at particular partial pressures of carbon dioxide.

The initial response to a rise in carbon dioxide is an increase in tidal volume followed by an increase in respiratory rate. Volatile anaesthetic agents are associated with reduced chemosensitivity. They depress ventilation which causes carbon dioxide levels to rise, but at the same time they reduce the ventilatory response to hypercarbia and also hypoxaemia. They also blunt the ventilatory response to acidaemia. Narcotic analgesic agents have similar effects.

Non-chemical control of breathing

A variety of mechanical and other receptors transmit information to the respiratory centre. These include the pulmonary stretch receptors which fire only when stretched and show little adaptation; irritant receptors which respond to noxious gases (including anaesthetic vapours) by causing spasm; muscle spindles in respiratory and skeletal muscle and J receptors which are thought to play a role in the sensation of dyspnoea.

Higher centres

Respiration is largely automatic but may be subject to voluntary control.

Neurophysiology

Sensory mechanisms

Postoperative pain is due to tissue damage resulting from the trauma of surgery. Cutaneous pain results from the stimulation of pain receptors in the epidermis by chemical irritants such as bradykinin, serotonin and histamine, also by potassium and hydrogen ions which leak out of damaged cells. Prostaglandins released into inflamed tissues sensitize the pain receptors to these substances and non-steroidal anti-inflammatory drugs act by reducing prostaglandin production. Pain originating from the viscera and blood vessels is transmitted along unmyelinated autonomic nerve fibres whilst pain impulses of cutaneous origin are transmitted along fast-conducting myelinated Aδ fibres and along slower conducting unmyelinated C fibres. These pain-conducting fibres synapse with interneurones in the substantia gelatinosa of the dorsal horn. The interneurones probably act as pain 'gates' as postulated by the Gate Control Theory of Melzack and Wall. The neurotransmitter between the small fibre terminals and the intermediate neurones is substance P. Enkephalins, which are naturally occurring opioid substances found in the substantia gelatinosa, inhibit the release of substance P. Opioid may act at a spinal level on the pain gates by mimicking naturally occurring enkephalins.

Pain impulses cross over to the opposite side of the spinal cord and are transmitted up in the contralateral spinothalamic tract to the sensory cortex. Visceral pain is transmitted in the ipsilateral spinothalamic tract. There are also descending inhibitory pathways which have the ability to control pain impulses as they enter the spinal cord.

Narcotic analgesics have their main action within the central nervous system, acting on enkephalinergic receptors in the brain. These aspects are discussed further in Chapter 18.

Motor mechanisms

Skeletal muscle consists of muscle fibres enclosed in a sarcolemmal sheath, each sheath contains many myofibrils. Muscle contracts in response to a stimulus delivered down its motor nerve.

Arrival of a nerve impulse at the motor nerve terminal results in the release and diffusion of acetylcholine across the synaptic cleft. Attachment of acetylcholine to the motor end-plate receptor produces an end-plate potential. The triggering of a muscle action potential occurs when the end-plate potential exceeds its threshold, this is followed by a wave of muscle contraction. Subsequently the acetylcholine concentration in the region of the motor end-plate receptor declines due to its breakdown by cholinesterases and diffusion out of the synaptic cleft (Fig. 2.8).

Muscle relaxants block this sequence of events. Muscle relaxants are divided into two broad categories: non-depolarizing (competitive) blocking drugs and depolarizing (non-competitive) blocking drugs. Non-depolarizers compete with acetylcholine for receptor sites on the motor end plate, but because the block is competitive some receptors will still be occupied by acetylcholine. Any end-plate potential generated will not reach the threshold necessary to fire off a propagating action potential, and so the fibre fails to contract. If a large number of fibres fail to contract the muscle is partially or totally paralysed. Reversal of paralysis is facilitated by the administration of anticholinesterase which prolongs the life time of acetylcholine at the end-plate receptor.

Depolarizing blockers compete with acetylcholine but produce end-plate depolarization which is prolonged. There is initial contraction of muscle

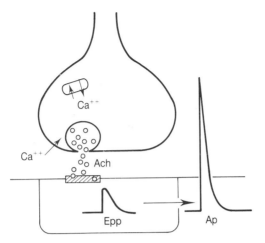

Fig. 2.8 Diagram of the neuromuscular junction showing the sequence of events associated with arrival of a nerve impulse. A nerve impulse approaching the nerve ending is associated with Ca^{++} entry and binding with the calcium-binding protein calmodulin. The formation of this complex enables vesicles to fuse with the axon terminal membrane and to discharge their components of acetylcholine (Ach) into the junctional gap. Postjunctionally binding of acetylcholine generates the endplate potential (Epp) which propagates to the muscle as an action potential (Ap).

with subsequent flaccid paralysis. The duration of paralysis is determined by the time taken for the drug to dissociate from the end-plate receptor and be metabolized by pseudocholinesterase. Chapter 3 contains a more detailed discussion of the pharmacology of muscle relaxants.

Autonomic nervous system
The autonomic nervous system is involved in the regulation of the circulation, respiration, visceral function and body temperature control. It is divided into sympathetic and parasympathetic nervous systems.

Sympathetic nervous system
Sympathetic nerve fibres which arise from the thalamus emerge from the thoracic and lumbar segments of the spinal cord (T_1–L_2). Preganglionic sympathetic fibres synapse with postganglionic fibres in the ganglia of the sympathetic chain which runs along the length of the spinal cord. Sympathetic transmission in the ganglia is cholinergic whilst postganglionic innervation of the end organs is noradrenergic, with the exception of the sweat glands and blood vessels in voluntary muscle (cholinergic). Preganglionic innervation of the adrenal glands releases adrenaline and noradrenaline into the circulation. Stimulation of the sympathetic nervous system results in increases in heart rate and blood pressure, vasoconstriction of cutaneous blood vessels (but vasodilatation in muscle blood vessels),

bronchial dilatation, reduction in gastrointestinal motility and sphincter constriction.

Parasympathetic nervous system

Parasympathetic fibres have a cranio-sacral origin, arising from cranial nerves III, VII, IX and X and from sacral roots S_2–L_3. Preganglionic parasympathetic fibres are longer than preganglionic sympathetic fibres and synapse at or near their target organ. Parasympathetic transmission in the ganglia is also cholinergic. Postganglionic nerves are shorter with cholinergic innervation of end organs. Parasympathetic stimulation results in a decrease in heart rate, bronchoconstriction, an increase in gastrointestinal motility and glandular activity with sphincter relaxation.

Nerve transmission

Cholinergic transmission results in two types of response: nicotinic or muscarinic. Of the two types of nicotinic receptors, type I is present at synapses of both sympathetic and parasympathetic ganglia. Type II nicotinic receptors are present at the neuromuscular junction where stimulation results in muscle contraction (see above). Muscarinic receptors occur at parasympathetic nerve endings on target organs and stimulation results in the parasympathetic responses outlined above.

Antagonism of nicotinic receptors on voluntary muscle results in muscle paralysis (see above). Antagonism of nicotinic receptors at autonomic ganglia can be used intraoperatively to reduce blood pressure acutely. Certain muscle relaxants, most notably tubocurarine, also affect ganglion-nicotinic receptors and cause falls in blood pressure (Table 2.1).

Table 2.1   Agonists and antagonists acting at the cholinergic receptor

Receptor type	Agonist	Antagonist
nicotinic I	nicotine	muscle relaxants
nicotinic II	nicotine	hexamethonium
		trimetaphan
		pentolinium
muscarinic	muscarine	atropine
		glycopyrrolate

The muscarinic effects of acetylcholine can be blocked by drugs such as atropine, hyoscine and glycopyrrolate, all of which will tend to produce dry mouth, tachycardia and decrease in gastrointestinal motility. Pethidine, chlorpromazine and promethazine also possess atropine-like actions.

Noradrenaline is the main transmitter substance in the postganglionic sympathetic neurones. There are two types of andrenergic receptor which may co-exist in the same effector organ: α and β. The β receptors may be further subdivided into β_1 (heart) and β_2 (lung). Stimulation of α receptors results in an increase in force of myocardial contraction with peripheral vasoconstriction, whilst stimulation of β receptors results in an increase in heart rate, bronchodilatation and muscle and kidney vasodilatation (Table 2.2).

Table 2.2 Agonists and antagonists acting at the adrenergic receptor

Receptor type	Agonist	Antagonist
α	adrenaline	phenoxybenzamine
	noradrenaline	phentolamine
	phenylephrine	tolazoline
	methoxamine	
β 1	dopamine	
β 2	salbutamol	β adrenoceptor
		antagonists
β 1 & 2	isoprenaline	
α & β	dobutamine	labetalol
	ephedrine	
	metaraminol	

Haematological system

Blood consists of red cells, white cells, platelets and plasma. Functions of blood include
- transport of metabolic substrates
- transport of metabolic waste
- transport of hormones, anti-infective agents etc.
- maintenance of the circulation
- haemostasis

Blood components

The normal red cell count is $5 \times 10^6/mm^3$ with each cell having a life span of 120 days. Erythrocyte production occurs in the bone marrow and is under the control of erythropoietin. Erythropoietin is a hormone produced in the kidney whose function is to maintain normal red cell mass. Cellular hypoxia is the main stimulus to erythropoietin production but anaemia also stimulates erythropoiesis.

Anaemias can be considered with respect to cell size (macro-, normo- or microcytic) and with respect to haemoglobin content (normo- or hypochromic). Anaemias occur as a result of insufficient red cell production, increased red cell destruction or blood loss.

Insufficient production occurs as a result of impairment of the stem cell line (e.g. marrow aplasia and renal failure) or impairment of differentiation. This in turn may be due to impairment of haemoglobin synthesis, either of the haem moiety (e.g. iron deficiency anaemia) or of the globin moiety (e.g. thalassaemia). Impairment of DNA synthesis may be due to deficiency of vitamin B_{12} or folate (needed for nucleiic acid and methionine synthesis). Prolonged exposure to nitrous oxide results in marrow suppression with impairment of methionine synthesis. Insufficient production may be due to multiple causes, as in the anaemia of chronic disease and marrow infiltration.

Increased red cell destruction can occur as a result of an intrinsic defect such as of cell shape (sickle haemoglobin) or an enzyme deficiency (e.g. glucose–6–phosphate dehydrogenase). Sickle haemoglobin is a variant commonly found in Afro-Caribbean patients in which an abnormality of the beta chain results in a shift of the oxygen dissociation curve to the right. The deoxy form of haemoglobin S is poorly soluble and crystallizes out at low partial pressures of oxygen (<5.5 kPa) resulting in sickling of the cell. Increased red cell destruction can also occur as a result of extrinsic abnormalities such as immune mechanisms, drug reactions, chemicals and bacteria.

Blood loss may be either acute or chronic.

Production of white cells (granulocytes, monocytes and lymphocytes) occurs in the bone marrow and in lymphoid tissue. White cells provide resistance to infection. Inhalational anaesthetic agents, especially halothane, inhibit cell-mediated immunity although the significance, particularly with respect to possible spread of malignancies, is unclear.

Haemostasis

Blood vessel damage sets in motion a train of events designed to limit blood loss. There are three distinct entities: local effects which result in vasoconstriction and blood diversion; platelet aggregation with formation of a platelet plug and release of vasoactive amines; and finally activation of the coagulation cascade.

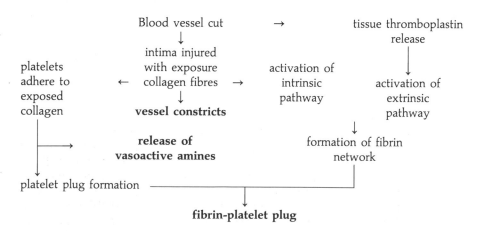

The integrity of the coagulation cascade can be assessed by measuring the partial thromboplastin time for the intrinsic pathway, the prothrombin time for the extrinsic pathway and the thrombin time for the common pathway. Platelets may be counted but no assessment of function is possible.

Anti-clotting mechanisms maintain a balance between abnormal coagulation and fibrinolysis. They include local liberation of endogenous anticoagulants (e.g. heparin), hepatic removal of activated clotting factors and the fibrinolytic cascade. The last named involves activation of plasminogen to form plasmin which in turn breaks down fibrin to form fibrin degradation products. Tissue injury promotes clot formation and at the same time activates the slower fibrinolytic process. Hypercarbia and venous stasis both promote fibrinolysis. Abnormal activation of the fibrinolytic cascade may occur in the presence of liver disease and cancers of the pancreas, lung and prostate. Prostatic surgery can release urokinase into the circulation which may in turn trigger the fibrinolytic cascade. The majority of anaesthetic agents and techniques have minimal effect on coagulation/fibrinolysis, except for epidural analgesia which enhances fibrinolysis.

Blood groups

Human red cells carry on their surface blood-group antigens which are genetically controlled; antibodies to these antigens develop and are present in the plasma. Blood grouping according to ABO and Rhesus antigens is the most important clinically but other groups exist (Table 2.3).

Table 2.3 Distribution of major blood groups in the UK

Blood group	Antigen	Antibody	Frequency
A	A	anti-B	42%
B	B	anti-A	8%
AB	A + B	nil	3%
O	neither	anti-A and B	47%

Eighty-five per cent of humans are rhesus positive and only 15 per cent are rhesus negative. Recipients of transfused blood should receive only blood of the same group as their own.

Blood transfusion

The administration of blood and blood products may be necessary to maintain oxygen transport, blood volume or clotting. Blood transfusion will normally be required for the correction of acute blood loss in excess of 15 per cent of the patient's circulating blood volume. Chronic blood loss and preoperative anaemias (depending on cause) can often be corrected with iron supplementation but may require transfusion. Stored blood should provide red cell survival rates of greater than 75 per cent 24 hours after transfusion; this equates with a storage life of roughly 35 days. Red cells in stored blood have decreased levels of 2–3 DPG and K^+ and the levels of clotting factors and platelets are much reduced. The incidence of transfusion reactions is 5 per cent (94 per cent due to immunological causes: febrile, allergic or haemolytic reactions; 6 per cent due to non-immunological causes: volume overload, citrate toxicity and transmission of infection including hepatitis).

Renal physiology

The main function of the kidneys is the control of the volume and composition of the extracellular fluid and the removal and excretion of waste products.

The kidneys receive approximately 20–25 per cent of the resting cardiac output. The normal glomerular filtration rate is 120 ml per minute with 99 per cent of the filtered load resorbed. The basic filtration unit of the kidney is the nephron which is subdivided into a Bowman's capsule, a proximal convoluted tubule, a loop of Henlé, a distal convoluted tubule and a collecting duct. The molecular threshold for ultrafiltration in the Bowman's capsule is 68000, thus substances with a molecular weight less than this value, such as sodium, potassium, glucose, urea and creatinine, will appear in the tubular lumen; whereas albumin, blood cells (red and white) and platelets will not. The appearance of albumin in the urine is an early indicator of renal damage. Reabsorption of substances can occur by active transport (e.g. sodium and glucose) or passive reabsorption (e.g. water, chloride, bicarbonate and urea). Tubular secretion of substances also occurs; this may be an active process (e.g. H^+ and K^+) or passive, involving diffusion down a concentration gradient.

Gastrointestinal physiology

The volume and acidity of hydrochloric acid secreted by gastric oxyntic cells is under neural and humoral control. Gastric acid secretion occurs in response to reflex stimulation of the vagi. Secretion also occurs in response to the excitatory hormone, gastrin, released from the pyloric antral mucosa as a result of stomach distension. The vagal innervation of the stomach maintains tone and motility. The normal pH of the stomach varies between 1.5 and 2.5. Histamine is a powerful stimulant to gastric acid secretion; it acts directly on oxyntic cells.

Trauma, pain, opiate administration and pregnancy all reduce motility and delay gastric emptying. Surgical vagotomy has a similar effect. Hence the need to perform a pyloroplasty at the same time.

Maintenance of tone in the gastro-oesophageal sphincter is important in preventing regurgitation of gastric contents and the adequacy of this sphincter is commonly reduced in pregnancy.

Atropine and other anticholinergic drugs block both vagally-mediated and gastrin-induced gastric acid secretion, as well as reducing gastric motility. Oral antacids can be used to buffer gastric acid and so raise pH but will increase gastric volume and some may release carbon dioxide which increases intragastric pressure, predisposing to regurgitation. Histamine H_2 antagonists reduce acid secretion and metoclopramide (an antidopaminergic agent) promotes gastric emptying by increasing peristalsis and relaxing the pylorus. Finally cisapride is a member of a new class of prokinetic agents which facilitates gastric motility by indirectly enhancing acetylcholine release from parasympathetic ganglia. It also increases the tone of the lower oesophageal sphincter and hence prevents acid reflux into the oesophagus.

Further reading

Adams A P, Hahn C E W. *Principles and practice of blood gas analysis*, 2nd edn. Edinburgh: Churchill Livingstone, 1982.

Covino B G, Fozzard H A, Rehder K, Strichantz G, (eds). *Effects of anaesthesia*. Clinical physiology series. American Physiological Society, 1985.

Melzack R, Wall P D. *The challenge of pain*. Harmondsworth: Penguin Books, 1982.

Schwieger I, Gamulin Z, Suter P M. Lung function during anaesthesia and respiratory insufficiency in the postoperative period: physiological and clinical implications. *Acta Anaesthesiologica Scandinavika* 1989; **33**: 527–34.

West, J B. *Respiratory physiology — the essentials*, 3rd edition. Baltimore: Williams and Wilkins, 1985.

3

Anaesthetic pharmacology
B.A. Astley

- Intravenous agents
- Inhalational agents
    anaesthetic gases
    volatile agents
- Muscle relaxants and their antagonists
    depolarizing muscle relaxants
    non-depolarizing muscle relaxants
    antagonists
- Opioids and their antagonists
    opioid agonists
    mixed agonist-antagonists
    opioid antagonists
- Anti-emetics
    anticholinergics
    the neuroleptic agents
    other antiemetics
- Benzodiazepines and their antagonists
    benzodiazepine antagonists
- Drug interactions

The preparation for and execution of successful anaesthesia is not dissimilar to cookery. The anaesthetist must be familiar with all the ingredients and be able to vary the quantities as necessary. Historically the classical triad of anaesthesia (narcosis, analgesia and muscle relaxation), was achieved by allowing the patient to breathe relatively high concentrations of the inhalational agents available at the time. Inevitably severe cerebral and cardiovascular depression often occurred, but with the advent of specific muscle relaxants and positive pressure ventilation in the 1950s it became possible to vary one component of the triad without incurring unacceptable cerebral depression ('Balanced Anaesthesia').

Fortunately for the anaesthetist (but not for the student!) new anaesthetic drugs are constantly being introduced and he should be familiar with their pharmacology and possible drug interactions.

Intravenous induction agents

These drugs all induce loss of consciousness rapidly after parenteral administration; this occurs as the brain receives a large percentage of the cardiac output and hence injected drug. Recovery of consciousness follows redistribution of the drug from the brain to the larger body compartments, muscle and fat, which also have a high affinity for these liposoluble drugs. These act as reservoirs from which the drug is eventually cleared by metabolism and excretion. Propofol is cleared rapidly and is therefore suitable for repeated injection or infusion to maintain anaesthesia, whereas a drug which is slowly cleared, e.g. thiopentone, would accumulate under these circumstances.

Thiopentone

A thio-barbiturate presented as a yellowish-white powder which is soluble in water and must be freshly prepared as a 2.5 per cent solution. The pH of the resulting alkaline solution is 11. Whilst it is not painful when injected intravenously, accidental injection into an artery causes intense pain and possible gangrene distal to the site of injection due to local vasospasm and thrombosis formation. It is still the most commonly used i.v. induction agent in the United Kingdom. Induction is rapid and smooth, but its metabolism in the liver is slow (10–15 per cent/hour) so that there is therefore some degree of hangover after administration. Thiopentone causes peripheral vasodilatation, direct myocardial depression and short-lived respiratory depression. These effects are proportional to the rate of injection and the amount given and the dose must always be titrated against the size and fitness of the patient. It was introduced in 1935 and the significance of its cardiovascular effects were realised during the Second World War when it was administered to shocked, hypovolaemic patients with disastrous results. It has no analgesic activity of its own. It is associated with histamine release and should be avoided in asthmatic patients. Anaphylactic reactions, although rare, are serious.

Methohexitone

An oxy-barbiturate presented as a white powder which is soluble in water and must be freshly prepared as a 1 per cent solution. Induction is rapid but is associated with excitatory central nervous system phenomena such as muscle movements and hiccups. Its use is contraindicated in patients with epilepsy as it may provoke convulsions. Injection into small veins may be painful so a large vein in the antecubital fossa should be chosen. Alternatively a very small dose of lignocaine may be given prior to injection of methohexitone, or any agent which causes pain. Clearance of methohexitone from the body is faster than that of thiopentone and it is therefore preferable to thiopentone for outpatient anaesthesia, when the patient is to return home the same day. It causes less cardiovascular depression than thiopentone.

Etomidate

An imidazole derivative unrelated to any other induction agent. Pain on injection occurs in 25–50 per cent of patients. Induction is rapid but spontaneous muscle movement occurs more commonly than with methohexitone. Recovery is rapid as the drug is metabolized in the liver and repeated doses are not cumulative. However, prolonged infusions have been associated with adrenocortical suppression and it is no longer used in this way. It does not cause significant cardiovascular depression.

Di-isopropyl phenol (Diprivan)

Introduced in 1977. It is insoluble in water and was originally solubilized in Cremophor-EL. Cremophor-EL is now known to be associated with anaphylactic reactions so that Diprivan is currently prepared in an oil and water emulsion containing 10 per cent soya bean oil. It is an opaque white liquid quite distinct in appearance from other induction agents. It produces rapid and smooth induction of anaesthesia but does cause pain on injection. In common with the barbiturates it depresses the cardiovascular system and respiratory system so care should be taken with hypovolaemic and elderly patients. Recovery is very rapid as the drug is metabolized, and it can be given repeatedly without cumulation. It is thus popular for day-stay surgery, and represents a most useful addition to the i.v. induction agents.

Ketamine

A derivative of phencyclidine which has the advantage of being able to be injected intramuscularly as well as intravenously. It produces dissociation, i.e. intense analgesia with only superficial sleep. It is the only induction agent with significant analgesic activity and can be used as the sole anaesthetic agent. It does not depress the cardiovascular or respiratory systems. It does not act as rapidly as thiopentone and causes hypertonus, salivation, postoperative nausea, emergence delirium and hallucinations. For these reasons the drug is not widely used for induction purposes in this country, although it is used as the sole anaesthetic agent in underdeveloped countries and in emergency situations.

Midazolam

A rapidly acting benzodiazepine which is discussed in more detail under the benzodiazepine section. It is mentioned here briefly because it can be used as an i.v. induction agent although there is a wide variation in response time which can be a disadvantage during a busy operating list.

All anaesthetic induction agents are potentially dangerous and should never be used by those without training in anaesthesia and resuscitation.

Inhalational agents

Desirable features of an inhalational agent:
• Low blood–gas solubility. Vapours which are insoluble in blood exert

higher partial pressures than soluble agents at the same blood concentration. The higher this partial pressure gradient the more easily the molecules pass across the blood–brain barrier at the start of anaesthesia, and across the alveolar membrane at the end of anaesthesia. Insolubility therefore confers quicker induction of and recovery from anaesthesia.
- High potency and volatility.
- Resistance to biotransformation. Some metabolites are harmful.
- Ether structure. This conveys cardiac stability with less chance of arrhythmias.
- Halogenation reduces flammability.

Nitrous oxide and cyclopropane are true anaesthetic gases. Their saturated vapour pressures (SVP) are above ambient pressure and therefore only exist as liquids under pressure. All the other inhalational agents are volatile liquids with SVPs below ambient pressure, and require specially calibrated vaporizers for their use.

Anaesthetic gases

Nitrous oxide
A non-irritant sweet-smelling gas supplied in blue colour-coded cylinders (or blue pipeline supply). It was first used in anaesthesia in 1844. It provides a smooth and rapid induction of anaesthesia as it has a low blood–gas solubility but it is a weak anaesthetic agent and cannot produce surgical anaesthesia when used alone with oxygen so that a more potent volatile agent or an intravenous opioid needs to be added. It is an excellent analgesic and the combination of 50 per cent nitrous oxide and 50 per cent oxygen (Entonox) is used during childbirth for the relief of pain. It does cause mild depression of the cardiovascular system and prolonged use is associated with megaloblastic changes in the bone marrow. This is not a problem in routine clinical use.

Cyclopropane
Supplied in an orange cylinder. It has a pleasant smell and provides the fastest induction of anaesthesia of the agents currently available in the United Kingdom. It is commonly used for induction of anaesthesia in babies and children where cannulation for intravenous induction may be difficult. It causes salivation, increased bronchial secretions and occasional bradycardia so that prior administration of atropine is advisable. It has sympathomimetic effects such that arterial pressure is maintained. However, its flammability and expense have contributed to its imminent demise.

Volatile agents
These are either halogenated hydrocarbons (halothane, trichloroethylene and chloroform) or ethers (enflurane, isoflurane, methoxyflurane and diethyl ether). They are listed in approximate order of popularity at present. All anaesthetic ethers and probably halothane have calcium channel-blocking properties which partly explains their actions on cardiac and vascular muscle as well as their ability to potentiate neuromuscular blockade.

Halothane
When halothane was introduced in 1956 it represented a true quantum leap in the safety of inhalational agents. It is well tolerated and provides a rapid and smooth induction of anaesthesia. It is potent and non-flammable. It produces a dose-related fall in blood pressure due to myocardial depression and sensitizes the heart to circulating catecholamines causing occasional arrythmias. It potentiates competitive muscle relaxants so that their dose may be reduced. Postoperative shivering in the recovery phase can be a nuisance and increase the patient's oxygen demand. Halothane is now thought to be associated with non-specific hepatotoxic damage. The incidence of this is 1:22000–35000 and it carries an 80 per cent mortality. Halothane undergoes significant metabolism in the liver (20–40 per cent) and the mechanism of hepatotoxicity is due to breakdown products, either causing damage directly or by acting as 'haptens' which set up an immunological toxic response. This liver damage occurs more commonly after repeated administration of halothane. The Committee of Safety of Medicines now recommends a 3-month period between repeat halothane administration. However, for such a rare complication its use should not be prejudiced and it remains a popular agent.

Enflurane
Introduced in 1978. It produces a rapid and smooth induction of anaesthesia. It is a stable compound which undergoes little biotransformation (2 per cent) and is non-flammable. It is approximately half as potent as halothane but depresses the cardiovascular and respiratory systems rather more. Hepatotoxicity after enflurane has been reported but the incidence is much lower than following halothane.

Isoflurane
An isomer of enflurane introduced in 1984. It is more insoluble in blood than halothane and in theory should produce a faster induction and recovery. In practice however (unlike halothane) it is irritant and causes coughing which slows induction. It is non-flammable. It potentiates neuromuscular blockers (a tendency with all ethers) and depresses the heart less than halothane. Only 0.2 per cent of isoflurane is metabolized so that hepatotoxicity after use is unlikely.

Trichloroethylene
A potent agent with considerable analgesic properties. It is cheap and non-flammable but has lost popularity owing to its prolonged induction and recovery time. It has now been withdrawn in the UK.

Diethyl ether
First used in anaesthesia in 1842. It is relatively soluble in blood and therefore provides a slow induction and recovery. It is a very volatile and potent agent. It is highly flammable which limits its use in the operating theatre, but it is safe, reliable and cheap, and is used extensively in developing countries which lack sophisticated apparatus.

Methoxyflurane
Is extensively metabolized and the fluoride ion produced causes dose-related nephrotoxic effects. In most countries it has now been withdrawn.

Chloroform
First used in anaesthesia in 1847. It enjoyed considerable popularity until increasing awareness of its toxic effects on the liver and myocardial irritability led to its replacement by safer agents.

Two new agents are currently undergoing trials before becoming available. *Sevoflurane* and *desflurane* are examples of the future inhalational anaesthetics. Both are non-flammable fluorinated ethers with solubilities lower than those of currently available inhalational anaesthetics so that induction and recovery should be even more rapid. Desflurane does not undergo hepatic degradation so that hepatotoxicity is unlikely.

Muscle relaxants and their antagonists

Muscle relaxants are traditionally classified into two groups, the depolarizing (non-competitive) agents typified by suxamethonium, and the non-depolarizing (competitive) acetylcholine antagonists typified by tubocurarine. The classical view of their mechanism of action holds that acetylcholine released by nerve impulses diffuses across the junctional gap and stimulates muscle fibres by acting on specific nicotinic receptor sites on the postjunctional membrane of the motor end-plate. These receptors are associated with an ion channel through which sodium and calcium ions flow and depolarize the membrane. The lifespan of acetylcholine is short since it is rapidly hydrolysed by the enzyme acetylcholinesterase. This is crucial otherwise the acetylcholine would exert a prolonged depolarizing effect and act as a neuromuscular blocker itself! There are also prejunctional nicotinic receptors, stimulation of which hastens mobilization of stored acetylcholine, thereby increasing transmitter output during high frequencies of stimulation.

Neuromuscular-blocking drugs act by blocking cholinoceptors at both sites. Block of the postjunctional receptors is responsible for the fall in amplitude of the muscle response, whereas block of the prejunctional receptors is responsible for the phenomenon of tetanic fade due to abolition of the usual positive feedback mechanism. Neuromuscular-blocking drugs may also act as ion-channel blockers (analogous to local anaesthetics).

Depolarizing muscle relaxants

Suxamethonium
The only depolarizing muscle relaxant in common use today. It appears to act by holding the ion channels open and preventing repolarization. The drug has a rapid onset of action and tracheal intubation can be performed within 60 seconds. The chief use of suxamethonium is for quick and reliable intubating conditions including the crash induction performed in emergency

surgery. Its duration of action is brief, about 3–5 minutes, because of its rapid hydrolysis to succinylmonocholine by plasma pseudocholinesterase. The features of a depolarizing block include an initial period of muscle fasciculation, absence of tetanic fade or post-tetanic potentiation and the block cannot be reversed by anticholinesterases (and indeed may be made worse). However, it does have a number of disadvantages:

- *Muscle pains*   This effect appears to be related to the initial fasciculations produced, and up to 50 per cent of patients experience pains after suxamethonium administration. The incidence can be lessened by prior administration of a very small dose of a competitive muscle relaxant.
- *Hyperkalaemia*   After suxamethonium administration the potassium gates remain open and there is a small leakage of potassium into the extracellular fluid. Patients suffering from tissue injury from trauma, burns or neurological injuries may exhibit larger changes in potassium flux which on occasion has resulted in cardiac arrest. For this reason suxamethonium is best avoided in such cases.
- *Raised intra-ocular pressure (IOP)*   Suxamethonium causes a transient rise in IOP. This is due in part to the contraction of the extra-ocular muscles and also to increases in arterial and venous pressures. This may be important if there is a penetrating eye injury; in such cases suxamethonium should be avoided if at all possible.
- *Bradycardia*   This occurs especially after repeated doses and may be a direct muscarinic effect of suxamethonium. Atropine must be available.
- *Malignant hyperpyrexia*   Suxamethonium in common with the volatile agents is a well-known trigger for this potentially lethal condition in susceptible subjects (Chapter 16).
- *Prolonged apnoea*   Deficiency or abnormality of the enzyme pseudocholinesterase will lead to a prolongation of the action of suxamethonium. The enzyme is synthesized in the liver and deficiency of it may accompany various forms of liver disease. The production of the enzyme is controlled genetically and there are four main variants. Patients with no cholinesterase activity will remain apnoeic for 4–6 hours. The management in this situation involves artificial ventilation of the lungs until recovery occurs. Cholinesterase activity can be assayed in the laboratory by blood tests in suspected cases.
- *Anaphylactoid reactions*   Reactions are rare but may be fatal; the anaesthetist must always be alert to such an emergency and be prepared to treat it immediately.

Non-depolarizing muscle relaxants
Competitive relaxants do not exhibit the disadvantages listed above associated with suxamethonium. However, many are eliminated by hepatic and renal routes, and the effects are prolonged by hepatorenal disease. Others show vagolytic effects resulting in a rise in heart rate and blood pressure, and some release histamine. All are potentiated by general anaesthesia. Features of competitive block include tetanic fade and post-tetanic potentiation, the ability of anticholinesterases to antagonize the block and an absence of initial fasciculations as seen after suxamethonium.

The onset time of neuromuscular block following competitive agents is longer than that following suxamethonium so that suxamethonium remains the drug of choice for an emergency crash induction where speed of intubation is of the essence.

Tubocurarine
The first competitive relaxant to be introduced into anaesthesia (1942) and although less used these days it still has its place and remains the drug by which the class are described. Like many classes of drugs, they all have similar sounding names (designed to confuse!). Tubocurarine tends to cause hypotension by a combination of histamine release and ganglion blockade. It is partly metabolized in the liver, the remainder being excreted in the urine.

Pancuronium
This has vagolytic effects resulting in an increase in heart rate and blood pressure. It is broken down in the liver and the effects are prolonged in patients with liver failure.

Alcuronium
This has a duration of action similar to these two drugs (>1h in clinically used doses) but is devoid of cardiovascular side-effects.

Atracurium and vecuronium
Two new competitive muscle relaxants introduced at the start of this decade. For the following reasons they are probably the most popular relaxants in this class: they have comparable onset times to the other competitive agents but a shorter duration of action when used in equipotent doses and are devoid of cardiovascular side-effects. Atracurium is unique in that it is not dependent on liver, kidney or enzymatic breakdown for its elimination. It undergoes Hofmann degradation at body pH and temperature, i.e. the molecule 'self-destructs' and is therefore non-cumulative. It can cause histamine release but major reactions are rare. Vecuronium does not cause histamine release but is broken down in the liver and tends to cumulate when given repeatedly. The significance of the shorter duration of action of these two drugs is that antagonism of neuromuscular block is more reliable.

Three new competitive muscle relaxants, *mivacurium*, *doxacurium* and *pipecuronium*, are undergoing clinical trials at the moment and may prove useful additions to our current list. The duration of action of mivacurium is only twice that of suxamethonium!

Antagonists
The anaesthetist must ensure that the patient has no residual neuromuscular blockade at the end of the operation. If there is, the patient may not be able to cough effectively (and is at risk of aspiration) or worse still may not be able to breathe adequately. Anaesthetists therefore administer anticholinesterases which act by prolonging the lifetime of acetylcholine at the neuromuscular junction so that it can compete with the relaxant for

occupation of the nicotinic receptors. However, acetylcholine is also effective at muscarinic receptors so that an antimuscarinic agent such as *atropine* or *glycopyrronium* must be given at the same time to prevent unpleasant muscarinic effects such as salivation, colic and bradycardia. The anticholinesterase most widely used for this purpose in the UK is *neostigmine*.

Awareness during anaesthesia is a potential problem when muscle relaxants are used. This is quite indefensible under normal circumstances and the anaesthetist must ensure that this does not occur.

Opioids and their antagonists

Pain is one of the commonest symptoms in medicine and methods of pain relief are discussed in Chapter 18. There are various classes of analgesics available of which the narcotic or opioid group is the most powerful. The term 'opiates' is misleading as it suggests that the drug is a derivative of opium. There are only three natural alkaloids of opium in clinical use, morphine, codeine and papaveretum (Omnopon). The remainder are semisynthetic e.g. diamorphine (heroin) or synthetic e.g. pethidine, fentanyl, alfentanil, pentazocine (Fortral). Hence the term 'opioid' is used.

The mechanism of action of morphine has been the subject of speculation for many years. Modern views on the subject date from 1973 when opioid receptors were discovered in the central nervous system. The fact that morphine attaches to a specific binding site suggested that there could be naturally occurring opioids which normally occupy such sites. In 1975 enkephalins and subsequently endorphins were discovered, both of which have analgesic activity. There are several different types of opioid receptor e.g. μ (mu), δ (delta), $\varkappa$ (kappa), ε (epsilon) and σ (sigma). Agonists at both μ and $\varkappa$ receptors mediate analgesia and opioid analgesics can be classified according to their primary action at these receptors.

Drugs acting at opioid receptors can possess two types of activity, agonist and antagonist, that is, they all have 'affinity' for opioid receptors but varying 'efficacy' once bound there. Morphine and diamorphine exhibit pure agonist actions (see below) whereas naloxone is a pure opioid antagonist. Naloxone possesses no analgesic properties and is capable of reversing all the effects of morphine. Between these extremes, drugs have partial agonist and partial antagonist properties e.g. buprenorphine. As with all drugs their potency is compared by the dosage needed to produce effect. Efficacy is the comparison of maximal effect. Opioids are used widely in anaesthesia in premedication, and for preoperative and postoperative analgesia.

Opioid agonists
Morphine is still the drug by which others in the class are compared.

Actions of morphine
- *Analgesia* By elevation of the pain threshold at spinal and thalamic levels and diminution of the emotional component of the limbic system.

- *Respiratory depression*   Direct depression of the medullary respiratory centre, the respiratory rate is reduced more than depth. Patients receiving high doses should have their respiration monitored.
- *Nausea and vomiting*   Most opioids are dopaminergic agonists on the medullary Chemoreceptor Trigger Zone (CTZ). Antidopaminergic drugs are therefore effective antiemetics.
- *Hypotension (mild)*   Due to a reduction in vasoconstriction tone and histamine release. Histamine release may trigger bronchospasm in asthmatics therefore it is safer to avoid morphine in such patients.
- *Pupillary constriction (miosis)*   Via stimulation of the Edinger-Westphal nucleus.
- *Cough suppression*   This may or may not be desirable.
- *Increase in smooth muscle tone and reduced gastrointestinal motility*   This results in delay in gastric emptying and constipation. Spasm of the Sphincter of Oddi and the ureteric sphincter occur, therefore avoid its use in biliary and renal colic.
- *Addiction*   Psychological and physical after long term administration.

Fate in the body

When morphine is administered orally most of it is taken up and metabolized in the liver (first-pass effect) so that a much larger dose is needed for a clinical effect. The maximal effect occurs within 2 hours and lasts for 6 hours. When it is administered i.v. or i.m., peak analgesia occurs in 20 and 90 minutes respectively and lasts for approximately 4 hours. Profound and prolonged analgesia can be produced by intrathecal or epidural administration (Chapter 12) which avoids the sympathetic and motor blockade associated with the use of local anaesthetics at these sites. There is, however, a real risk of respiratory depression after intrathecal or epidural use as well as following intravenous infusion so that the patient should be nursed in a high dependency unit where the respiratory rate can be monitored. All opioid analgesics except pentazocine are subject to the Controlled Drugs Regulations and must be signed for in a register and checked by a doctor or sister with special authority to handle such drugs.

Examples of agonists

Papaveretum
An extract of opium containing 50 per cent morphine. The average dose for an adult is 10–20 mg. It is used widely in premedication with hyoscine. The hyoscine acts as a drying agent and an antiemetic (20 per cent of patients feel nauseated after opioid premedication). It is also used preoperatively to supplement inhalational agents.

Codeine
A weaker analgesic than morphine. An efficient antitussive agent.

Diamorphine
Twice as potent as morphine and causes more euphoria.

Pethidine
Anticholinergic actions and 10 times less potent than morphine with less euphoria. It is thought not to release histamine in significant amounts.

Fentanyl
100 times as potent as morphine. Its duration of action is relatively short therefore it is suitable as i.v. adjunct to inhalational anaesthesia. Respiratory depression may be profound.

Alfentanil
A derivative of fentanyl with higher lipid solubility and faster onset of action. Its duration of action is shorter than fentanyl hence it is suitable for day case surgery and continuous intravenous infusion.

Mixed agonists-antagonists

Buprenorphine
A powerful agonist and partial antagonist that can be given sublingually to avoid first-pass metabolism by the liver. Receptor binding is so strong that naloxone may not reverse its effects. Doxapram (a non-specific respiratory stimulant) can be used.

Pentazocine
A powerful analgesic which produces dysphoria. Can antagonize respiratory depression caused by fentanyl yet allow continuing analgesia and is sometimes used at the end of surgery for this action.

Opioid antagonists
Naxolone has pure antagonist qualities. It binds to opioid receptors without effect and it has no efficacy at these receptors. It is used for the reversal of opioid-induced respiratory depression. It has a rapid onset of action (within 60 sec of i.v. administration) and a duration of action of 30 minutes. Care must therefore be taken with longer acting opioids as dangerous respiratory depression may return. Nalmefene is a new pure opioid antagonist with a longer duration of action which may prove useful.

Nalorphine and levallorphan both have mixed agonist and stronger antagonist properties. Both of these have been superseded by naloxone.

Antiemetics

Nausea and vomiting are unpleasant symptoms at the best of times and do occur after anaesthesia. This is especially likely after ether, cyclopropane, trichloroethylene and halothane (in decreasing order). Premedication with, or the intraoperative use of, opiates also causes nausea. It tends to be more common in children, females, and patients who are prone to nausea anyway. It is less common if the stomach is empty and occurs particularly after abdominal surgery especially if the gastrointestinal tract has been handled. Inhibition of nausea and vomiting can be achieved by:

- depression of the (motor) emetic centre (anticholinergics, antihistamines);
- depression of the dopaminergic (sensory) CTZ (phenothiazines, butyrophenones);
- depression of CTZ and hastening cholinergic-mediated gastric emptying (metoclopramide, domperidone).

All these drugs apart from the anticholinergics are dopamine antagonists. This explains the occurrence of extrapyramidal side-effects sometimes seen after their use.

Anticholinergics

Hyoscine
The only drug which possesses antiemetic qualities and is useful in the treatment of motion sickness as well as opioid-induced nausea. It is an effective antisialogogue and is used frequently in combination with an opioid e.g. papaveretum in premedication. It produces amnesia and sedation in most patients. Care must be taken in the elderly as excitement may occur.

The neuroleptic agents
Neurolepsis is described as a drug-induced behavioural state produced by phenothiazines and butyrophenones. These drugs produce a cataleptic immobility such that the patient becomes dissociated from his surroundings but remains responsive. In combination with nitrous oxide, oxygen and a powerful opioid, 'neuroleptanaesthesia' is produced, which as a technique has the advantage of cardiovascular stability, with analgesia and tranquillity extending into the postoperative period. Neurolepts are structurally similar to GABA and probably act by stimulating GABA receptors.

Properties of phenothiazines
- neurolept properties
- antiemesis
- antihistamine effects
- sedation
- depression of temperature regulation
- extrapyramidal effects (antidopaminergic)
- anti α_1-adrenergic/anticholinergic effects
- cholestatic jaundice. A rare sensitivity reaction.

Chlorpromazine
Used in psychiatry and for intractable vomiting.

Perphenazine
Very potent antiemetic but extrapyramidal effects common if doses are repeated too freely. It is being withdrawn in the UK.

Prochlorperazine
Good antiemetic. Less sedative effects than other phenothiazines.

Promethazine
Has sedative antiemetic and anticholinergic effects. Useful in premedication.

Trimeprazine
Used as sedative/premedication especially in children.

Butyrophenones
These are the most potent inhibitors of vomiting. They exhibit mild α-adrenergic-blocking activity but do not cause significant falls in blood pressure. Extrapyramidal side-effects do occur. Examples in use include *droperidol* and *haloperidol*.

Other antiemetics
Metoclopramide and *Domperidone*
Metoclopramide has little sedative or antihistamine effect. It hastens gastric emptying and increases the tone of the lower oesophageal sphincter. It can cause extrapyramidal side-effects. Domperidone is similar to metoclopramide.

Benzodiazepines and their antagonists

Benzodiazepines are classed as minor tranquillizers and are the most commonly prescribed drugs in the western world. They produce sedation, hypnosis and emotional modification by depressing the excitability of the limbic system. They act at specific receptors in the central nervous system (demonstrated in 1977). This receptor interaction stimulates the activity of the inhibitory transmitter, gamma aminobutyric acid (GABA).

Properties of benzodiazepines
- anxiolysis
- sedation/hypnosis
- amnesia and production of anterograde amnesia i.e. loss of memory for events occurring subsequent to administration
- muscle relaxation
- anticonvulsant activity

They do not cause significant enzyme induction (cf. barbiturates). They exhibit a greater margin of safety compared to many central nervous system depressants and in most subjects are relatively safe in overdosage. They do not cause significant depression of either the cardiovascular or respiratory systems. Most are metabolized to active compounds, some of which have long half-lives e.g. desmethyldiazepam. They possess no analgesic properties. Prolonged oral administrations can result in withdrawal symptoms.

In anaesthesia benzodiazepines are used in premedication, for induction of anaesthesia and for intravenous sedation for procedures not requiring full general anaesthesia e.g. dental work, radiographic procedures, endoscopy, cardioversion etc. They are not used specifically as muscle relaxants although for procedures such as endoscopy the muscle relaxation is helpful.

Diazepam
This is insoluble in water and therefore needs to be formulated in an organic solvent or emulsifying agent. The former formulation causes far more pain on injection and occasional thromboembolism so that the latter preparation, Diazemuls, has gained in popularity. The major active metabolite, desmethyldiazepam, has an elimination half-life of about 24 hours so that the patient may remain drowsy well into the postoperative period. Diazepam can be given orally or intramuscularly 1–1.5 hours preoperatively as a premedication. Alternatively it may be given intravenously to induce anaesthesia (but postoperative drowsiness is a problem) and in sub-anaesthetic doses as i.v. sedation.

Lorazepam
This has similar actions to diazepam but has a longer onset and duration of action. For premedication it can be given orally 2 hours preoperatively and appreciable blood levels persist for 24–48 hours. In fact, owing to its long duration of action it can be given simultaneously to patients on an operating list several hours before the start! It is a powerful amnesic.

Temazepam
This has a significantly shorter onset and duration of action than diazepam or lorazepam (half-life 4–10 hours). It is used orally in premedication and night sedation.

Midazolam
A water-soluble benzodiazepine which does not cause pain on injection. Although it can be used as an i.v. induction agent it has a slower induction time than thiopentone with marked variation in response. It has a much more rapid onset of action than diazepam and a quicker recovery. Its chief therapeutic use is for i.v. sedation and the production of amnesia for short procedures. The drug is injected slowly, titrating the dose against the response of the patient.

Benzodiazepine antagonists

Flumazenil
This has been developed as a benzodiazepine antagonist. Its use should probably be limited to reversal of anaesthesia or sedation. Evaluation of the precise definition of the receptor and hence the development of drugs with greater specificity of action is bound to follow in the future.

Drug interactions

Interactions can occur between drugs administered to the patient whilst in hospital and drugs that the patient takes on a regular basis at home. When the effect of one drug is inhibited by another, antagonism occurs. The effect of one drug may be enhanced by another resulting in addition or potentiation of effect. The reduced anaesthetic requirement for halothane when nitrous oxide is used is an example of a therapeutically useful drug interaction, as is potentiation of muscle relaxants by the inhalational agents. Potentiation of competitive muscle relaxants by calcium channel blockers e.g. verapamil, nifedipine and by aminoglycoside antibiotics may surprise the clinician who is not aware of these interactions.

Interactions may affect drugs before absorption. For example, if thiopentone and suxamethonium are mixed together a precipitate is formed. Antacids can bind digoxin in the stomach, reducing the amount available for absorption.

Binding to plasma proteins occurs with most drugs. As only the unbound form is active, reduced binding will enhance drug action. Thus highly protein-bound drugs such as salicylates, sulphonylureas, sulphonamides and phenylbutazone will increase the effects of drugs that are less bound e.g. warfarin. This can result in spontaneous haemorrhage.

Drug metabolism occurs in the liver and drugs which induce the microsomanenzymes e.g. barbiturates, analgesics and inhalational agents, can reduce the efficacy of other drugs. Conversely enzyme inhibition can occur reducing the metabolism of drugs. Monoamine oxidase inhibitors elevate the levels of catecholamines and enhance the effects of indirectly acting sympathomimetics e.g. ephedrine. Procainamide inhibits plasma cholinesterase and may interfere with the duration of action of suxamethonium.

Actions of drugs at receptors may be altered by competition e.g. antagonism of tubocurarine by anticholinesterases (used therapeutically). Treatment of opioid overdose by naloxone is another example of competitive antagonism at the receptor level. There are many more examples of interactions but this section serves only to outline the mechanisms of drug interaction and make the reader aware of the possible pitfalls of multiple drug therapy.

Further reading

Atkinson R S, Rushman G B, Lee J A. *A synopsis of anaesthesia*. Bristol: Wright, 1987.
Astley B. Recovery from neuromuscular blockade. In: Kaufman L, (ed). *Anaesthesia Rev. 4*. London: Churchill Livingstone, 1987: 180–93.
Bowman W C. *Pharmacology of neuromuscular function*, 2nd edn. Bristol: Wright, 1990.
Prys-Roberts C, (ed). *Current opinion in anaesthesiology*, vol 2. London: Current Science, 1989.
Smith G, Aikenhead A R, (ed). *Textbook of anaesthesia*. London: Churchill Livingstone, 1985.
Vickers M D, Schneider H, Wood-Smith F G. *Drugs in anaesthetic practice*. London: Butterworths, 1984.

4

The process of anaesthesia
P. M. Yate

- The induction room
    setting up
    objectives of surgical anaesthesia
    induction and maintenance of general anaesthesia
- Management of the patient in the operating theatre
    maintenance of general anaesthesia
    special considerations in the choice of anaesthetic agents
    the nature of surgery
- Care of the patient on the operating table
    maintenance of tissue oxygenation
    maintenance of blood flow
    control of circulating volume
    maintenance of lung ventilation
    management of body temperature
    positioning the patient on the table
    management of a regional anaesthetic
    termination of the anaesthetic
- The recovery room
    respiratory problems
    cardiovascular problems
    other problems in recovery
    discharge to the ward

By the time the patient reaches the anaesthetic room the process of anaesthesia has already begun. He has been seen and assessed by members of the surgical and anaesthetic teams. Any medical problems have been evaluated and where possible treated to optimize the patient's physical state; for example cardiac failure treated, hypertension controlled and anaemia corrected. Additionally, plans have been made for the management of specific medical problems over the period of anaesthesia and surgery, such as the setting up of a glucose, potassium and insulin infusion to control diabetes. To allay anxiety and to prepare the patient, the anaesthetic has been discussed during the anaesthetist's visit, informing the patient what to expect in the anaesthetic room and during the postoperative period. This is particularly important when complicated procedures in the anaesthetic room are envisaged prior to the induction of general anaesthesia such as invasive monitoring or when regional anaesthesia is planned. It is also important if special circumstances apply in the recovery period, for example when the patient is to be artificially ventilated, has to remain in an abnormal position or suffers some form of sensory impairment such as bandaged eyes. Finally, some form of pharmacological premedication may have been prescribed and this is usually given 1–2 hours prior to the planned induction of anaesthesia.

The object of this chapter is to describe the sequence of events taking place during an anaesthetic, from the time the patient arrives in the anaesthetic room until the patient is fully recovered.

The induction room

Whilst waiting for the patient to arrive in the anaesthetic room, the anaesthetist will check the anaesthetic equipment (Chapter 8), draw up any drugs required (Chapter 3), label the syringes and check that any blood ordered is in the theatre suite. The patient should be escorted to the theatre suite by a nurse, ideally one with whom the patient is familiar to provide a friendly companion. In the case of children a parent should be encouraged to accompany their child to theatre and remain with the child until anaesthesia is induced. Immediately the patient arrives in the anaesthetic room, his or her identity is checked with the operating list and the patient's notes, the nature and if appropriate the side of the operation is also confirmed and the patient's consent form checked.

Setting up
For all cases monitoring equipment is attached prior to the induction of anaesthesia and base line readings obtained (Chapter 5). Pre-anaesthetic monitoring should consist of
- pulse oximeter
- blood pressure recording device
- continuous electrocardiogram

Intravenous access is essential and depending on the nature of the case may be either a small 21 or 23 gauge cannula inserted into a vein on the back of the hand or, if an intravenous infusion is required, a large diameter 14 to 16 gauge cannula which is usually inserted into a forearm vein with the help of local anaesthesia. At this point the patient is now ready for the induction of anaesthesia.

Objectives of surgical anaesthesia
The provision of surgical anaesthesia today has progressed from simply rendering the patient unconscious during the period of surgery, to all aspects of patient care during surgery. Objectives include a rapid, smooth and painless induction of anaesthesia followed by maintenance of reliable surgical anaesthesia. This may be achieved with general or regional anaesthesia which should be performed to minimize upset of body systems

and permit a quick, smooth pain-free recovery from anaesthesia. Other objectives include the provision of good surgical conditions, for example muscle relaxation, and prevention of the deleterious effects of surgery by, for example, replacing fluid loss. The management of all normal bodily functions will have to be taken over as the patient will be unable to care for him or herself and such functions as temperature regulation and bronchial toilet will have to be managed. As the patient will be unable to prevent physical damage resulting from positioning, care has to be taken to prevent pressure damage to skin and nerves, excessive traction on joints and nerves and damage to the eyes.

Induction and maintenance of general anaesthesia

Depth of anaesthesia

Ideally, anaesthesia should rapidly achieve a depth appropriate for surgery. Anaesthesia which is too light is associated with movement, muscle rigidity, cardiovascular instability and worse, patient awareness. The latter may cause serious distress at the time and in the long term lead to chronic psychological disturbance. Awareness under anaesthesia may vary from the patient recalling sounds heard (hearing is the last of the sensations to disappear under anaesthesia) to the patient experiencing the pain of surgery. All forms of inadvertent awareness under anaesthesia are unacceptable. The risk of awareness has been made substantially greater in recent years by the increasing use of neuromuscular blocking agents thus removing one of the key signs of inadequate anaesthesia — movement. Likewise excessive anaesthesia can be harmful producing depression of the cardiovascular and respiratory systems and prolonging the recovery period. Thus, the signs of anaesthetic depth are very important. An early attempt to define depth of anaesthesia was the description of four planes of anaesthesia. Although these planes were specifically designed to apply to ether anaesthesia the principles still apply today, with some modification, in the era of polypharmacy.

Stages of anaesthesia

Stage I *Analgesia*
The period of analgesia until loss of consciousness. The patient's ventilation is irregular and of small volume, the pupils are small and reflexes are still intact.

Stage II *Excitement*
The period from loss of consciousness to the establishment of rhythmic ventilation. Characteristically the ventilation is of large volume and irregular, the pupils are large and divergent, the eyelash reflex is lost, but others, particularly the laryngeal reflexes, remain intact. The patient may be very restless during this period.

Stage III *Surgical anaesthesia*
Ventilation is now regular but may become depressed in both rate and volume as anaesthesia is deepened. Initially the pupils are pin point, central, and non-reacting, then as anaesthesia is deepened they dilate but

remain fixed. Marked reflex depression occurs although deeper levels of surgical anaesthesia are required to totally suppress laryngeal and anal sphincter reflexes.

Stage IV   *Apnoea*

Respiration ceases, muscular relaxation is intense, the pupils are fixed and dilated. This is excessive anaesthesia and the patient is endangered.

Today, anaesthesia is usually induced by the intravenous route and is so rapid that the excitement stage is usually bypassed, although it may still be observed during a gaseous induction. The use of neuromuscular blocking agents has removed those signs related to striated muscle activity i.e. muscle tone, ventilatory pattern and eye movements. The most valuable indicator today is the intensity of sympathetic nervous system activity. Thus, *light anaesthesia* would be identified by a tachycardia, hypertension, dilated reactive pupils and sweating; *excessive anaesthesia* would be identified by marked hypotension, bradycardia and dilated non-reacting pupils. Unfortunately, many of these signs can be influenced by factors other than anaesthetic depth; tachycardia may be provoked by blood loss, bradycardia by traction on the eye or viscera. This has led to the development of more sophisticated measures of anaesthetic depth. Most of these monitors, none of which are in widespread use, depend upon processing the electro-encephalogram.

Induction of anaesthesia

As it is pleasant for the patient, induction is most commonly performed intravenously via a previously sited intravenous cannula (Table 4.1). The agents used are varied and on occasion more than one will be used, but the principles of administration are similar.

Table 4.1   Agents commonly used during the intravenous induction of anaesthesia

Type of compound	Names of drugs	Average dose/kg
Rapid onset ⎫ routine barbiturates ⎬ induction Alkyl phenols ⎭ agents	Thiopentone Methohexitone Propofol	4.5 mg 1.5 mg 2.5 mg
Benzodiazepines	Midazolam	0.2 mg
Opioids	Fentanyl Morphine Alfentanil	⎧ Need very ⎨ high doses ⎩ if used alone
Phencyclidene derivatives	Ketamine	2 mg (or 10 mg i.m.)

After asking the patient to breathe 100 per cent oxygen through a face mask ('pre-oxygenation'), the drug is injected by slow i.v. injection whilst observing the effect locally at the site of injection and titrating it against central effects, remembering that the arm–brain circulation time is at least 15 seconds and may in elderly patients be 60 seconds or more. The patient will be observed and asked if the injection is painful as this may indicate extravasation of the injected drug into the subcutaneous tissues or intra-arterial injection. As the patient goes to sleep involuntary movements such as twitching or hiccups may occur. The injection is stopped when the patient loses consciousness. This is identified by failure of the patient to respond to commands, relaxation of muscles and loss of the eyelash reflex. The eyelash reflex is detected by stroking the eyelash and observing whether the patient blinks or not.

If the anaesthesia is for relatively minor surgery a spontaneous ventilation technique using a face mask is common. This usually employs an inhalational anaesthetic vapour such as isoflurane. The vapour is carried either in an oxygen/air or oxygen/nitrous oxide mixture. The vapour is introduced slowly starting with a low concentration and gradually increasing the inspired concentration at a rate of 0.5–1.0 per cent about every three breaths taken by the patient. If the introduction of the anaesthetic vapour is too rapid it may irritate the patient's respiratory tract resulting in coughing, bronchospasm and/or apnoea. The inspired concentration is raised considerably above that required to maintain anaesthesia to produce a concentration gradient from the anaesthetic machine to the patient's brain. As the patient exhibits signs of surgical anaesthesia, that is automatic respiration, absence of movement, small pupils and a stable cardiovascular system, the inspired vapour concentration is reduced and anaesthesia can be considered induced. Some assistance in maintaining the patient's airway may be achieved by inserting an artificial airway.

Intubating the trachea

There are two main methods of managing the airway during anaesthesia: intubation or by a face mask. The choice of technique is determined by the nature of the surgery, the patient and anaesthetic factors. The undoubted advantage of intubation in securing the airway always has to be balanced against the risks of technique such as dental damage and sore throat.

Indications for intubation

• surgical factors	• head and neck surgery
	• major surgery
	• long operations
• patient factors	• anatomically difficult airway
	• risk of aspiration
• anaesthetic factors	• technique involving artificial ventilation
	• convenience during long operations

The decision to intubate or not is now further complicated by the development of the laryngeal mask which represents a half-way stage and can replace the endotracheal tube, particularly where convenience is the main indication.

Intubation may be performed prior to induction of anaesthesia using topical anaesthesia. This is usually achieved with the help of a fibreoptic laryngoscope. This reduces the risk of aspiration of stomach contents during induction of anaesthesia and may be useful in the management of patients in whom a difficult intubation is envisaged, such as someone with an intra-oral tumour or a gross spinal deformity of the cervical spine which restricts neck movement. However, awake intubation is a time-consuming procedure and for routine anaesthesia intubation is usually performed with the patient asleep. It may be done under inhalational or i.v. anaesthesia alone, however, as very deep anaesthesia is required it is more commonly facilitated by the use of a neuromuscular blocking agent. If it is intended that the patient should breathe spontaneously after intubation or if rapid intubation is required, suxamethonium is given immediately after the induction agent. When suxamethonium is used some anaesthetists administer a small dose of a non-depolarizing neuromuscular blocking agent given either immediately prior to, or mixed in with, the intravenous induction agent. This may prevent the fasciculations and severe postoperative muscle pains caused by suxamethonium.

The onset of neuromuscular blockade occurs in about 60 seconds. If a non-depolarizing agent is given the onset of the intense neuromuscular blockade required for intubation may take up to 4 minutes. During the period from administration of a neuromuscular blocking agent until intubation, anaesthesia and oxygenation are maintained by mask ventilation with oxygen and a vapour (with or without nitrous oxide), or more rarely anaesthesia is maintained by incremental doses of an intravenous anaesthetic agent. Following the onset of neuromuscular blockade laryngoscopy is performed, the larynx, trachea and pharynx may be sprayed with lignocaine to provide topical analgesia which reduces the intense stimulation of intubation. The mask is then reapplied and ventilation continued for

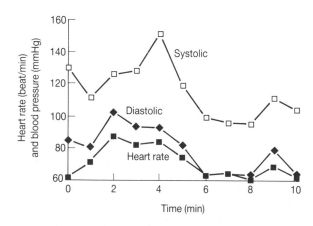

Fig. 4.1   Cardiovascular changes occurring during induction of anaesthesia in a 51-year-old man.   1 Thiopentone 350 mg and suxamethonium 75 mg injected 2 Laryngoscopy   3 Endotracheal intubation   4 Commencement of surgery.

another 30–60 seconds to allow time for the lignocaine to work. Laryngoscopy is repeated and the trachea intubated. The position of the endotracheal tube is confirmed by direct vision of the tube entering the larynx, auscultation of the chest and, if available, demonstration of expired carbon dioxide by capnography. Intubation is associated with intense cardiovascular stimulation, resulting in transient tachycardia and hypertension (Fig. 4.1). This may be harmful in some patients with intracranial pathology or ischaemic heart disease. In these high-risk subjects a variety of techniques are used to modify this cardiovascular response. Spraying with lignocaine has already been mentioned. Other techniques include pretreatment with beta adrenoceptor antagonists, administration of large doses of opioids at induction and the i.v. injection of a further dose of the induction agent immediately prior to intubation. Following successful intubation the tracheal cuff on the endotracheal tube is inflated gradually to a pressure adequate to prevent an air leak on gentle ventilation. The tube is then secured in place, either by strips of elastoplast or by a tie around the head.

Patients at risk for aspiration of gastric contents

If the patient is considered to be at risk of aspirating stomach contents during induction, the above routine needs to be modified.

Risk factors for aspiration of gastric contents at induction

- delayed gastric emptying
  - pregnancy
  - trauma
  - alcohol
  - opioids
  - ileus

- incompetent gastro-oesophageal sphincter
  - hiatus hernia
  - pregnancy
  - nasogastric tube

- increased intra-abdominal pressure
  - intra-abdominal masses
  - obesity
  - suxamethonium

Preoperative management should include attempts to empty the stomach and antacid prophylaxis. Intubation may either be performed awake or by a routine known as 'crash induction' or 'rapid-sequence induction'. In the latter case the objective is to pass the endotracheal tube quickly and accurately to minimize the risk of aspiration. First, equipment is prepared as before but with special care taken to have duplicates of all items close at hand, a selection of endotracheal tubes available and suction tested and running with the sucker tip under the patient's pillow. The patient is then pre-oxygenated with 100 per cent oxygen using a close-fitting face mask to wash all the nitrogen out of the lungs. By this time, the lungs will contain approximately 3 litres of oxygen which will maintain oxygenation even if the patient is apnoeic for 5 minutes. A predetermined dose of an induction agent is injected rapidly followed by suxamethonium. Simultaneously, the trained assistant will apply 'cricoid pressure' (p. 58). This compresses the oesophagus between the trachea and cervical spine thus preventing passive regurgitation and is maintained until the trachea is intubated and the cuff inflated to isolate the airway. Finally, before the patient is ready to be transferred into the operating theatre, additional monitoring may be instituted, for instance the insertion of a central venous pressure catheter or intra-arterial or urinary catheters. For intraoral or intranasal surgery when blood or fluid is expected to accumulate in the mouth, a throat pack is usually inserted to prevent soiling of the trachea. A label marked 'throat pack' is affixed to the patient to reduce the possibility of it being inadvertently retained at the end of the operation.

Management of the patient in the operating theatre

Maintenance of general anaesthesia

Originally anaesthesia was maintained by the use of one drug, frequently ether, which was used to produce unconsciousness, muscular relaxation and to suppress haemodynamic stimulation due to painful stimuli. However, this usually requires very deep levels of anaesthesia. More recently the concept of 'balanced anaesthesia' has developed and polypharmacy is used to achieve the different effects. These can roughly be divided into hypnosis, relaxation and analgesia (Table 4.2).

Table 4.2   Drug activity

	Hypnosis	Relaxation	Analgesia
Thiopentone	+++	+	o
Methohexitone	+++	+	o
Propofol	+++	+	o
Etomidate	+++	+	o
Ketamine	+++	o	+++
Benzodiazepines	++	+	o
Suxamethonium	o	+++	o
Atracurium	o	+++	o
Halothane	+++	++	o
Enflurane	+++	++	(+)
Isoflurane	+++	++	(+)
Nitrous oxide	++	o	++
Opioids	+	o	+++
Local anaesthesia	o	(++)	+++

The combination of drugs used varies widely depending on the individual patient, the surgery to be performed and the duration of surgery. However, certain principles apply; hypnosis is essential, the degree of relaxation required is variable and depends on the nature of the surgery and an analgesic component is desirable.

Spontaneous ventilation techniques are usually used for minor procedures of relatively short duration which only involve body-surface surgery. For more major procedures, particularly those requiring muscle relaxation to facilitate surgical access for intra-abdominal or intrathoracic procedures, *controlled ventilation* with neuromuscular blockade is usually used.

When using spontaneous-ventilation anaesthetics hypnosis is usually maintained after induction by a mixture of an anaesthetic vapour and nitrous oxide. The analgesia is provided by the nitrous oxide and may be supplemented by opiate premedication or by the administration of small i.v. doses of opioids preoperatively. However, the use of opioids in this technique is limited due to the inevitable ventilatory depression associated with large doses. An alternative approach is to supplement the general anaesthesia with a regional block, for example an epidural for a prostatectomy.

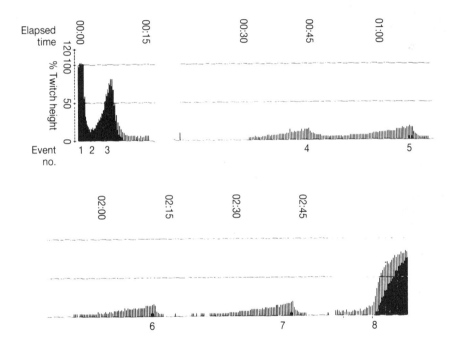

Fig. 4.2 Segments of a recording of the evoked electromyogram recorded from the adductor pollicis muscle after stimulation of the ulnar nerve with repeated train-of-flow stimuli. They demonstrate the management of neuromuscular blockade in a 56-year-old man undergoing orthopaedic surgery.

The trace prints the first and fourth twitch recorded from each train of four stimuli. At 1 suxamethonium is given and rapid depolarizing block occurs permitting intubation at 2, then recovery of neuromuscular function occurs until at 3 a loading dose of atracurium is given and non-depolarizing neuromuscular blockade develops, note the development of fade. Block is maintained with a twitch height for the first twitch kept at approximately 5–15 per cent of initial control level, by the administration of incremental doses of atracurium at 4, 5, 6, and 7. Neuromuscular blockade is reversed by neostigmine at 8.

When using controlled ventilation the patient is paralysed with a non-depolarizing relaxant, hypnosis is then maintained with a small concentration of inhalational vapour in 66 per cent nitrous oxide, and analgesia is supplemented with an i.v. opiate. 'Top-up' doses of relaxant are usually given either by the clock, on clinical observation of increasing muscle tone or when indicated by a neuromuscular transmission monitor (Fig. 4.2). The degree of neuromuscular blockade required depends on the indication. If used purely to facilitate ventilation, only modest degrees of block are required as spontaneous ventilation will be largely suppressed by opiate administration. For other situations, such as closure of a laparotomy incision, intense neuromuscular blockade is required to avoid the need for very deep levels of anaesthesia. Supplementary doses of opioids may be given, again either by the clock or on indication of inadequate analgesia i.e. hypertension, tachycardia or sweating.

A more recent technique is the replacement of the inhalational component of the anaesthetic by an i.v. infusion of a short-acting i.v. agent, such as propofol, to produce hypnosis. This is usually combined with incremental doses or even infusions of an opioid analgesic. This mode of anaesthesia, known as total i.v. anaesthesia (TIVA), offers several advantages, the major one being the avoidance of polluting the operating theatre environment with waste anaesthetic gases.

Special considerations in the choice of anaesthetic agents

Patients with hepatic and/or renal failure
In this situation drugs should be chosen whose excretion does not depend on the damaged organ. Thus, inhalational agents which are excreted through the lungs are particularly suitable. Of the muscle relaxants, atracurium offers significant advantages; because of its spontaneous break-down by Hoffman degradation it is therefore independent of both hepatic and renal function.

The nature of surgery
Modern anaesthetic drugs enable the anaesthetist to help make surgery easier. The use of neuromuscular blocking agents or regional nerve block to provide intense muscle relaxation revolutionized access to the thorax and abdomen. Furthermore, manipulation of the patient's physiology may be an advantage.

Induced hypotension
Most forms of anaesthesia are associated with a modest fall in blood pressure which to a certain extent reduces peroperative bleeding and improves surgical vision. In some situations, such as surgery using an operating microscope, a more drastic approach may be required. This form of anaesthesia is known as hypotensive anaesthesia and the mean blood pressure may be reduced to as low as 50 mm Hg. This is not without risk and patient selection needs to be careful and the indications good. Pharmacologically this is tackled in much the same way as treating hypertension, either by reducing myocardial contractility and heart rate with beta-blocking

drugs or by reducing peripheral resistance with such drugs as sodium nitroprusside.

Local reduction of bleeding
This can be achieved by careful patient positioning, such as head-up tilt for surgery on the middle ear, or by preparation of the operative site by local infiltration of a vasoconstrictor. The latter may be particularly effective for body-surface surgery, for example infiltration of a solution containing 1:200 000 adrenaline into the nose can reduce bleeding as effectively as profound hypotension.

Reducing intracranial pressure and volume
For neurosurgical procedures surgical access can be improved by reducing the cerebral blood flow and pressure. This can be done by lowering arterial pressure, hyperventilation with CO_2 washout, and using i.v. anaesthetic agents such as barbiturates to reduce cerebral blood flow.

Care of the patient on the operating table

The crucial task is to care for the patient both during the operation and afterwards in the recovery period.

Maintenance of tissue oxygenation
The key objective in the management of the patient during surgery is the maintenance of adequate tissue oxygenation. A balance must be kept between oxygen demand (which is around 250 ml/min in an adult) and oxygen supply which can be summarized by the oxygen flux equation:

available oxygen=cardiac output×oxygen content
(Oxygen content=per cent saturation×haemoglobin+dissolved oxygen. Dissolved oxygen=PaO_2 kPa×0.0225)

All these variables can be affected by anaesthesia and surgery, and may be manipulated by the anaesthetist to maintain tissue oxygenation. A simple estimate of the oxygen flux can be obtained by the measurement of haemoglobin saturation by a pulse oximeter and of the circulation by observation of the patient's blood pressure and heart rate.

Maintenance of blood flow
Most anaesthetic agents depress the cardiovascular system. Virtually all anaesthetics are direct myocardial depressants and some are also vagotonic, for example, halothane. These effects on the heart are often combined with a degree of peripheral vasodilatation, leading to reduced venous return. The overall effect being a reduction in blood pressure and cardiac output. This is compounded by the general lack of sympathetic stimulation associated with hypnosis. These effects are balanced out to some extent by the intense stimulation of surgical pain. This results in normotension or more commonly a mild degree of hypotension.

Falls of up to 20 per cent of preoperative blood pressure values are routinely accepted. Greater falls may indicate excessive anaesthesia and the hypotension can be easily reversed by reducing the inspired concentration of vapour. However, in some situations, to avoid the risk of patient awareness the blood pressure is elevated either by fluid administration or by administration of a vasopressor, such as ephedrine or metaraminol. Certain periods of an anaesthetic are particularly associated with cardiovascular instability, for example hypotension frequently occurs following induction of anaesthesia due to the cardiovascular effects of a large bolus of an induction agent. These effects can be minimized in high-risk patients by very slow i.v. injection of the induction agent which enables the anaesthetist to carefully titrate the dose required. Another cause of peroperative hypotension is the absence of surgical stimulation such as the period spent waiting for the result of histology.

More serious causes of hypotension include hypovolaemia, myocardial failure due to ischaemia or arrhythmias. The latter being particularly associated with halothane anaesthesia and with certain forms of surgery, notably oral surgery. Likewise, bradycardia tends to occur as a reflex after certain intense stimuli such as dilatation of the cervix, traction on the vas deferens and during ophthalmic surgery (oculocardiac reflex). Bradycardia may be minimized in these circumstances by prophylactic treatment with an anticholinergic drug such as atropine.

Control of circulating volume

The maintenance of an adequate circulating volume and haemoglobin concentration for oxygen transport requires careful perioperative fluid balance. Allowance has to be made for the fact that the patient may have been starved for up to 12 hours prior to surgery. During abdominal surgery large volumes of fluid may be lost from exposed bowel and up to 10 ml/kg per h may be required as replacement. The converse of hypovolaemia may occur during endoscopic-urological surgery. If a large amount of bladder irrigation fluid (glycine) is used, substantial fluid may be absorbed leading to water overload which in turn leads to cardiovascular and neuropsychological problems, the so called TURP (Trans Urethral Resection of Prostate) syndrome.

The methods of estimating blood loss during surgery are highly inaccurate being based on a combination of experience, measurement of loss and observation of the patient's cardiovascular system. Aids to the assessment of blood loss include the weighing of swabs (this will tend to underestimate the loss), observation of the suction bottles, and an extra 30 per cent should be allowed for blood on the surgical drapes. Patient indicators of blood loss include hypotension and tachycardia, poor peripheral perfusion and oliguria. Central venous pressure (CVP) is a particularly useful indicator of the adequacy of volume replacement and thus of hypovolaemia.

The decision to replace blood loss with blood rather than crystalloid or synthetic colloid is multifactorial. In view of the potential complications of transfusion it is avoided whenever possible. However, it usually becomes necessary in adults when the blood loss exceeds 20 per cent of the patient's blood volume or when the blood loss is even less in children. This decision may be influenced by the patient's preoperative haemoglobin, the ability of the patient to withstand anaemia and the total anticipated loss; if it is expected to be massive, transfusion is often started early to avoid 'getting behind'.

Maintenance of lung ventilation

The care of the patient's respiratory system to facilitate adequate oxygenation and carbon dioxide removal is a key area of an anaesthetist's expertise. This can be considered as:

- provision of an adequately oxygenated gas mixture
- maintenance of the patency of the airway from the anaesthetic machine to the alveoli
- ensuring adequate ventilation.

The provision of an adequate gas mixture requires both an appropriate fresh gas flow and increased oxygen concentration. An inspired oxygen concentration of less than 0.3 is rarely used thus allowing a margin of safety for impaired gas exchange due to increased V/Q inequalities and hypoventilation.

For many patients spontaneous ventilation will prove adequate although some degree of respiratory depression is inevitable with most techniques, particularly if narcotics are administered either as part of premedication or preoperatively. The indications for controlled rather than spontaneous ventilation technique range from absolute to debatable. Absolute indications are:

- muscle relaxation required to facilitate surgery
- cardiothoracic surgery involving an open chest
- anaesthetic technique likely to induce unacceptable respiratory depression
- hypocapnia induced to reduce intracranial volume.

Controlled ventilation is usually achieved with the assistance of a mechanical ventilator. For anaesthesia simple machines are adequate and are usually set with a large tidal volume and a slow respiratory rate. Modest hyperventilation to cause mild hypocapnia is common, this suppresses the respiratory stimulant effect of carbon dioxide.

Mechanical ventilation of the lungs is not without its hazards. Cardiovascular depression has been mentioned and maldistribution of ventilation occurs leading to V/Q mismatch. The latter is responsible for the need for a large minute volume. However, the most serious risk is that associated with technical failure; disconnection from the ventilator can be fatal and thus careful monitoring of ventilation is mandatory. Throughout the period of artificial ventilation a disconnection alarm is used, and tidal volume, inflation pressures and the end–tidal carbon dioxide concentration are monitored.

Management of body temperature

A fall in body temperature is an almost inevitable occurrence during any reasonably long surgical procedure (Fig. 4.3). The aetiology of this is partly environmental due to the relatively low ambient temperature surgeons often choose to work in, the use of cold surgical solutions and evaporation from exposed visceral surfaces. Anaesthesia may also contribute through the administration of cold i.v. fluids, the reduction in metabolic activity and the prevention of shivering and vasodilatation. Although in many patients modest hypothermia is of little consequence, it may be harmful, particularly in children and neonates, because of the metabolic effort required in the immediate postoperative period to raise the body temperature. Hence, the desirability to monitor core temperature peroperatively and to take active steps to maintain body temperature. Simple manoeuvres to achieve this include the administration of warmed i.v. fluids by using a blood warmer, the maintenance of a warm ambient temperature and the use of heated mattresses.

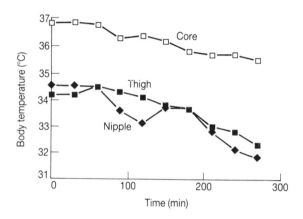

Fig. 4.3   Changes in body temperatures in a 45-year-old female undergoing resection of a mandibular tumour.

Positioning the patient on the table
Approximately 0.01 per cent of all patients suffer some form of temporary nerve damage peroperatively. This is often due to faulty positioning on the operating table. To prevent this care should be taken to avoid excessive extension or flexing of joints; for example the shoulder should not be abducted beyond 90° on an arm board, there should be no direct pressure on nerves by armrests at the elbow or by lithotomy poles pressing on the peroneal nerve. If the patient is placed prone, the brachial plexus is at risk from traction on the arm.

Eyes must be protected; they should be closed during anaesthesia (p. 261). If the patient is placed prone, pillows should be placed under the patient's chest and pelvis to facilitate abdominal movement for ventilation.

Management of a regional anaesthetic
Regional anaesthesia offers several advantages; postoperative confusion is unusual, respiratory complications are reduced in the immediate postoperative period and the patient's cerebral status can be monitored throughout surgery. A block can sometimes be continued into the postoperative period

to provide analgesia and some patients prefer regional blockade to general anaesthesia. The patient may find lying still for a long period of time difficult. In some cases small doses of an i.v. sedative such as midazolam are given to produce sedation although this may achieve the opposite effect and produce disinhibition and restlessness. Other problems are detailed in Chapter 12. Although the sole use of regional anaesthesia does not involve loss of consciousness, because of the potential problems many of the principles underlining the conduct of a general anaesthetic still apply. The patient should still be starved on arrival in theatre, and cardiovascular monitoring and the arranging of i.v. access prior to the induction of anaesthesia are essential.

Termination of the anaesthetic

Towards the anticipated end of surgery the administration of anaesthetic drugs is reduced with the aim of awakening the patient soon after the end of surgery, but not before the last stitch. Immediate recovery from anaesthesia can be a pleasant experience for the patient if carefully managed. Within a short time the patient may be expected to emerge from being deeply anaesthetized, possibly intubated and artificially ventilated, to being aware, caring for their own airway and self-ventilating. To do this the patient needs:

- to be awake
- the neuromuscular blockade reversed
- to be free of pain, whilst avoiding excessive doses of opioids because of the risk of secondary respiratory depression.

Hyperventilation washes out CO_2 from the body stores; this produces the syndrome of posthyperventilation hypoxaemia in the first hour of recovery. This condition may be avoided by restoring Pa_{CO_2} concentration towards normal during the final phase of anaesthesia by adjustments to the fresh gas flow and/or ventilator as appropriate for the anaesthetic system used.

Consciousness is achieved by gradually reducing anaesthetic administration towards the end of the procedure, continuing the nitrous oxide until the end of surgery.

Persisting neuromuscular blockage should be antagonized by the administration of an anticholinesterase/anticholinergic combination such as neostigmine and atropine (Chapter 3). Care is taken not to attempt to reverse profound neuromuscular blockade as it is unlikely that adequate reversal will be achieved. This situation is avoided by not attempting to reverse the block within 10 minutes of an increment of a neuromuscular blocking agent, or when no evoked muscular activity can be detected by a nerve stimulator. Clinical signs of inadequate reversal are twitching or jerky movements by the patient ('tracheal tug'), rapid shallow ventilation, inability to sustain a 5-second head lift, hand grip or protrusion of the tongue, inability to cough or clear the airway or obvious patient distress. The patient may even whisper 'I can't breathe'. Failed or inadequate reversal may be detected by the use of a nerve stimulator (p. 76).

Analgesia should be maintained into the postoperative period, it is very much easier to maintain analgesia than to gain control of pain later. Indications of excessive opioid administration are apnoea or bradypnoea and the presence of adequate muscle tone. The patient may even be awake and not breathing. Another important clue is the presence of pin-point pupils. Opioid-induced respiratory depression can be reversed by cautious administration of the opiate antagonist naloxone, given in small divided doses so as not to totally reverse the analgesia. An alternative approach to postoperative analgesia is the peroperative insertion of a regional nerve block, or local infiltration of a local anaesthetic into the wound site. Virtually all forms of surgery are amenable to this approach and the quality of recovery can be greatly improved by providing analgesia without opioid analgesics with their inevitable associated respiratory depression, nausea, vomiting and dysphoria.

Postoperative nausea and vomiting can be reduced by the peroperative prophylactic administration of an antiemetic, although despite this about 20 per cent of all patients will still vomit in the postoperative period. Before extubating the patient adequate spontaneous ventilation should be established. If a nasogastric tube is *in situ* this should be aspirated. The larynx and pharynx should be inspected with the help of a laryngoscope and any blood, saliva, foreign bodies or throat packs removed. The patient is then turned on one side, usually the left, the tracheal cuff is deflated and the patient extubated after several breaths of 100 per cent oxygen. Immediately after extubation using gentle positive pressure the patient should be given 100 per cent oxygen to breathe via a face mask. The trolley may be tipped head down if there is any suspicion that the patient may vomit or regurgitate, or if there is blood present in the oropharynx.

The recovery room

The immediate recovery period is the most dangerous, however, full recovery from anaesthesia may take several days. Most patients spend ½–1 hour in a special postoperative area within the theatre suite. Here, their vital signs can be serially monitored by specially trained nurses who have instant access to members of the surgical and anaesthetic team. Observations are made of the patient's well-being, colour, blood pressure, respiratory and pulse rates as well as other physiological parameters. Drainage from surgical drains is recorded and the surgical wound regularly inspected for signs of haemorrhage. The nursing staff are trained to identify airway obstruction and in simple measures to clear obstruction. All patients should be given supplemental oxygen via a disposable plastic face mask to treat at least the modest hypoxia which would otherwise inevitably occur after anaesthesia (Chapter 7).

The recovery from anaesthesia is not always smooth and various problems may be encountered. The most common serious problems are those related to obstruction of the upper respiratory tract and respiratory and cardiovascular depression.

Respiratory problems
Recovery-room respiratory problems are the most common. Airway obstruction may occur if the patient is still unconscious and is usually treated by holding the patient's chin forward to pull the tongue away from the

posterior pharyngeal wall. Maintaining a clear airway is aided by keeping patients on their side in the recovery position. In this position the chin and tongue will tend to fall forward and any fluid accumulating in the patient's mouth such as blood, saliva or vomit will tend to drain out of the mouth rather than down the trachea. Additionally, if the patient regurgitates stomach contents and aspirates, only the dependent lung will be soiled. Laryngospasm is a frightening complication which may occasionally occur in semiconscious patients when the larynx is irritated by blood or secretions. It is characterized by a rapidly developing inspiratory stridor, quickly followed by cyanosis. Treatment involves suction, holding the chin forward and administration of 100 per cent oxygen using a face mask under positive pressure, this usually proves adequate until the spasm passes.

Hypoventilation is common and may be due to:
- opioid overdose characterized by a slow respiratory rate
- persisting neuromuscular blockade characterized by difficult breathing and an irregular respiratory rate.

If cyanosis occurs, check the **A**irway, check the **B**reathing and check the **C**irculation and then treat as indicated (**ABC**).

Cardiovascular problems

Minor cardiovascular problems are common due to the persisting effects of the anaesthetic agent. The vagotonic effects of drugs such as halothane and propofol may persist into the recovery period causing bradycardia which is easily treated with i.v. atropine. Tachycardia may indicate pain, hypovolaemia or rarely a primary cardiac problem. Brief periods of modest hypotension may occur and may either be the result of continued effects of anaesthetic agents on the cardiovascular system or of hypovolaemia due to blood loss. It may be precipitated by the administration of opioid analgesics and the consequent vasodilatation. Hypotension is usually easily treated by tipping the patient's head down and administering i.v. fluid.

Other problems in recovery

Restlessness may occur in the recovery room and some patients may become delirious and pull on surgical drains and intravenous cannulae or try to get out of bed. This may be an emergence phenomena which is commoner in older patients, especially alcoholics, or it may indicate genuine pathology. Pain is the commonest cause; more seriously, *restlessness may indicate hypoxia* or inadequate reversal of neuromuscular blockade. These must be excluded before the administration of a tranquillizer is even considered.

Some patients may be hypothermic and rewarming can be assisted by holding the patient in a warm area, providing adequate blankets and using an aluminium space blanket.

Discharge to the ward

Transfer of the patient from the recovery room to the ward is governed by simple discharge criteria. The patient should probably remain in recovery for at least 30 minutes, cardiovascular and respiratory observations should be stable and there should be no evidence of bleeding. The patient should be awake, this can be determined by simple questions, for example asking the patient his name, date of birth and name of his hospital ward. Vomiting and pain should be controlled and a plan for the further management of the patient's pain made.

In some patients the criteria will not be met. Unconscious or unstable patients should not be transferred from the recovery room to the general ward without detailed arrangements for their care being made. If the criteria are met the patient is now transferred back to the ward. The patient should be accompanied by a nurse, an anaesthetic record chart which details all anaesthetic drugs given, peroperative cardiovascular and respiratory changes, monitoring used, fluids administered, an estimate of blood loss and details of any untoward events. This can prove invaluable, not only if problems are encountered in the postoperative period, but also in the management of any future anaesthetic.

5

Monitoring
A.P. Adams

- Monitoring the anaesthetic machine
- Monitoring the patient
- Continuous monitoring devices
    pulse oximetry
- Intermittent monitoring devices
- Invasive and specialized monitoring
- Operations or procedures of brief duration
- Recovery from anaesthesia
    transfer of patients
- Medico-legal considerations
    product liability
    monitoring standards

The anaesthetist cares for his patients before, during and after the operation, and he or she does this by appropriate history taking, perusal of the case notes and examination of the patient preoperatively. In addition, the anaesthetist prescribes and administers whatever medication is appropriate. This section is mainly concerned with 'assessing' or 'monitoring' the patient's condition during anaesthesia itself, this is then continued into the recovery period. In addition to monitoring the anaesthetic delivery and the patient, good records must be kept at the time the observations are made. This may be done either by the anaesthetist's handwritten record or by direct hard-copy printouts appropriately annotated.

It is helpful to describe monitoring in two categories; firstly the anaesthetic machine and, secondly, the patient. The equipment used in both cases has alarm systems with limits which should be set to approximate values for the patient concerned and the anaesthetic technique being used.

First and foremost the anaesthetist must stay with his patient all the time during the administration of the anaesthetic. During the course of an anaesthetic he must not leave the patient, e.g. to answer a telephone call or have a cup of coffee, unless another competent anaesthetist takes over direct care. If he does, and should a disaster befall his patient, then he is open to serious charges. If the patient should survive in a brain damaged condition, as happens from time to time, the damages awarded may run into many thousands of pounds, indeed over a million or so. This is apart from the intense tragedy of the situation and the distress to families, relatives and the doctor concerned. The duty of the anaesthetist is to be in the room with his patient for any general anaesthetic, local or regional anaesthetic block or sedative technique which he has initiated and for which he is responsible and to make sure that the depth of anaesthesia is appropriate and the physiological condition of the patient is satisfactory.

The anaesthetist is there to care for his patient by observing what is going on, taking action as appropriate, and keeping a written record of what is happening (recording the vital signs). The control of an anaesthetic may not be delegated to someone else such as a nurse or a technician. Sometimes it is unavoidable for a change of anaesthetist to be made during the course of the operation. It is essential to tell the surgeon what is proposed, not only as a matter of courtesy but also for safety considerations. Should this be necessary it is imperative that the outgoing anaesthetist checks and agrees with the incoming anaesthetist what the present and previous condition of the patient is, the drugs and techniques that have been employed and the state of blood loss and fluid replacement. It is essential that they agree the correct name and hospital identity number of the patient, for it is not uncommon for a surgeon to ask the anaesthetist to give a drug, such as an i.v. antibiotic, and the new anaesthetist needs to check that his patient is not specially sensitive or allergic to such a drug. Again, severe blood loss may occur later and the new anaesthetist needs to check each unit of blood against the patient's transfusion form and identity label.

All relevant events occurring in the operating theatre are recorded on an anaesthetic record or chart. The format of such forms differs from hospital to hospital. Those more recently introduced are capable of being analysed by computer for data analysis, quality control, accounting and so on. Some anaesthetic charts incorporate the patient's *consent to operation*; this is a very useful feature as the 'consent' is kept in the notes attached to the relevant anaesthetic chart. In some hospitals the drugs used for premedication may be prescribed on this chart but it is usually better to do this on the main drug chart. It can be laborious to enter a lot of handwritten information on the chart, and it can also distract the anaesthetist's attention from his patient, therefore the best anaesthetic charts are those that require the least time to complete, for example checking boxes against a prepared checklist of drugs, techniques, types of equipment and so on.

Particular attention must be paid to time so that an accurate record is made of both when events occur and the routine observations. These observations include the times drugs are given and physiological changes such as a rise or fall in blood pressure, heart rate etc. It is becoming increasingly common for physiological variables (*the vital signs*) such as heart rate, arterial pressure, central venous pressure, body temperature, oxygen saturation, and also the concentrations of end-tidal carbon dioxide (capnography) and any anaes-thetic gases or vapours, to be recorded automatically on a convenient paper recorder or printer. Other changes which may also be recorded are those which relate to the delivery of the concentrations of oxygen, anaesthetic gases and vapours. The behaviour of devices such as ventilators and other forms of breathing machine can also be monitored by recording the pressures delivered, the frequency and the inspiratory/expiratory ratio.

It is most important that the recording of events should be made at the actual time they occur. Nevertheless, the anaesthetist is not expected to write down everything at a busy or crucial time because he must not be distracted from the care of his patient. Thus the events relating, say, to the induction of anaesthesia may be written down, not at the time the initial drugs are given, but as soon as possible afterwards when induction is complete and the anaesthetist is fully satisfied that all is well with his patient. Should a cardiac arrest occur there is a protocol which includes arranging, when possible, for one person, usually a junior nurse or medical student, to note the time and doses of drugs used, the electrical energy and number of attempts at defibrillation, the siting of intravascular cannulae, and the patient's responses; these are called out to her by the person(s) involved.

Retrospective changes should never be made to hospital notes and this includes anaesthetic charts. If corrections or additions need to be made the procedure is to make a legible fresh note which explains why a correction is required. This entry should be signed, and the date and time at which it was made also recorded. The person making such a correction should print his name legibly in capital letters under his signature and add his designation, e.g. senior house officer, registrar in anaesthetics, etc. Not very long ago a junior anaesthetist was convicted and fined under the Forgery and Counterfeit Act 1968. His crime was to destroy his anaesthetic record in the postoperative period and attempt to substitute a new one because he feared he had inadvertently administered a drug which should have been diluted before use. If he had followed the commonsense advice given above he would have been spared a very harrowing time, unwelcome publicity and the ensuing loss of his job.

Monitoring in the operating theatre may be considered as the monitoring of the anaesthetic machine and apparatus such as the lung ventilator, and the monitoring of the patient. These two considerations are often inter-related. It is absolutely essential for safe practice that monitoring equipment should be designed and used as ergonomically as possible. For instance, all monitors should be viewed within one field of vision, which should ideally include visualization of the patient and anaesthetic apparatus. The 'Christmas tree effect', i.e. the stacking of monitors in a somewhat haphazard fashion, is to be deplored: it is hazardous because of the risk of damage to the apparatus as well as being ergonomically unsound because the anaesthetist has difficulty in scanning the monitors.

Specific basic monitors and measurements used in anaesthesia are
- oxygen analyzer (to monitor gases issuing from anaesthetic machine
- ECG (electrocardiograph, also gives heart rate)
- NIBP (non-invasive blood pressure)
- Pulse oximetry (also gives pulse rate)
- capnography (continuous display of end-tidal P_{CO_2})
- expired tidal/minute volume
- ventilator failure alarm (disconnection, under- or over-pressure, cycling of machine)

- body temperature, hypothermia or hyperthermia (malignant hyperthermia syndrome)
- peripheral nerve stimulator (use with muscle relaxants)

Monitoring the anaesthetic machine

The anaesthetic machine may be considered in two categories: the oxygen supply and the breathing system. The oxygen supply may be from cylinders of oxygen on the anaesthetic machine or from an outside oxygen source, i.e. an oxygen pipeline. The pipeline is supplied either from a liquid-oxygen tank in the grounds of the hospital (the vacuum-insulated container) or from a bank of cylinders arranged with their reducing valves set so that when one cylinder is exhausted the next automatically comes into line (Chapter 8).

Each system requires a warning should the supply fail or be interrupted for any reason. In the case of an oxygen-pipeline supply there are audible alarms and a warning lamp on a central display panel. Ideally there should be an audible alarm just outside the operating theatre itself to alert of impending oxygen-supply failure, so that all who work there can hear it. The anaesthetic machine must always have at least one checked full cylinder of oxygen attached to it (with a spanner or ratchet for turning it on) so it can be put into use if necessary. It may seem obvious that the place to site the central alarm unit and display panel is where those whose duty it is to take action can promptly observe it. Not long ago an instance occurred where the pipeline oxygen ran out. However, because the hospital had instituted financial cuts in an effort to save money, there was no one in the porters' central station to observe the warnings; the porters had been deployed by management to another part of the building. There have been various instances where bulk-liquid tanker drivers have succeeded in circumventing the antifouling connections to the liquid-oxygen plant. In two hospitals they refilled the liquid-oxygen reservoir not with more liquid oxygen but with liquid air in one case and with liquid nitrogen in the other. Nevertheless the safety of a supply of oxygen from a liquid-oxygen source is greater than when the supply is from cylinders fitted to the anaesthetic machine.

The anaesthetic machine must be fitted with a low-pressure warning device so that if the oxygen supply fails there will be an audible alarm. This will then take care of the situation irrespective of whether the supply is from a pipeline or from cylinders attached to the machine.

There is a need for careful monitoring of the breathing system or anaesthetic 'circuit'. These are of various types (Chapter 8). The individual components of breathing systems can fall apart especially where there is a 'make-or-break' connection and the likelihood of this is great enough for it to be one of the very first things one should check when anything appears wrong. Other things to check for are oxygen failure, kinked or obstructed airways, cardiac failure or a blocked gas exit valve leading to pneumothorax.

During spontaneous breathing observation of the reservoir or breathing bag in the system may reveal a leak, disconnection, overpressure or hyperventilation due to rebreathing. These faults are best detected by a combination of the continuous monitoring of the expired tidal and minute volume and the end-tidal carbon dioxide concentration. There must also be a high-airway pressure alarm to alert for the development of a high-airway pressure because of the risk of pulmonary barotrauma.

During mechanical ventilation of the lungs using methods such as IPPV (intermittent positive pressure ventilation), it is essential to monitor the pressure in the airway. Alarms are fitted with adjustable low- and high-pressure limits which should be set by the anaesthetist according to the requirements of the patient. These devices give an illuminated and an audible alarm to indicate violation of the set threshold for both lower and upper pressure limits.

Monitoring the patient

The patient is monitored by the use of:
- direct clinical monitoring by the anaesthetist
- non-invasive monitoring equipment
- invasive monitoring methods (when specifically indicated)

The anaesthetist must keep a continuous check on the condition of his patient and the most important way of doing this is by making full use of his own senses. He is the only member of the team who has the specific experience and training for this task. The anaesthetist's attention is directed to keeping a check on the colour of his patient. Cyanosis should never be allowed to develop, and if it does the cause needs to be instantly identified to permit adequate remedial action to be taken. A patient died recently under extraordinary conditions; a venturi injector device was connected at one end to a cylinder containing oxygen at a pressure of 15–20 p.s.i. and at the other end to a sized 5.0 cuffed microlaryngeal tube which was placed in the trachea. Puffs of oxygen were delivered to the patient by intermittent operation of a pistol-grip type of trigger. Unfortunately, with such a dangerous system there was no room left around the tube for the patient to exhale out to the atmosphere and a pneumothorax developed. The anaesthetist took the development of cyanosis to mean that the patient needed more oxygen and continued to operate the trigger over a period of time. The patient 'blew up' as a result of the pneumothorax, causing massive surgical emphysema, and oxygen was forced under pressure into most of the tissues of the body, causing respiratory and cardiac failure and death. The picture displayed was of the Michelin man of the tyre advertisements.

Thus it is paramount to make clinical observations during every anaesthetic by looking, feeling and listening. Firstly, *looking* to see the chest *rise and fall with every breath*; movement should be even and synchronous on both sides of the chest and also with the reservoir bag in the breathing system; if they are not, airway obstruction in some form or other is usually present. Tracheal tug is a sign in which the larynx is pulled down or 'tugs' during spontaneous respiration. This sign is associated with incomplete recovery from the effects of muscle relaxants (partial curarization), and with metabolic acidosis. If the endotracheal tube is placed too far down the trachea so that it enters one bronchus, then one side of the chest (i.e. the opposite side to that intubated endobronchially) will move less or not at all.

The anaesthetist should be looking closely for cyanosis as a sign of hypoxia; the mucous membranes of the mouth and lips, and the nail beds of the fingers are easily observed for the first signs of it. Cyanosis is always an indication that hypoxia is present and can never be considered as a normal part of any anaesthetic. There are rare exceptions to this rule, e.g. when methaemoglobinaemia is present due to the use of dyes such as methylene blue for certain diagnostic surgical procedures (e.g. to identify the parathyroid glands), or as a manifestation of prilocaine toxicity. If cyanosis should develop the cause must be immediately identified and rectified before any surgical or diagnostic procedure is started or continued.

The anaesthetist must be on the look out for inadequate anaesthesia especially 'awareness' which really means the patient is not anaesthetized adequately. This can happen for a variety of reasons; if the anaesthetist forgets to turn on the supply of anaesthetic gases or vapours, if a leak develops in the delivery of gases from the anaesthetic machine to the breathing system (diversion), if the nitrous oxide cylinder has run out, if the vaporizer has run dry and needs to be refilled, or if the emergency oxygen-bypass valve (flush valve) has been accidentally locked 'on' so that the additional oxygen dilutes the anaesthetic gas mixture. Clinical signs which may indicate awareness include any movement by the patient (e.g. of the limbs of partially paralysed or non-paralysed patients), but it may be detected earlier by movements of the face (facial nerve), the eye or by frowning (frontalis muscle). Other indicative signs are the formation of tears, sweating, dilated pupils, and rises in blood pressure and heart rate.

Secondly, *feeling*. An excellent test to detect lung ventilation is to place the fingers of each hand on the patient's chest over the first rib on each side. Since movement of the first rib is not great under normal conditions it provides a guide to the whole movement of the chest wall. If the anaesthetist is not positioned at the head of the table (e.g. he may be by the patient's side during operations on the ear, eye, nose, or head and neck), keeping a hand on the abdomen to feel the movement of the diaphragm is the standard method. The anaesthetist should also feel the pulse to obtain important beat-to-beat information as to the rate and rhythm of the heart; the amplitude of the pulse volume felt by the fingers indicates conditions such as hypovolaemia (a fast and thready pulse) or hypervolaemia (a full bounding pulse).

Thirdly, *listening*. The anaesthetist should always confirm correct placement of an endotracheal tube as previously described and in addition must also use his stethoscope to listen for the entry and exit of air to and from the chest. He should also routinely use his stethoscope to listen over the left hypochondrium to hear whether the sound of gas entering the stomach can be heard. If this is heard it indicates oesophageal intubation. If access to the chest is denied (e.g. because of the need for surgical access) an oesophageal stethoscope can be used; this device consists of a small-bore catheter fitted with a floppy balloon at its distal end which is positioned in the oesophagus behind the heart. It is thus easy to listen for both breath and heart sounds simultaneously. If desired the proximal end of the catheter can be fitted to a small individually moulded earpiece placed in one ear to allow what is going on in the operating theatre also to be heard. This arrangement is more comfortable for the anaesthetist than the nuisance of continuously wearing the conventional binaural stethoscope headpiece, and since his end of the long tube is usually fastened to his shirt by a safety pin it has the advantage of anchoring him to his patient! Use of an oesophageal stethoscope is also a recognized method of detecting venous air embolism as a heart murmur develops if this occurs.

There is always the risk of misplacing the endotracheal tube in the oesophagus and this should be taught the very first time the student learns to intubate. Experienced anaesthetists may also on occasion inadvertently intubate the oesophagus. However, the anaesthetist who is paying attention will recognize this fact at once by using the above clinical tests and can swiftly reposition his tube long before any possible harm has been done. A normal capnogram (Fig. 5.1) provides an excellent check on the correct position of the endotracheal tube. Accidental inflation of the oesophagus and stomach, besides allowing hypoxia to develop, produces gastric distension with the risk of damage to tissues, mediastinal emphysema, regurgitation and aspiration of gastric juice, and splinting of the movement of the diaphragm.

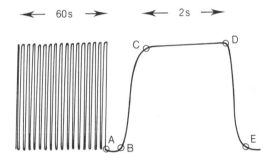

Fig. 5.1 The normal capnogram at slow and fast recording speeds. A-B denotes the exhalation of gas from the anatomical deadspace (containing no CO_2); B-C denotes the exhalation of mixed expired gas; C-D is the alveolar or end-tidal 'plateau'; D denotes the onset of inspiration and D-E denotes the return of the CO_2 trace to the baseline as fresh gas is inspired.

The anaesthetist is accustomed to the rhythmic sounds of his equipment in the operating theatre. Alterations in the frequency and amplitude of sounds should immediately put him into a state of extra alert. For instance, a rise or fall in heart rate, evident from a change in the rhythmic 'blip blip' of the ECG monitor, immediately alerts the anaesthetist even if the change is no more than a few beats per minute. Again, disturbance of the rate or rhythm of the gently hissing expiratory valve will indicate a change in the volume of gases in the breathing system, perhaps one gas has 'run out'. Some mechanical ventilators (e.g. those of the minute-divider type and those electrically time-cycled) continue to cycle when a disconnection from the patient has occurred, so apparently reassuring noises may continue to be heard. However, the experienced anaesthetist will be aware of this and will always ensure that he has the back-up of a ventilator-disconnection alarm which has been checked and turned on; some models of alarm function without the need for controls or switches.

The sounding of audible alarms on monitors indicate that a default or preset parameter has been violated. The default is the alarm setting(s) built into the monitor by the designers in their attempts to anticipate what the 'average' anaesthetist requires as a norm. The fact that such default settings vary between monitors from different manufacturers indicates that anaesthetic techniques, anaesthetists and their patients all vary. There can be too many different alarms in the operating theatre and one of the reasons for a cacophony of sounds is the failure of an anaesthetist to predetermine the approximate upper and lower limits of the various alarms according to the particular condition of his patient. One of the difficulties is that there is, at present, little agreement amongst manufacturers to standardize alarm sounds. However, it is hoped that a standard will shortly be published on this subject. It has not been unknown for an anaesthetist to be bewildered by an alarm only to find that one of the surgical team has taken his pager or 'bleep' into theatre in the pocket of his trousers.

Continuous monitoring devices

Whenever possible clinical skills must be backed-up by specific monitoring devices to provide a continuous observation of the pulse volume, arterial pressure, arterial oxygen saturation (pulse oximetry) and end-tidal CO_2 concentration (capnography), together with an ECG. However, intimate knowledge of the correct functioning of any monitoring device, whether continuous or intermittent, is absolutely fundamental to safe anaesthetic practice.

A combination of devices to monitor expired tidal or minute volume, end-tidal carbon dioxide tracing (capnography) and airway pressure should be used to ensure that ventilation is adequate during both spontaneous and mechanical ventilation. The UK is one of the few countries in the world where some anaesthetists continue to use carbon dioxide gas. Several instances of inadvertent administration of CO_2 have occurred such that the Department of Health and the Association of Anaesthetists of Great Britain & Ireland (AAGBI) have issued a warning that cylinders of the gas should not remain on the anaesthetic machine unless the anaesthetist specifically requires it for that particular patient. End-tidal CO_2 monitoring provides a useful safeguard.

Continuous monitoring of body temperature using an electrical thermometer (thermistor or thermocouple) is advised; the sensor may be placed in the axilla, nasopharynx or in the oesophagus behind the heart. A 'triple-oesophageal tube' is often used in the USA as a routine: this monitors the ECG and core temperature and enables auscultation of heart and breath sounds.

Monitoring must be continued from before the induction of anaesthesia, during anaesthesia and into the recovery period. Although it is recognized that a normal ECG tracing may be present when the circulation is grossly inadequate, the ECG may provide early warning of impending circulatory failure due to myocardial ischaemia, conduction defects or arrhythmias. It should therefore be displayed from before induction until a point in the recovery period when further surveillance is considered unnecessary.

Pulse oximetry

Cyanosis and bradycardia are late signs of hypoxaemia, and pulse oximetry represents a very significant advance in patient safety because even astute clinicians can fail to detect cyanosis early enough.

The basis of pulse oximetry is to shine light of known intensity and given wavelength through a tissue such as the nail bed of a finger or toe, the lobe or pinna of the ear, or even the tongue. The amount of light which is transmitted through the tissue is measured. In the red region of the spectrum, at a wavelength of 650 nm, there is a large difference in optical absorption between reduced haemoglobin and oxyhaemoglobin. When haemoglobin is oxygenated the transmission of light is increased. In the near infra-red region of the spectrum, at 805 nm, there is an isobestic point. There are several of these points and they represent wavelengths at which the optical absorption of fully reduced and fully oxygenated haemoglobin are equal. Hence, a measurement at this wavelength determines the total amount of haemoglobin present, and the difference in output between the measurements at the two wavelengths (650 nm and 805 nm) is an index of the oxygen saturation of the blood. However, when light is shone through a substance or tissue it is reflected and scattered as well as being transmitted and the physical law involved (Lambert–Beer) is to be regarded as entirely empirical.

A pulse oximeter analyses the changes in the transmission of light through any pulsating arterial vascular bed. The amount of light transmitted depends on the amount absorbed by the various structures present, such as skin, muscle, bone, venous and capillary blood, etc. The path length that the light has to travel through, say, the finger, is constant until it is changed (increased and decreased) due to expansion and relaxation caused by the entry and exit of pulsing arterial blood into the system; this produces the familiar plethysmographic waveform. The amount of light absorbed and transmitted will then alter. This 'pulse added' signal (Fig. 5.2) is subtracted from the background transmission signal by a microprocessor-controlled empirical algorithm, computed hundreds of times per second; the saturation is averaged over a short time interval of 3–6 s to produce a rapid response. The algorithm is created by measuring pulse-added absorbances in healthy, awake volunteers breathing various gas mixtures. These absorbances are then correlated with actual oxygen saturations obtained by arterial sampling and a standard *in vitro* method. The differing light absorption characteristics of oxygenated and non-oxygenated blood are thus used to continuously compute the oxygen saturation of the arterial blood.

The probe of the pulse oximeter houses two narrow band light emitting diodes (LEDs) functioning at wavelengths in the red and infra-red part of the spectrum. Although skin, flesh, bone and venous blood reflect and absorb a

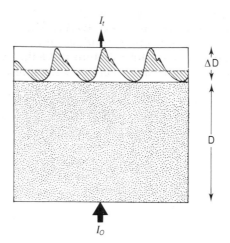

Fig. 5.2   Principle of pulse oximetry. D is the fixed absorbance of light shone through the non-pulsating structures (e.g. bone, muscle, skin, veins) of a tissue; ΔD is the 'pulse added' component, or variable absorbance of light as a result of the pulsating arterial system in the tissue. Io is the intensity of the incident light and I_t is the intensity of the transmitted light emerging from the tissue.

constant amount of light, arterial blood, by contrast, absorbs varying amounts of light because of the pulsatile blood flow. Because only two wavelengths are used the pulse oximeter cannot distinguish between more than two forms of pigment, i.e. reduced and oxyhaemoglobin. An error will occur with a two-wavelength oximeter if a third pigment such as carboxy-haemoglobin (COHb) is present. Each LED switches on and off at about 720 Hz (red on, red off and IR on, both off, etc.) and a single broad-band photodiode detects the amount of light transmitted. The photodetector produces outputs for the transmitted light from each of the diodes and also for any ambient light detected during the off periods in the 720 Hz cycle.

Intermittent monitoring devices

Every patient receiving general anaesthesia, local or regional anaesthesia, or i.v. sedation must have their heart rate and arterial pressure measured and recorded every 5 minutes. If clinical circumstances preclude such measurements this must be noted on the anaesthetic record.

Whenever a general anaesthetic is administered which involves the use of muscle relaxant drugs a means of assessing the state of the patient's neuromuscular function by way of supramaximal stimulation of a peripheral motor nerve should be available. Commonly used sites are the ulnar nerve at the wrist (observation of the adductor pollicis), the common peroneal at the lateral side of the knee, or the facial nerve in front of the ear.

Invasive and specialized monitoring

Special anaesthetic techniques such as deliberate hypotension demand additional monitoring (e.g. arterial cannulation for blood pressure measurement).

Additional monitoring is needed for operations on the heart and lungs or central nervous systems, and in any situation where major blood loss is expected. The monitoring required includes invasive procedures such as direct measurement of arterial pressure, central venous or pulmonary artery pressures, urine output and blood loss. Relevant haematological and biochemical analyses (including pH, serum electrolytes and tests of blood coagulation) should also be available. Additional monitoring will be required in special circumstances where there is a pre-existing medical disease (e.g. serum glucose concentrations during operations on severe diabetics or exploration for insulinomas).

Operations or procedures of brief duration

The same standards of monitoring must be applied for brief operations or procedures. Many an anaesthetist has been caught by a surgeon's promise of a 'quick one'. This applies whether in the hospital or at other sites where anaesthetics may be given for dental procedures, cardioversion, electroconvulsive therapy, etc. Pulse oximetry is especially useful in these circumstances and indeed no anaesthetic should be given without this form of monitoring. Every anaesthetist has stories to tell of how use of pulse oximetry has revealed unexpected and otherwise unobserved problems. Moreover, pulse oximetry detects significant hypoxia well before the best-trained observer can detect cyanosis even in optimal conditions of lighting, etc. Pulse oximetry is essential in all dark-skinned patients and in patients with sickle cell trait or disease, as well as being of great help in a wide variety of problems.

Recovery from anaesthesia

At the end of anaesthesia the anaesthetist must see that all his records are up-to-date. He must give verbal and written instructions for postoperative monitoring and continuing care to the person responsible for the recovery of the patient. Usually this person is the recovery nurse. The monitoring used in the recovery room should be appropriate to the patient's condition and the anaesthetic used and a full range of monitoring devices, as employed during anaesthesia, should be available.

Transfer of patients
Disasters have befallen patients because inexperienced persons have been left to accompany them from one hospital to another, or indeed between one part of the hospital and another — commonly between such areas

or departments as X-ray, accident & emergency, wards, recovery room or operating theatre. Similar requirements and monitoring standards pertain here as well as in the operating theatre and anaesthetic room.

Medico-legal considerations

The anaesthetist, like any other doctor, has a duty of care for his/her patient and the standard of care s/he must provide is one which a reasonably careful and competent anaesthetist would have observed. If a patient is paralysed with muscle relaxant drugs then the anaesthetist has a duty of care to keep the patient breathing and oxygenated lest they die. If s/he makes a mistake s/he may be accused of negligence; if s/he adopts a 'couldn't care less' attitude and his/her patient dies then s/he may be accused of manslaughter. In the UK anaesthetics may only be administered by fully registered practitioners who have been trained in the specialty.

Product liability
Since product liability has recently been introduced into the EEC the anaesthetist should write down what equipment or products he is using. This is because if a product applied or attached to a patient proves defective and causes injury, the patient has recourse to the manufacturer of the equipment and may be able to prove liability and thus recover damages. An instance of this sort of problem occurred in the 1970s when a batch of i.v. infusion fluids was found to be contaminated with micro-organisms during the manufacturing process. If the anaesthetist has not noted the equipment he has used on the patient he then throws himself open to a claim for damages should harm befall his patient.

Monitoring standards
The hospitals which comprise the Harvard Medical School in Boston decided to introduce standards of monitoring in 1987. This had the effect of improving standards of patient care and also within a short time reduced the premiums for malpractice insurance for anesthesiologists. The standards were soon adopted by the American Society of Anesthesiologists and similar standards have been introduced in some states with the full force of law (e.g. New York and New Jersey). Now, many countries throughout the world have adopted the same, similar or even more stringent standards for anaesthetic practice. The Association of Anaesthetists of Great Britain & Ireland (AAGBI) published their *Recommendations for Standards* in 1988. Some of the recommendations in this chapter differ slightly from those originally issued by the AAGBI because of developments with the passage of time; the result here is to alter the emphasis of the AAGBI document in several areas to 'must' rather than 'should', as advocated by a leading UK barrister who specializes in anaesthetic malpractice law, and to clear up some situations which were previously a little vague. The result should represent a beneficial effect in terms of patient safety. The cost of full monitoring is really quite small, about £2 per patient (1990 values).

Further reading

Adams A P. Capnography and pulse oximetry. In Atkinson R S, Adams A P, (eds). *Recent advances in anaesthesia and analgesia* 16th edn. London: Churchill Livingstone, 1989: 155–75.

Buck N, Devlin H B, Lunn J N. *The report of a confidential enquiry into perioperative deaths.* London: The Nuffield Provincial Hospitals Trust, 1987.

Eichhorn J H, Cooper J B, Cullen D J, Maier W R, Philip J H, Seeman R G. Standards for patient monitoring during anesthesia at Harvard Medical School. *Journal of the American Medical Association* 1986; **50(12):** 9–15

Hanning C D. 'He looks a little blue down this end.' Monitoring oxygenation during anaesthesia. *British Journal of Anaesthesia* 1985; **57:** 359–60.

Morgan-Hughes J O. Lighting and cyanosis. *British Journal of Anaesthesia* 1968; **40:** 503–507.

Powers M J, Gore G. Medicolegal aspects of anaesthesia. In: Nunn J F, Utting J E, Brown B R, (eds). *General anaesthesia* 5th edn. London: Butterworths, 1989: 1370–83.

Recommendations for standards of monitoring during anaesthesia and recovery. London: The Association of Anaesthetists of Great Britain & Ireland, 1988.

Checklists for anaesthetic machines. A recommended procedure based on the use of an oxygen analyser. London: The Association of Anaesthetists of Great Britain & Ireland, 1990.

Saunders M T. *Product Liability.* London: The Medical Defence Union, 1989.

Sykes M K. Essential monitoring. *British Journal of Anaesthesia* 1987; **59:** 901–902.

Symposium on complications and medico-legal aspects of anaesthesia. *British Journal of Anaesthesia* 1987; **59:** 813–927.

6

Fluids, electrolytes and acid-base balance
W. Aveling

- Fluid compartments
  - the capillary membrane
  - the cell membrane
  - movement of water between compartments
- Normal water and electrolyte balance
- Prescribing fluid regimens
  - basal requirements
  - continuing loss
  - correction of pre-existing dehydration
  - intraoperative fluid balance
- Acid-base balance
  - terminology and definitions
  - interpretation of acid base changes
  - treatment of acid base disturbances

Fluid compartments

Every student knows that man is mostly water. Any understanding of fluid and electrolyte balance depends on a knowledge of the various fluid compartments. An adult male is 60 per cent water, a female, having more fat, is 55 per cent water, newborn infants are 75 per cent water. The most important compartments are in the intracellular fluid (ICF) — 55 per cent of body water, and the extracellular fluid (ECF) — 45 per cent. Extracellular fluid is further subdivided into the plasma (part of the intravascular space), the interstitial fluid, the transcellular water (e.g. fluid in the gastrointestinal tract, the CSF and aqueous humour) and water associated with bone and dense connective tissue which is less readily exchangeable and of much less importance. The partitioning of the total body water (TBW) with average values for a 70 kg male, who would contain 42 litres of water, is shown in Fig. 6.1.

The key to understanding fluid balance is a knowledge of which compartment or compartments fluid is being lost from in various situations, and in which compartments fluids will end up when administered to the patient. For practical purposes we need only consider the plasma, the interstitial space, the intracellular space and the barriers between them.

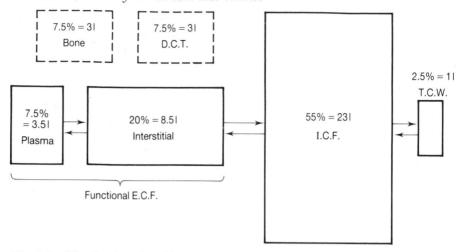

Fig. 6.1 Distribution of total body water in a 70 kg man. ECF=extracellular fluid, ICF=intracellular fluid, DCT=dense connective tissue, TCW=transcellular water.

The capillary membrane

The barrier between the plasma and interstitium is the capillary endothelium which allows the free passage of water and electrolytes (small particles) but restricts the passage of larger molecules such as proteins. These large molecules are known as the colloids. The pore size of an average capillary is 4–5 mm, the kidney and liver have larger pores and brain capillaries are relatively impermeable. The osmotic pressure generated by the presence of colloids on one side of a membrane which is impermeable to them is known as the colloid osmotic pressure (COP). Albumin (molecular weight 69 000) does not normally cross from the plasma to the interstitial space in any quantity and is mainly responsible for the difference in COP between the plasma and the interstitium. The COP is normally about 25 mmHg and tends to draw fluid into the capillary while the hydrostatic pressure difference between capillary and interstitium tends to push fluid out. This balance was first described by Starling.

The cell membrane

The barrier between the extracellular and intracellular space is the cell membrane. This is freely permeable to water but not to sodium ions which are actively pumped out of cells. Sodium is therefore mainly an extracellular cation while potassium is the main intracellular cation. Water will move across the cell membrane in either direction if there is any difference in osmolality between the two sides. Osmolality expresses the osmotic pressure across a selectively permeable membrane and depends on the number of particles in the solution, not their size. Normal osmolality of ECF is 280–295 mOsmol/kg. Since each cation is balanced by an anion, an estimate of plasma or ECF osmolality can be obtained from the formula:

Osmolality (mOsmol/kg)=2 $(Na^+ + K^+)$+glucose+urea (mmol/litre)

The difference between osmolality and osmolarity needs explanation: osmolality is expressed per kg of solvent (usually water) whereas osmolarity is expressed per litre of solution. The presence of significant amounts of protein in the solution, as in plasma, means that the osmolality and osmolarity will not be the same. Note that the colloids contribute very little to total osmolality as the number of particles is small, although as we saw above they play an important role in fluid movement across the capillaries.

Movement of water between compartments

Consider what happens when a patient takes in water, either by drinking or in the form of a 5 per cent glucose infusion whose glucose is soon metabolized. It will rapidly distribute through the ECF with a resultant fall in ECF osmolality. Since osmolality must be the same inside and outside cells, water will move from ECF to ICF until the osmolalities are the same. Thus a litre of water, or 5 per cent glucose, given to a patient will distribute itself throughout the body water. By a converse argument we can see that someone marooned on a life raft with no water will lose water from all compartments.

Normal saline (0.9 per cent) contains Na^+ and Cl^- 150 mmol/litre and has an osmolality of 300 mOsmol/kg. If this is infused into a patient it will stay in the ECF, and because the osmolality matches that inside the cells there is no movement of water into the cells. Conversely a patient losing electrolytes and water together, as in severe diarrhoea, loses the fluid from the ECF and not the ICF.

Finally, consider the infusion of human plasma protein fraction (4.5 per cent albumin). The electrolyte and protein content are like that of plasma, so there is no change in colloid osmotic pressure and the solution stays in the plasma compartment (there are, of course, circumstances in which it can leak out). A burned patient losing plasma loses it from the vascular compartment and initially there is no shift of fluid from the interstitial space. As blood pressure falls, hydrostatic pressure in the capillary falls and if colloid osmotic pressure is maintained, the Starling forces will draw water and electrolytes into the vascular compartment from the interstitium. Because there are only 3.5 litres of plasma, losses from this compartment lead to hypoperfusion and reduced O_2 transport to tissues and are potentially life threatening.

Since the plasma is part of the ECF any loss of ECF results in a corresponding decrease in circulating volume and is potentially much more serious than a loss of an equivalent volume from the total body water. For example, compare a man losing 1 litre of water a day because he is marooned on a life raft, with a man losing 1 litre of water and electrolytes a day due to a bowel obstruction. The man on the life raft will lose 7 litres in a week from his total of 42 litres of body water, i.e. a 17 per cent loss. The plasma volume will fall by 17 per cent which is survivable. The man with a bowel obstruction, on the other hand, loses his 7 litres from the functional ECF of 12 litres, i.e. a 58 per cent loss. Losing more than half of the plasma volume is not compatible with life. This is why people on life rafts can survive much longer than patients in surgical wards who are incorrectly treated.

Normal water and electrolyte balance

We take in water as food and drink, we also make about 350 ml per day as a result of the oxidisation of carbohydrates to water and carbon dioxide, and known as the metabolic water. This has to balance the output. Water is lost through the skin and from the lungs, these insensible losses amount to about 1 litre a day. Urine and faeces account for the rest. A typical balance is shown in Table 6.1.

Table 6.1   Average water balance for a sedentary adult in temperate conditions

Input (ml)		Output (ml)	
Drink	1500	Urine	1500
Food	750	Faeces	100
Metabolic	350	Lungs	400
		Skin	600
TOTAL	2600	TOTAL	2600

The precise water requirements of a particular patient depend on their size, age and temperature. Surface area (1.5 litres of water per m^2) is the most accurate guide but it is more practical to use weight, giving adults 30–40 ml/kg. Children require relatively more water than adults as set out in Table 6.2.

Table 6.2   Water requirements for children

Weight	Water requirements
0–10 kg	100 ml/kg
10–20 kg	1000 ml + 50 ml/kg for each kg >10
> 20 kg	1500 ml + 25 ml/kg for each kg >20

The average requirements of sodium and potassium are 1 mmol/kg daily of each. Human beings are very efficient at conserving sodium and can tolerate much lower sodium intakes but they are less good at conserving potassium. There is an obligatory loss of potassium in urine and faeces and patients who are not given potassium will become hypokalaemic. As potassium is mainly an intracellular cation there may be a considerable fall in total body potassium before the plasma potassium falls.

Prescribing fluid regimens

In prescribing fluid regimens for patients, we need to consider three aspects
- basal requirements
- continuing abnormal losses over and above basal requirements
- pre-existing dehydration and electrolyte loss

Intraoperative fluid balance needs special consideration as all three of the above apply. Normally nourished patients who are 'nil by mouth' for a few days during surgery, do not need feeding intravenously. Only in special circumstances is i.v. feeding required and that is outside the scope of this chapter.

Basal requirements

We have seen above the daily requirements of water and electrolytes. If we look now at the various crystalloid solutions that are available (Table 6.3), we can design fluid regimens for basal requirements.

Table 6.3 Content of crystalloid solutions

Name	Known as	Na$^+$	Cl$^-$	K$^+$	HCO$_3^-$	Ca^{++}	calculated
				mmol/litre			mOsmol/litre
Sodium chloride 0.9%	Normal saline	150	150				300
Sodium chloride 0.9%, potassium chloride 0.3%	normal saline+ KCl	150	190	40			380
Sodium chloride 0.9%, potassium chloride 0.15%	normal saline+ KCl	150	170	20			340
Ringer's lactate	Hartmann's	131	111	5	29 1(as lactate)	2	280
Glucose 5%	5% dextrose	40	40				280
Glucose 5%, potassium chloride 0.3%	5% dextrose+ KCl						360
Glucose 5%, potassium chloride 0.15%	5% dextrose+ KCl		20	20			320
Glucose 4%, sodium chloride 0.18%	dextrose saline	30	30				286
Glucose 4%, sodium chloride 0.18%, potassium chloride 0.3%	dextrose saline+ KCl	30	70	40			366
Glucose 4%, sodium chloride 0.18%, potassium chloride 0.15%	dextrose saline+ KCl	30	50	20			326
Sodium chloride 0.45%	half normal saline	75	75				150
Sodium chloride 1.8%	twice normal saline	300	300				600
Sodium bicarbonate 8.4%	—	1000			1000		2000
Sodium bicarbonate 1.4%	—	167			167		334

Normal saline, Hartmann's, 5 per cent dextrose and dextrose saline are the most commonly used. Note that their osmolalities are similar to that of ECF, i.e. they are isotonic with plasma. The purpose of the glucose is to make the solution isotonic, not to provide calories, although a small amount of glucose does have a protein-sparing effect during the catabolism that follows major surgery and trauma.

Our standard 70 kg patient can be provided with the 24-hour basal requirements of 30–40 ml/kg water and 1 mmol/kg of sodium in any of the ways shown in Table 6.4.

Table 6.4 Basal water and sodium regimens for a 70 kg patient on i.v. fluids

Solution	Volume ml	Na$^+$ mmol	K$^+$ mmol
5% glucose	2000	—	
0.9% saline	500	75	
5% glucose	2000	—	—
Hartmann's	500	65.5	2.5
4% glucose	2500	75	—
0.18% saline			

Potassium
None of these regimens supply significant amounts of potassium. Potassium chloride is usually added to the bags and is supplied as ampoules of 20 mmol in 10 ml or 1 g (=13.5 mmol) in 10 ml. Bags of crystalloid can be obtained with potassium already added, usually labelled red. It cannot be stressed enough that potassium can be very dangerous because hyperkalaemia causes cardiac arrhythmias and asystole. It should never be injected as a bolus. There have been a number of tragedies reported to the medical defence organisations in which potassium chloride ampoules were mistaken for sodium chloride and used as 'flush' with fatal consequences. Hyperkalaemia may also occur if potassium supplements are given to anuric patients. For this reason one usually waits until one is certain of reasonable urine output before adding potassium to the regimen postoperatively. Safe rules for giving potassium are:
- urine output at least 40 ml/hr
- not more than 40 mmol added to 1 litre
- no faster than 40 mmol/hr

Continuing loss
Patients with continuing losses above the basal requirements need extra fluid. The commonest example in anaesthetic and surgical practice is the patient with bowel obstruction. Fluid can be aspirated by a nasogastric tube to assess both volume and electrolyte content. Saline with added potassium should be given to replace it. Dextrose saline is not an appropriate fluid for this purpose because it only contains 30 mmol/l, and 5 per cent glucose is even worse. Hyponatraemia will result if these solutions are used to replace bowel loss.

To keep track of the fluids, a fluid-balance chart should be kept. This records all fluid in (oral and i.v.) and all fluid out (urine, drainage, vomit, etc.). Every 24 hours these are totalled, allowance made for insensible losses and the balance, positive or negative, recorded. Any patient on i.v. fluids should have a daily balance, daily electrolyte measurements and a new regimen prescribed every day. The instruction 'and repeat' should never be used in fluid management and has led to disasters in the past.

Correction of pre-existing dehydration

Patients who arrive in a dehydrated state clearly need to be resuscitated with fluid over and above their basal requirements. Usually this will be done intravenously. The problems are:

- to identify from which compartment or compartments the fluid has been lost
- to assess the extent of the dehydration

The fluid used to resuscitate the patient should be similar in composition and volume to that which has been lost.

From what we know about the movement of fluid between compartments (see above) and using the patient's history one can usually decide where the losses are coming from. As we have seen, bowel losses come from the ECF while pure water losses are from the total body water. Protein-containing fluid is lost from the plasma and there may sometimes be a combination of all three types of loss.

Assessment of deficit

To estimate the extent of the losses, history, clinical examination, measurement and laboratory tests all play a part. A dehydrated patient will be thirsty, have dry mucous membranes, sunken eyes and cheeks, loss of skin elasticity and weight loss. They will feel weak and in severe cases will be mentally confused. The cardiovascular system responds with tachcardia and peripheral vasoconstriction so that the patient feels cold. Eventually, blood pressure and cardiac output fall, at which point the vital organs, brain, liver and kidneys, which up to now have been protected, are affected. Clouding of consciousness and oliguria are signs of severe dehydration. Weight, pulse, blood pressure and urine output are essential and simple measurements in the assessment and treatment of fluid loss.

Venous pressure

Equally important and a little more complex is the measurement of central venous pressure (CVP). An i.v. catheter is inserted into a central vein. The tip should lie within the thorax, usually in the superior vena cava or right atrium. In this position, blood can be aspirated freely and there is a swing in pressure with respiration. The pressure is usually measured by an electronic transducer but can be done quite simply by connecting the patient to an open-ended column of fluid and measuring the height above zero with a ruler (Fig. 6.2).

The zero point for measuring CVP is the fifth rib in the mid-axillary line with the patient supine (this corresponds to the position of the left atrium). The normal range for CVP is 3–8cmH$_2$O (1mmHg=1.36cmH$_2$O). A low reading, particularly a negative value, confirms dehydration, but CVP measurements are more use as a guide to the adequacy of treatment. The response of the CVP to a fluid challenge of 200ml 5 per cent glucose tells more about the state of the circulation than a single reading. A dehydrated patient's CVP will rise in response to the challenge but then fall as the circulation vasodilates to accommodate the fluid. If the CVP rises and does not fall again this indicates overfilling or a failing myocardium.

The CVP reflects the function of the right ventricle, usually this parallels left ventricular function. In cardiac disease there may be disparity between

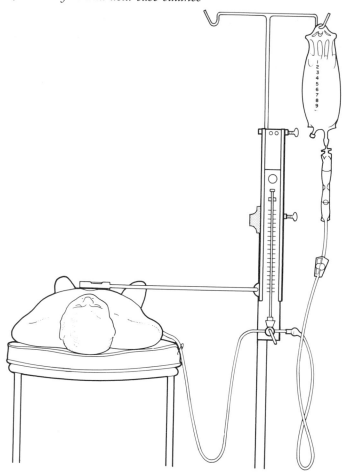

Fig. 6.2 Measurement of central venous pressure by the use of a fluid filled manometer.

the function of the two ventricles. The left ventricular function can be assessed by the use of a balloon-tipped catheter (Swan–Ganz) in a branch of the pulmonary artery. When the balloon is blown up to occlude the vessel the pressure measured distally gives a good guide to the left atrial pressure. This is called the pulmonary capillary wedge pressure (PCWP) and is normally 5–12 mmHg. For the assessment of volume replacement in patients who have normal cardiac function CVP is quite adequate and PCWP is unnecessary and expensive.

Quantification of plasma and ECF loss

If plasma is lost from the circulation, the plasma remaining still has the same albumin concentration though the volume is diminished. Since no red cells are lost they become concentrated, resulting in a rise in haematocrit. Plasma is, of course, part of the ECF so that losses of fluid and electrolytes without protein loss will cause a rise in haematocrit but also a rise in plasma–protein concentration (Fig. 6.3). Changes in plasma albumin and haematocrit thus provide a good guide to ECF losses, while only haematocrit is of use in monitoring plasma loss.

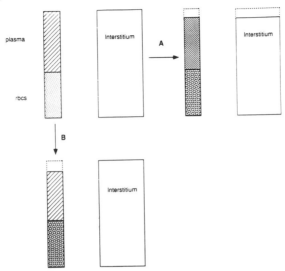

Fig. 6.3 A: loss of ECF leading to rise in albumin and haematocrit. B: loss of plasma leading to rise in haematocrit but no change in albumin concentration.

In ECF depletion the total amount of albumin stays the same although its concentration goes up. If Pr_1 is the initial albumin concentration and Pr_2 is the concentration after dehydration it can be shown that

$$\left[\text{\% fall in ECF volume} = \left(1 - \frac{Pr_1}{Pr_2}\right) \times 100\right]$$

$$\left[\begin{array}{c}\text{e.g. if the albumin rises from 35 to 45 g/l} \\ \text{fall in ECF volume} = \left(1 - \frac{35}{45}\right) \times 100 = 22\%\end{array}\right]$$

By a similar argument one can calculate the fall in plasma volume as follows

$$\left[\text{\% fall in plasma volume} = 100\left[1 - \frac{Hct_1}{100 - Hct_1} \times \frac{100 - Hct_2}{Hct_2}\right]\right]$$

$$\left[\begin{array}{c}\text{e.g. Haematocrit (Hct) rises from 40 per cent to 50 per cent and} \\ \text{fall in plasma volume} = 100\left[1 - \left(\frac{40 \times 50}{60 \quad 50}\right)\right] = 33\%\end{array}\right]$$

Haematocrit and plasma albumin are thus very useful in the assessment of ECF and plasma losses, much more so than the sodium which, though being lost, does not change in concentration.

Water and electrolyte replacement

Once the amount of deficit has been assessed as discussed above, we come to the question of what to give to restore the situation. A look at the composition of various body fluids (Table 6.5) shows us that ECF losses of water and electrolytes should be replaced with either normal saline or ringer-lactate with added potassium (see above: basal requirements).

Table 6.5   Electrolyte content and daily volume of body secretions

	Na$^+$	K$^+$	Cl$^-$	Daily volume
		mmol/litre		in litres
Saliva	15	19	40	1.5
Stomach	50	15	140	2.5
Bile, pancreas, small bowel	130–145	5–12	70–100	4.2
Insensible sweat	12	10	12	0.6
Sensible sweat	50	10	50	variable

The only hypotonic secretions are saliva and sweat. The sodium content of sweat varies and responds to aldosterone. Gastric secretion though having a sodium content of only 50 mmol/litre is isotonic with ECF because of the hydrogen it contains. Where the losses are primarily of gastric secretions, e.g. pyloric stenosis, one might think it necessary to supply hydrogen ions. In fact, the kidney compensates by retaining hydrogen and excreting sodium and bicarbonate so that the net effect is a loss of sodium and chloride. Normal saline with potassium should therefore be used in rehydration.

Plasma replacement and plasma substitutes

When we need to replace lost plasma there is a choice between giving plasma prepared from donated blood or one of the synthetic plasma substitutes. Human plasma protein fraction (HPPF) is prepared by separating red cells from donated blood. A bottle contains plasma from several donors and has been pasteurized to prevent the transmission of disease (e.g. hepatitis or HIV). It contains 4.5 per cent albumin, has no clotting factors and is stable at room temperature. The main disadvantage is its cost (£40 in UK, 1990) which reflects its limited availability.

A number of solutions containing molecules large enough to stay within the capillaries and generate colloid osmotic pressure are available as plasma substitutes (Table 6.6).

Dextrans
The dextrans are glucose polymers available in preparations of different molecular weights. There is a large range of molecular weights in the solution. Dextran 70 is so called because the average molecular weight is supposed to be 70 000. In fact, the number average molecular weight which is much more relevant to the colloid osmotic pressure is 38 000 (see legend to Table 6.6). Dextran 40 has smaller molecules and can be nephrotoxic. Dextran 110 has larger molecules. Neither of these will be considered further. Dextran 70 is quite a good plasma substitute but has declined in popularity because of its adverse effects on coagulation and cross matching and the relatively high incidence of allergic reactions.

Table 6.6 Characteristics of colloid solutions

Name	Brand name	No. average* molecular wt.	MW range	Na⁺ Na⁺	K⁺	Ca⁺⁺ mmol/litre	t½ in plasma	Adverse reactions Mild %	Adverse reactions Severe %	Effect on coagulation	Cost UK1990
Human plasma protein fraction	HPPF	69000	69000	150	2	—	20 days	0.02	0.004	none	£40
Dextran 70 in saline 0.9% or glucose 5%	Macrodex Lomodex 70 Gentran 70	38000	10000–250000	150	—	—	12 hr	0.7	0.02	inhibit platelet aggregation factor VIII interfere with crossmatch	£3.60 £4.10
Polygeline (degraded gelatine)	Haemaccel	24500	5000–50000	145	5	6.25	2.5 hr	0.12	0.04	none	£3.80
Succinylated gelatine	Gelofusin	22600	10000–140000	150	0.4	0.4	4 hr	0.12	0.04	none	£3.10
Hydroxy ethyl starch 6% in saline (Hetastarch)	Hespan	70000	$10000-10^6$ 10^6	154	—	—	25 hr	0.09	0.006	>1.5g/kg per day can cause coagulopathy	£15.30

*Number average molecular weight should not be confused with weight average molecular weight which is usually quoted by the manufacturers. No. average MW is more appropriate.

Gelatins

Gelatin solutions are prepared by the hydrolysis of bovine collagen. They have the advantage over dextrans of not affecting coagulation and having a low incidence of allergic reactions. Being of smaller average particle size they stay in the intravascular space a shorter time. Haemaccel contains potassium and calcium ions which can cause coagulation if mixed with citrated blood in an infusion set. Haemaccel stays a short time in the circulation, 30 per cent of the molecules being dispersed to the interstitial tissues in 30 minutes. Gelofusin is probably preferable from this point of view.

Hetastarch

6 per cent hetastarch in saline has become available in the last few years. It has the largest average molecular weight of any of the plasma substitutes and therefore stays in the circulation longer. The dose should be limited to 1500 ml/70 kg, more can cause coagulation problems. About 30 per cent of a dose is taken up by the reticuloendothelial system without apparent detriment to its function. Smaller molecules (<50 000 MW) are filtered by the kidneys. Larger ones are broken down by plasma amylase until small enough for renal excretion.

Choice of solution for plasma expansion

The intravascular space can be expanded by the use of crystalloid solutions, e.g. saline, but because the fluid spreads throughout the ECF, 4 litres of crystalloid are needed to expand the plasma by 1 litre. In an emergency crystalloid is useful. All the battle casualties in the Falklands War were resuscitated in the field with Hartmann's solution.

For most patients with acute hypovolaemia the best combination of advantages at low cost is offered by succinylated gelatin (Gelofusin). Being relatively short acting it is particularly useful as a holding measure until blood becomes available.

In continuing hypovolaemia, hetastarch gives more prolonged expansion and its larger molecules are better retained in the circulation when the capillaries are leaky, e.g. in septicaemic shock.

Blood loss and blood transfusion

So far we have talked about plasma loss and plasma expansion. Most of what has been said about the assessment and replacement of plasma volume applies to blood loss. Transfusion of donated blood is possible in most circumstances but has several disadvantages to be weighed against the fact that only haemoglobin carries oxygen. With a haemoglobin of 14 g/dl evolution has equipped us with spare capacity as far as oxygen carrying capacity is concerned. Indeed, as haematocrit falls, the decrease in oxygen carrying is compensated for by better tissue perfusion due to reduced blood viscosity. It has been shown that the best balance between oxygen carrying and viscosity occurs around a haematocrit of 30 per cent (see Chapter 2). It is also suspected that blood transfusion at the time of surgery for certain cancers leads to immunological suppression and poorer long-term survival. Since the AIDS scare there is greater reluctance on the part of the public to accept blood transfusions. There are also hazards associated with transfusions; these can be summarized as:

- Hazards of any transfusion
  - transfusion of disease, e.g. AIDS, malaria (donor blood screened for HIV, hepatitis, syphilis)
  - bacterial contamination
  - pyrogenic reactions (antibodies to white cells)
  - incompatibility reactions
  - ±haemolysis (clerical error commonest cause)

- Hazards of massive transfusion
  - hypothermia
  - hyperkalaemia
  - citrate toxicity
  - acidosis
  - air embolism
  - microaggregate embolism, 'shock lung'
  - accidental overload
  - dilution and consumption of clotting factors

For all these reasons as well as the expense of blood and the rarity of some blood groups, one is reluctant to transfuse blood. In practical terms operative blood loss up to 500 ml can be replaced with crystalloid, remembering that four times as much will be needed (see above), or plasma substitutes. Only if more than 1 litre of blood has been lost should one consider giving blood.

Rather than supply whole blood, it is more efficient for the transfusion service to separate it into the following components

- plasma-reduced blood (packed cells)
- washed red cells: if transfusion reaction a problem
- plasma protein fraction (HPPF)
- fresh frozen plasma (FFP): contains clotting factors more dilute than the concentrates below
- cryoprecipitate: rich in factor VIII
- factor VIII concentrate: even richer in VIII
- factor II, VII, IX, X concentrate
- factor XI concentrate
- fibrinogen
- platelet concentrate

Blood cross-matched for patients undergoing surgery usually comes as plasma-reduced blood ('packed cells'). This is more viscous than whole blood and needs to be given with appropriate amounts of crystalloid or colloid solution to restore the volume.

The quantity of blood lost is assessed clinically as outlined above, and at operation by watching the suction bottle and weighing swabs, but this generally underestimates the loss. In operations like transurethral resection of the prostate, measurement of haemoglobin in the irrigating fluid gives an accurate measure of blood loss. In acute blood loss haematocrit and haemoglobin concentrations do not change until the blood remaining in the patient has been diluted by shift of fluid from the interstitial space or i.v. infusion. Plasma-reduced blood and whole blood more than a day old (which it almost always is) contain no viable platelets and few clotting factors. The same applies to plasma–protein fraction. In massive transfusion both dilution and consumption of clotting factors make it necessary to send blood for a clotting screen and give platelets and fresh frozen plasma (FFP) according to the results. As a rule one gives a unit of FFP for every 4–6 units of stored blood transfused.

Intraoperative fluid balance
During an operation everything we have discussed so far may be going on at the same time. The patient is starved for 6–12 hours, there may be blood loss, plasma loss, ECF loss and evaporation of water from exposed bowel. As part of the stress response to surgery the patient retains water and sodium. The importance of careful monitoring in major surgery will be obvious, this includes accurate assessment of blood loss, haemodynamic variables and urine output.

As a rule of thumb, in intra-abdominal surgery Hartmann's solution 5 ml/kg per h may be given up to 2 litres. This will compensate for starvation, ECF loss, evaporation and some blood loss. Blood or colloids may have to be given in addition.

For the first 36 hours postoperatively there is water retention and there is sodium retention lasting 3–5 days. Obligatory potassium loss of 50–100 mmol/day continues. If additional sodium is given it is simply retained although the urine may show an increase in sodium 'output. Provided that intraoperative losses have been replaced, by the end of the operation one should give the basal requirements (30–40 ml/kg H_2O+1 mmol/kg Na^+ and K^+) plus additional blood or colloid if there is significant wound drainage. Remember not to start potassium until urine output is established, the operation of inadvertent bilateral ureteric ligation is not unknown.

Acid-base balance

Claude Bernard was the first to recognize that to function effectively the body needs a stable 'milieu interieur'. The hydrogen ion concentration is a most important part of this. An acid is a hydrogen ion (proton) donor and a base accepts hydrogen ions. Throughout life the body produces hydrogen ions and they must be excreted or buffered to keep the internal environment constant.

Terminology and definitions

Hydrogen ion activity
Hydrogen ion activity is traditionally expressed in pH units, pH being the negative $\log_{10}$ of the hydrogen ion concentration:

$$\left[pH = -\log_{10}[H^+] = \log_{10}\frac{1}{[H^+]} \right]$$

Hydrogen ion concentration can also be expressed directly in nanomoles/litre and you will find both systems in use in medicine (Table 6.7).

Table 6.7 Conversion table for pH units and hydrogen ion concentration

pH unit	H^+ nmol/litre
8.00	10
7.70	20
7.44	36
7.40	40
7.36	44
7.10	80
7.00	100

Note that the pH is a logarithmic scale so that each 0.3 unit fall in pH represents a doubling of hydrogen ion concentration.

Acidosis and alkalosis

The normal ECF pH is 7.36–7.44 (44–36 nmol/litre). Acidaemia is a blood pH below this range and alkalaemia above it. Acidosis is a condition that leads to acidaemia or would do so if no compensation occurred, but the terms acidosis and acidaemia are often used loosely to mean the same thing which is not strictly correct. Alkalosis and alkalaemia are defined in a similar way.

Respiratory acidosis
A fall in pH resulting from a rise in the P_{CO_2} is a respiratory acidosis, e.g. narcotic overdose leading to hypoventilation causes a rise in P_{CO_2}.

Respiratory alkalosis
A rise in pH due to a lowering of the P_{CO_2} such as occurs in hyperventilation.

Metabolic acidosis
A fall in pH due to anything other than CO_2 (sometimes referred to as non-respiratory acidosis). There is a primary gain of acid or loss of bicarbonate from ECF.

Metabolic alkalosis
A rise in pH from non-respiratory causes. There is either a gain in bicarbonate or a loss of acid from the ECF.

Compensatory changes
If the initial problem is respiratory, the result is called a *primary* respiratory acidosis or alkalosis. If the respiratory problem persists for more than a few hours the kidney will excrete or retain bicarbonate to try and compensate for

the respiratory disturbance. This is referred to as *secondary or compensatory* metabolic acidosis or alkalosis.

Thus a *primary* respiratory acidosis may be accompanied by a *secondary* metabolic alkalosis. For example, chronic obstructive airways disease leads to a rise in the Pco_2: *primary respiratory acidosis*. To compensate for this the kidney retains bicarbonate leading to a rise in ECF bicarbonate: *secondary or compensatory metabolic alkalosis*.

In the same way primary respiratory alkalosis (e.g. the hyperventilation that occurs at high altitude) will be compensated by a secondary metabolic acidosis.

Where the first disturbance is metabolic, e.g. the build up of acid in diabetic ketoacidosis, the primary metabolic acidosis will cause hyperventilation (secondary respiratory alkalosis) which will tend to restore the pH to normal. This respiratory compensation for a metabolic change happens much more rapidly than the metabolic compensation for a respiratory problem.

The fourth possible combination of changes is to have a metabolic alkalosis (e.g. loss of H^+ in pyloric stenosis) compensated by a respiratory acidosis. However, hypoventilation (respiratory acidosis) leads to a fall in Po_2 which stimulates ventilation so that in practice compensatory respiratory acidosis is not usually seen.

In deciding which is the primary and which the secondary change it is important to realize that the compensatory changes do not bring the pH back to normal, they bring it back *towards* the normal range. In other words, even after compensation, the measured pH is altered in the direction of the primary problem (acidosis or alkalosis). Compensatory mechanisms merely make the disturbance in pH less than it otherwise would have been. It is also important to consider the history. Examiners may give students blood gas results to interpret but in real life blood gases come from patients. Knowing that a patient is an unconscious diabetic breathing spontaneously, rather than an anaesthetized patient on a ventilator, certainly helps one's interpretation.

Buffers

Buffers are substances which, by their presence in solution, minimize the change in pH for a given addition of acid or alkali. Three-quarters of the buffering power of the body is within the cells, the rest is in the ECF. Proteins, haemoglobin, phosphates and the bicarbonate system are all important buffers. The particular importance of the bicarbonate system is that CO_2 is excreted in the lungs and can be regulated by changes in ventilation. Bicarbonate excretion in the kidney can also be regulated. The lungs are responsible for the excretion of 16000 mmol/day of acid and the kidneys for only 40–80 mmol/day. The formation of carbonic acid from CO_2 and water is catalysed by carbonic anhydrase (present in red cells). The reaction may go in either direction:

$$\left[H^+ + HCO_3^- \rightleftharpoons H_2CO_3 \rightleftharpoons H_2O + CO_2 \right]$$

The Henderson-Hasselbach equation is derived from this and expresses the relationship between the bicarbonate concentration the CO_2 and the pH:

$$\left[pH = pK + \log_{10} \frac{HCO_3^-}{H_2\,CO_3} \right]$$

The carbonic acid can be expressed in terms of CO_2 so that a more useful form of the equation is:

$$\left[pH = pK + \log_{10} \frac{(HCO_3^-)}{0.03\,Pco_2} \right]$$

As this is a buffer system which minimizes changes in pH, we can see that if the CO_2 rises so will the bicarbonate to keep $\dfrac{HCO_3^-}{Pco_2}$ constant. Similarly a fall in bicarbonate will be accompanied by a fall in Pco_2 to prevent a change in pH.

Interpretation of acid-base changes

As the patient's acid-base status varies, three things are changing at once: pH, HCO_3^- and Pco_2. Blood gas machines measure directly Po_2, pH and Pco_2. The actual bicarbonate HCO_3^- is calculated from the Henderson-Hasselbach equation. They also derive other variables which help in the interpretation of the acid-base status. These are:

Standard bicarbonate (SBC)

This is the concentration of bicarbonate in the plasma of fully oxygenated blood at *37°C at a Pco_2 of 5.3 kPa (40 mm Hg)*. In other words, it tells you what the bicarbonate would be if there was no respiratory disturbance. Looking at the standard bicarbonate therefore tells what is happening on the metabolic side. Normal standard bicarbonate is 22–26 mmol/litre. Values above this indicate metabolic alkalosis and those below, metabolic acidosis.

Base excess (BE)

This is the amount of strong base or acid that would need to be added to whole blood to titrate the pH back to *7.4 at a Pco_2 of 5.3 kPa and 37°C*. It tells you the same thing as standard bicarbonate, namely the metabolic status of the patient. Normal base excess is obviously 0 (±2 mmol/litre). Positive base excess occurs in metabolic alkalosis and negative base excess (sometimes called base deficit) indicates metabolic acidosis. The base excess is an *in vitro* determination in whole blood. It is also known as the actual base excess (ABE) or the base excess (blood) (BE b).

Standard base excess (SBE)

This is an estimate of the *in vivo* base excess and takes into account the difference in buffering capacity between the patient's ECF and the blood that was put in the blood–gas machine. Interstitial fluid, having less protein and no haemoglobin, has a lower buffering capacity than blood. SBE is therefore ±1–2 mmol/litre greater than BE but this makes very little difference in practice. SBE is sometimes called base excess ecf (BE ecf).

Total CO_2 (TCO_2)

This is the total concentration of CO_2 in the plasma as bicarbonate and dissolved CO_2.

$$\left[TCO_2 = [HCO_3^-] + (PCO_2 \times solubility) \right]$$

Oxygen saturation (O_2 sat)

The percentage saturation of haemoglobin by oxygen is derived from the haemoglobin oxygen dissociation curve and the measured Po_2. Normal value >95 per cent.

Po_2 and inspired oxygen (F_iO_2)

To interpret the Po_2 one needs to know the age of the patient and the F_iO_2. Normal arterial Po_2 declines with age. Roughly speaking $Po_2 = (100 - \underline{age\ in\ years})$ mmHg or $(13.3 - 0.044 \times age)$ kPa. The expected
$\qquad\qquad\qquad\qquad 3$
alveolar Po_2 (PAo_2) can be predicted from the inspired oxygen by the simplified alveolar gas equation: $PAo_2 = P_iO_2 - \underline{PACO_2}$ where R is the
$\qquad\qquad\qquad\qquad\qquad\qquad\qquad\qquad\qquad R$
respiratory exchange ratio (normally 0.8). In dry gas P_iO_2 in kPa=fractional inspired oxygen (F_iO_2) per cent. Alveolar gas is saturated with water vapour (6.3 kPa) for which allowance must be made. If the F_iO_2 was 40 per cent and the Pco_2 5.3

$$\left[PAo_2 = (40 - \underline{40 \times 6.3}) - \underline{5.3} = 30.85\ kPa \right]$$
$$\qquad\qquad\quad 100 \qquad\ 0.8$$

As an approximate rule of thumb 10 may be deducted from the F_iO_2 per cent to give the expected PAo_2 in kPa, e.g. F_iO_2 50 per cent, therefore approx. $PAo_2 = 40$ kPa. The difference between the estimated PAo_2 and the measured arterial Po_2 is called the $(A-a)\Delta Po_2$ gradient. It is normally 0.5–3 kPa.

Table 6.8 Print-out from a blood-gas machine with normal values

Temperature	37°C
pH	7.36–7.44 (44–36 nmol/litre)
Pco_2	4.6–5.6 kPa (35–42 mmHg)
Po_2	10.0–13.3 kPa (75–100 mmHg)
HCO_3^-	22–26 mmol/litre
TCO_2	24–28 mmol/litre
SBC	22–26 mmol/litre
BE	$-2+2$ mmol/litre
SBE	$-3+3$ mmol/litre
O_2 Sat	>95%
Hb	11.5–16.5 g/dlitre

Without considering the inspired oxygen it is not possible to comment sensibly on the observed PAo_2. A rough calculation of the $(A-a)$ Po_2 gradient should be made when commenting on blood gas results. Some machines even calculate this for you as well!

A blood-gas machine usually prints out the variables shown in Table 6.8. There is often a haemoglobin measurement and the temperature of measurement (37°C) is quoted.

Temperature correction

The blood-gas machine operates at 37°C. Because gases are more soluble in liquid at lower temperatures (as drinkers of cold lager will know) the blood gases would be different if measured at another temperature. Blood-gas machines are programmed to correct the gases if you tell the machine the patient's actual temperature. However, there has been much debate as to whether it is appropriate to correct for temperature. Suffice it to say that the protagonists of not correcting for temperature (the alpha-stat theory) hold sway and one should probably act on the blood gases as measured at 37°C and not the temperature-corrected values.

The anion gap

For electrochemical neutrality of the ECF the number of anions must equal the number of cations. The main cations are sodium and potassium and the main anions are chloride, bicarbonate, proteins, phosphates, sulphates and organic acids.

Normally only Na^+, K^+, HCO_3^- and Cl^- are measured in the laboratory. Thus, when we add the normal values for these they do not balance:

cations		anions	
Na^+	140	Cl^-	105
K^+	5	HCO_3^-	25
Total	145	Total	130

The difference is known as the anion gap and represents the other anions not usually measured.

$$\left[\text{anion gap} = (Na^+ + K^+) - (HCO_3^- + Cl^-) = 11 - 19 \, \text{mmol/litre} \right]$$

Its significance is that in certain metabolic acidoses, e.g. keto-acidosis or lactic-acidosis, the anion gap will be increased by the presence of organic anions. However, in metabolic acidosis in which chloride replaces bicarbonate, e.g. bicarbonate loss due to diarrhoea, the anion gap will be normal.

Plan for interpreting blood gases

- Check for internal consistency. Remember that the machine only measures pH, Pco_2 and Po_2. If it measures any of these wrongly, which is not infrequent, the derived variables will also be wildly abnormal. If the results do not fit with the clinical picture, suspect the machine.

Example: a patient on a ventilator in theatre with an end-tidal CO_2 of 5 per cent has the following gases:

Po_2	13.0
pH	7.64
Pco_2	5.1
HCO_3^-	37.5
TCO_2	38.5
SBC	39.0
BE	+15
SBE	+16
O_2Sat	99 per cent

It is much more likely that the pH has been measured wrongly than that the patient has a gross metabolic alkalosis.

- Look at the pH. Remember the pH change is always in the direction of the primary problem, acidosis or alkalosis.
- Look at the Pco_2. Abnormality of the CO_2 indicates the respiratory component.
- Look at the base excess or standard bicarbonate. Both give the same information, i.e. the metabolic acid-base status after correcting for the Pco_2.
- Calculate the anion gap.
- Look at the Po_2 and calculate the A–a gradient.

Examples of abnormal blood gases

Example 1

pH	7.51	The alkalaemia is due to primary respiratory
Pco_2	3.7	alkalosis (low Pco_2). There is no metabolic
Po_2	29	compensation (normal base excess). The Po_2
HCO_3^-	22.1	expected if breathing 40 per cent oxygen:
TCO_2	23.6	$F_iO_2-10=(40-10)=30$. The patient is
SBC	25	hyperventilating.
BE	+1.1	
SBE	+2	
O_2 Sat 100 per cent		
(F_iO_2 40 per cent)		

Example 2

pH	7.28	A respiratory acidosis with high Pco_2 due
Pco_2	7.33	to hypoventilation. Again no metabolic
Po_2	9.21	compensation (normal SBC and BE). Low Po_2
HCO_3^-	25.2	due to hypoventilation
TCO_2	28.4	
SBC	22.3	
BE	−1.9	
SBE	−2.5	
O_2 Sat 91 per cent		
(F_iO_2 air)		

Example 3

pH	7.35
Pco_2	9.33
Po_2	7.11
HCO_3^-	39.1
TCO_2	41.2
SBC	32.4
BE	+8.2
SBE	+9.1

O_2 Sat 85 per cent
(F_iO_2 air)

Again a respiratory acidosis (high Pco_2) but this time compensated by metabolic alkalosis (high SBC and positive base excess). This is typical of chronic obstructive airways disease with renal compensation.

Example 4

pH	7.21
Pco_2	4.0
Po_2	13.3
HCO_3^-	11.5
TCO_2	12.8
SBC	9.3
BE	−15.2
SBE	−16.4

O_2 Sat 99 per cent
(F_iO_2 air)

The acidaemia (low pH) is primarily due to a metabolic acidosis (low SBC, base excess −15). Compensatory respiratory alkalosis (low Pco_2) does not return the pH to normal. Po_2 normal.

Example 5

pH	7.36
Pco_2	4.21
Po_2	10.49
HCO_3^-	17.6
TCO_2	18.5
SBC	17.8
BE	−6.2
SBE	−6.9

O_2 Sat 96 per cent
(F_iO_2 60 per cent)

The pH is in the normal range despite low Pco_2 (respiratory alkalosis) and low standard bicarbonate (metabolic acidosis). The important thing here is the Po_2. It is apparently in the normal range but not when breathing 60 per cent O_2. The (A−a) Po_2 gradient is roughly 40 kPa. These gases are typical of a patient with adult respiratory distress syndrome.

Treatment of acid-base disturbances

As in any other field of medicine, treatment should be directed at the underlying cause. Correcting the Pco_2 is usually possible by taking over the patient's ventilation and adjusting the minute volume to give the desired Pco_2.

Treatment of a metabolic acidosis is more controversial. It was traditional to treat a metabolic acidosis by giving sodium bicarbonate according to the formula: (base excess×body weight in kg÷3) mmol starting by giving half the dose. 8.4 per cent sodium bicarbonate contains 1 mmol/ml.

It is now argued that, particularly in a hypoxic state such as exists at cardiac arrests, bicarbonate administration may do more harm than good. The bicarbonate generates CO_2 which crosses easily into cells making the intracellular acidosis worse. If ventilation is impaired the CO_2 generated is unable to escape via the lungs. The traditional practice of giving 50–100 mmol of bicarbonate at a cardiac arrest is probably unjustified.

There is still a place for bicarbonate therapy in acidosis due to diarrhoea, renal tubular acidosis and uraemic acidosis. As outlined above, the base excess is used to calculate the dose. 8.4 per cent sodium bicarbonate is hyperosmolar and must be given into a large central vein. Accidental subcutaneous administration can cause tissue necrosis. Also bear in mind that each mmol of HCO_3^- is accompanied by Na^+ and it is easy to overload the patient with sodium. Frequent blood gas and electrolyte analyses must be made during treatment with bicarbonate.

Further reading

Adams, A P, Hahn CEW. *Principles and Practice of Blood-Gas Analysis*, 2nd edition. London: Churchill-Livingstone, 1982.

Graf H, Arieff A I. Use of sodium bicarbonate in the therapy of organic acidosis. *Intensive Care Medicine* 1986; **12**: 285–8.

Hillman K. (1990). Fluids and Electrolytes. In: Scurr C, Feldman S, Soni N, (eds). *Scientific Foundations of Anaesthesia. The Basis of Intensive Care*, 4th edition. London: Heinemann.

Linton R A F. Pulmonary gas exchange and acid base status. In: Churchill-Davidson H C, (ed). *A Practice of Anaesthesia*, 5th edition. London: Lloyd Luke, 1984.

Robarts W M, Parkin J V, Hobsley M. A simple clinical approach to quantifying losses from the extracellular and plasma compartments. *Annals of the Royal College of Surgeons of England 1979;* **61**: 142–6.

Webb A R, Barclay S A, Bennett E D. In vitro colloid osmotic pressure of commonly used plasma expanders and substitutes. *Intensive Care Medicine* 1989; **15**: 116–20.

Willatts, S M. *Lecture notes on fluid and electrolyte balance*, 2nd edition. Oxford: Blackwell Scientific Publications, 1987.

7

Oxygen therapy
J.N. Cashman

- Types of hypoxia
- Assessment of hypoxia
- Indications for oxygen therapy
- Oxygen therapy
    adjuncts to oxygen therapy
    apparatus
- Humidification
- Hazards of oxygen therapy
    fire risk
    drying of secretions
    oxygen toxicity

Oxygen is necessary for all cellular metabolism, however following anaesthesia and surgery, oxygen delivery to the tissues may be markedly impaired. Additional oxygen (30–40 per cent) is therefore administered routinely to all patients postoperatively in order to prevent tissue hypoxia.

Types of hypoxia

Hypoxia is a state in which aerobic metabolism is reduced as a result of a fall in the partial pressure of oxygen within the mitochondria.

Hypoxia is classified as hypoxic, anaemic, stagnant or histotoxic. Hypoxic hypoxia may be the result of a reduction in the partial pressure of oxygen in the inspired air, alveolar hypoventilation, ventilation-perfusion mismatch, a diffusion defect at the alveolar-capillary membrane or venous admixture (sometimes called shunt hypoxia). Anaemia results in a reduced oxygen-carrying capacity of the blood, but it is also important to realize that anaemic hypoxia can occur in the presence of a normal haemoglobin if there is competition for the haemoglobin oxygen binding sites e.g. carbon monoxide poisoning. Stagnant (or ischaemic hypoxia) occurs when there is inadequate perfusion of tissues, as occurs in low-output states. Histoxic hypoxia occurs when there is poisoning of cellular-enzyme pathways e.g. cyanide poisoning. Finally, in exceptional circumstances such as very severe exercise there may be over-utilization of oxygen.

Assessment of tissue hypoxia

Tissue oxygen availability is dependent on three factors: the haemoglobin concentration, the haemoglobin oxygen saturation and cardiac output. The relationship between the partial pressure of oxygen in the blood (Po_2) and haemoglobin oxygen saturation is given by the haemoglobin oxygen-dissociation curve (Fig. 7.1).

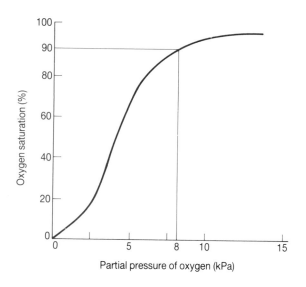

Fig. 7.1 Oxygen haemoglobin dissociation curve.

Measurement of arterial Po_2 is a reasonable indicator of oxygenation, provided that the oxygen-carrying capacity of blood is normal and cardiac output is not reduced. A reduction in arterial Po_2 to 8 kPa (60 mmHg) is equivalent to an oxygen saturation of 90 per cent, assuming a normal haemoglobin oxygen-dissociation curve. A fall in arterial Po_2 to this level is not associated with any significant reduction in oxygen delivery to the tissues. Greater falls may be associated with compensatory signs, including a shift in the haemoglobin oxygen-dissociation curve, polycythaemia, and an increase in cardiac output, all of which can be measured and their value assessed.

Acute cyanosis is not clinically obvious if there is less than 5 g/dl of reduced haemoglobin, this corresponds to an oxygen saturation of 75 per cent or an arterial Po_2 of 5 kPa (37.5 mmHg) in a normal patient.

Probably the best indicator of tissue oxygenation is the mixed venous Po_2 (obtained from the pulmonary artery via a Swan–Ganz catheter). A fall to less than a 4.6 kPa (35 mmHg) is a good indicator of tissue hypoxia.

Indications for oxygen therapy

In theory oxygen therapy is indicated whenever Po_2 falls below the normal level. In practice oxygen therapy is instituted if there is a potentially harmful degree of hypoxia (Po_2 <8 kPa; 60 mmHg or haemoglobin-oxygen saturation <90 per cent).

Although the aetiology of postoperative hypoxia is multifactorial there are three broad areas of physiological alteration responsible for postoperative respiratory impairment. These are:

- decreased alveolar ventilation and $\dot{V}/\dot{Q}$ mismatching
- airways closure and lung collapse (atelectasis)
- interstitial oedema

Most anaesthetic drugs can cause temporary alveolar hypoventilation, as can pain from the operative site especially after upper abdominal and thoracic surgery. Airway obstruction results in alveolar hypoventilation, and postoperative oxygen requirements may be increased by shivering and restlessness. Ventilation-perfusion abnormalities are amongst the most frequent causes of hypoxia. Changes which may occur in the pulmonary circulation due to falls in cardiac output may result in underperfusion of the apices of the lungs and altered $\dot{V}/Q$ relationships.

Functional residual capacity is reduced by surgery whilst the supine position causes the airways to close more easily within the tidal range. Smoking and obesity exacerbate these changes. Atelectasis may result from accumulation of bronchial secretions or from aspiration.

Pulmonary oedema causes a decrease in lung compliance with increased airway resistance and altered regional blood flow. Interstitial and alveolar oedema may be precipitated by cardiogenic factors such as fluid overload and left heart failure, or non-cardiogenic causes such as oxygen toxicity (see below) and septicaemia.

Additional factors contributing to postoperative respiratory impairment include preoperative lung disease such as chronic obstructive airways disease and asthma, and impairment of the normal mucociliary clearance by anaesthetic vapours.

Oxygen therapy

The majority of patients requiring oxygen therapy will have had normal respiratory control preoperatively, and oxygen may be administered in such concentrations as is necessary to achieve a satisfactory arterial oxygen partial pressure. But it must be remembered that even in the normal patient the inhalation of 100 per cent oxygen can reduce minute ventilation by approximately 10 per cent. A proportion of patients will rely on their hypoxic drive for respiratory control. In such patients respiratory narcosis may result from too high an inspired concentration of oxygen.

Adjuncts to oxygen therapy

Correct positioning of the patient markedly improves the mechanical functioning of the lungs. Sitting the patient upright increases lung volume, relieves the splinting of the diaphragm by abdominal contents and maximizes the contribution of the accessory muscles. This is particularly important in patients who have undergone thoracic surgery. Obviously the patient must first be awake and protecting his own airway before being sat upright. The unconscious patient must always be nursed in the coma position.

Humidification of inhaled gases is particularly important in asthmatics and children in order to avoid drying and inspissation of bronchial secretions. The provision of adequate pain relief is also important as this enables the patient to breathe more deeply, particularly during physiotherapy.

Apparatus

Delivery of oxygen is achieved using either masks or nasal catheters. In specific circumstances (e.g. paediatrics) oxygen tents or head boxes may be used. Oxygen delivery systems can be classified as fixed-performance devices and variable-performance devices.

Fixed-performance devices   These devices allow accurate control of oxygen concentration. Most types of standard anaesthetic breathing systems, as well as the Entonox mask used for pain relief in labour, are examples of fixed-performance devices. However, the most practical system for ward use is the Vickers Ventimask, a device based on the venturi or air-entrainment principle (Fig. 7.2). A constant amount of air from the room is entrained through side holes by a specific oxygen-supply flow rate, resulting in a fractional inspired oxygen concentration (F_iO_2) which is related to the relative proportions of air and oxygen. The high flow rate delivered to the patient exceeds the patient's own peak inspiratory flow

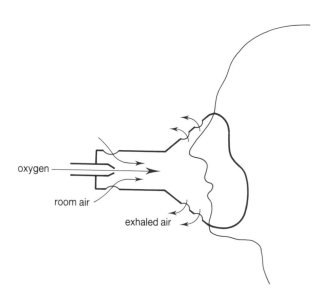

oxygen

room air

exhaled air

Fig. 7.2 Venturi system of oxygen delivery.

rate and eliminates rebreathing by ensuring that only premixed gas is inhaled. The main advantage of the venturi system is that it can deliver accurately low concentrations of oxygen (24, 28 and 35 per cent). This is particularly useful in patients who are reliant on their hypoxic respiratory drive.

Variable-performance devices In these devices a fixed flow rate of oxygen at less than the patient's minute volume enters the mask (Fig. 7.3). The final inspired concentration of oxygen depends on the relationship between the patient's minute volume and the oxygen flow rate. However, some control is allowed by varying oxygen flow rate. Variable-performance devices are of three types: no-capacity systems, small-capacity systems and large-capacity systems.

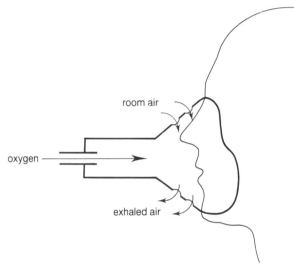

Fig. 7.3 Low-capacity oxygen delivery system.

Nasal 'specs' are an example of a *no-capacity system*. They have the advantage of being comfortable for the patient. The nasal cavities act as a reservoir, thus helping to reduce rebreathing. At low flows (less than 3 litres/min) the F_iO_2 is increased very little, whilst a flow rate of 6 litres/min provides a F_iO_2 of 30–40 per cent. At higher flow rates the gas stream becomes uncomfortable and is poorly tolerated.

The two commonest *small-capacity systems* used are the MC (Mary Catterall) and Hudson masks. In these systems some oxygen is stored in the mask, however, the internal capacity of the mask should ideally be small since this volume represents additional dead space. The rebreathing caused by this additional dead space can result in a significant increase in ventilation which may be deleterious, especially in the patient with respiratory failure. Adjustment of the flow rate from 2 to 10 litres/min produces a F_iO_2 ranging from 30 to 70 per cent. However, with respiratory depression the inspired oxygen progressively increases as ventilation falls. The main advantage of this type of mask is that being of an aviation style they are comfortable to wear.

Large-capacity systems, of which the Polymask and Oxyaire are examples, are not used much nowadays. They have a 'rebreathing' bag attached to the mask. The fresh gas flow is supplied to the mask at a rate which exceeds the minute volume. The performance, reliability and dead space of these types of mask are very variable.

Humidification

The major site of humidification of inspiratory gases is the upper airways (nasopharynx and oropharynx) ensuring that air reaching the trachea has a relative humidity close to 100 per cent (43 mg of water per litre of gas) at 37°C. At less than 75 per cent relative humidity, the action of the cilia lining the respiratory tract is significantly reduced. Humidification devices should aim therefore to provide greater than 75 per cent relative humidity. It is essential to humidify inspired gas whenever the upper respiratory tract is bypassed, for example, endotracheal intubation or tracheostomy and even when nasal 'specs' are used. However, it is not generally necessary to humidify additional oxygen delivered by facemask unless the patient is particularly at risk (such as due to excessive or thick secretions) or if oxygen therapy is to be continued for a prolonged period of time. Humidification of inspired gases can be achieved by heat-and-moisture exchangers ('artificial nose'), cold-water humidifiers, hot-water humidifiers or by droplet humidifiers.

Heat-and-moisture humidifiers (e.g. the Pall Ultipore) retain heat and moisture from exhaled air on a filter and the dry gas of a subsequently inhaled breath is warmed and humidified as it passes through the filter. This type of humidifier cannot provide greater than 80 per cent relative humidity and tends to become clogged up with prolonged exposure. The main advantage is that they are disposable and simple to use.

Cold-water humidifiers are inefficient and provide little humidification unless the gas flow is passed through a sintered plate to produce a stream of small bubbles of gas. This results in gas which is completely saturated at the temperature of the water, but the relative humidity will be reduced as the gas is heated to body temperature. Cold-water humidification is not suitable when the upper airway has been bypassed.

In hot-water humidification, gas is passed over water heated to 40–60°C, and the relative humidity approaches 100 per cent as the gas cools to 37°C as it passes along the delivery tubing. The gas temperature must be monitored at the patient-end of the delivery tubing. This system is not suitable for administration by facemask as heated gas delivered to the patient is uncomfortable and may even produce a scald, particularly if there is a thermostat failure.

Droplet humidification is a highly efficient means of humidification which works by producing a cloud of small water droplets. The ideal droplet size necessary to ensure uniform deposition throughout the airways is 2–10 μm. Gas-driven humidifiers produce droplets of 5–20 μm in size. However, the mist produced by ultrasonic nebulizers (droplet size 1–4 μm) may contain up to four to five times the amount of water needed to produce full saturation. As a result substantial deposition of water can occur in intubated patients resulting in water intoxication. However, in non-intubated patients very few water droplets reach the trachea or bronchi.

Hazards of oxygen therapy

The main hazards of oxygen therapy are related to the physical properties of oxygen and to the pathological effects of oxygen on the organism.

Fire risk
Extreme care should be exercised in ensuring that no source of ignition is present in the vicinity of an oxygen-enriched environment, and especially if hyperbaric oxygen is being used. Particular attention should be paid to electrical safety.

Drying of secretions
The breathing of dried gases has a detrimental effect on the respiratory tract (see above). Humidification of inspired gases is necessary if the upper respiratory tract is bypassed.

Oxygen toxicity
High tensions of oxygen appear to be damaging to biological tissues. An inspired concentration of greater than 80% applied to the lung for longer than two days frequently results in a pathological process similar to 'respiratory distress syndrome'. Also paraesthesia may accompany prolonged breathing of high inspired concentrations of oxygen. In premature infants, exposure to excessively high concentrations of oxygen can cause blindness due to retrolental fibroplasia. Finally in adults the risk of absorption atelectasis is increased by breathing high concentrations of oxygen, particularly in patients with a history of chronic obstructive airways disease.

8

Anaesthetic apparatus
P K Barnes

- The anaesthetic machine
    - gas supply
    - pressure and flow regulation
    - addition of volatile anaesthetics
    - safety features
- Anaesthetic breathing systems
- Automatic ventilation

The anaesthetic machine

The anaesthetic machine enables the anaesthetist to deliver a known concentration of oxygen and anaesthetic agents to a patient. The modern anaesthetic machine has evolved from the original 'Boyle's' machine designed by H E G Boyle in 1915. It differs greatly in detail but adheres to the basic principles of the original design. The anaesthetic machine will be considered under the following headings

- supply of anaesthetic gases
- regulation of the pressure and flow of the gases
- the addition of vaporized liquid anaesthetics
- safety features

Gas supply
The gases supplied to the anaesthetic machine are oxygen, nitrous oxide, carbon dioxide and cyclopropane. Oxygen and nitrous oxide are used in the majority of general anaesthetics. Carbon dioxide is sometimes added to the inspired gas mixture in order to maintain arterial-carbon-dioxide partial pressure at a normal value during artificial ventilation or in order to stimulate respiration. Cyclopropane is an explosive gas and although it is a useful and powerful anaesthetic agent, it is being phased out due to lack of use and because of the risk of explosion.

Oxygen is supplied to the anaesthetic machine in two ways: from a pipeline directly attached to the anaesthetic machine, or from a cylinder. In most hospitals a sufficiently large amount of oxygen is used to justify the installation of a large container of liquid oxygen which can supply the whole hospital. The pipeline supply to the anaesthetic machine is taken from this source. The pipeline is permanently attached to the anaesthetic machine and a pressure gauge indicates the pipeline pressure which is 4 bar (Fig. 8.1). Although the pipeline is the main source of supply to the anaesthetic machine, oxygen cylinders are mounted on the machine as a back-up if there is failure in the pipeline supply. The cylinders contain gaseous oxygen and a pressure gauge mounted on top of the cylinder registers the pressure in a full cylinder which is 137 bar at room temperature (Fig. 8.2). The contents of the cylinder are in the gaseous form so the gauge pressure will fall linearly as the cylinder empties.

Nitrous oxide is also supplied to the anaesthetic machine from a pipeline which comes from a bank of large cylinders situated outside the operating theatre. In addition the machine also has housings for two nitrous oxide cylinders. These can be switched on if the anaesthetic machine is used in a situation without a pipeline supply or if the pipeline fails. Nitrous oxide cylinders contain liquid nitrous oxide. The space above the liquid contains nitrous oxide vapour. The pressure gauge mounted on the nitrous oxide cylinder registers a pressure of 51.7 bar at 20°C. This is the saturated vapour pressure of nitrous oxide at room temperature. When the cylinder is opened, gaseous nitrous oxide escapes and is replenished by vaporization of the liquid nitrous oxide. The reason nitrous oxide is in liquid form in the cylinder is because at room temperature nitrous oxide is below its critical temperature and it is therefore liquefied when under pressure, as it is in the cylinder. The vaporization of liquid nitrous oxide requires latent heat of vaporization. The liquid nitrous oxide therefore cools and the saturated vapour pressure falls. The pressure registered on the gauge may therefore fall slightly from 51.7 bar. However, when the cylinder valve is closed, the liquid will reach room temperature again and the pressure on the gauge will be restored to 51.7 bar. When all the liquid nitrous oxide has been used up, the pressure registered by the gauge will fall in linear fashion as the nitrous oxide gas is used.

Pressure and flow regulation

The pressure of oxygen and nitrous oxide entering the anaesthetic machine from cylinders is higher than that entering from the pipelines. For this reason a pressure-regulating valve is mounted close to the housing of the cylinders (Fig. 8.2), the gas pressure leaving the valve is 4 bar. The gases then enter the flowmeter bank. There are separate flowmeters for oxygen, nitrous oxide, carbon dioxide and cyclopropane. At the base of each flowmeter is a control knob that allows gas to enter the flowmeter by opening a needle valve. In essence, anticlockwise rotation of the control knob moves a pin out of an orifice allowing gas to pass into the flowmeter. The controls are colour coded and the oxygen control is much larger and projects further than the others so that it can be easily recognized. The flowmeter tubes are conical in shape, although this is not obvious at first sight (Fig. 8.3). When gas flows through the flowmeter an aluminium bobbin rises in the flowmeter tube and rotates to indicate that it has not become stuck. The upper rim indicates the flow of gas passing through the flowmeter. The flowmeters are accurately calibrated during manufacture.

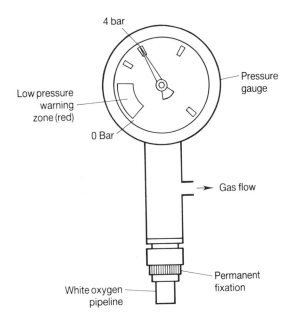

4 bar

Pressure
gauge

Low pressure
warning
zone (red)

0 Bar

Gas flow

Permanent
fixation

White oxygen
pipeline

Fig. 8.1

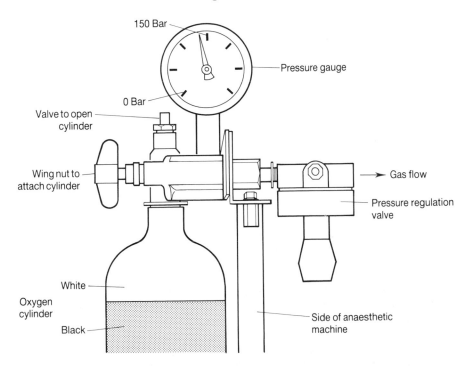

150 Bar

Pressure gauge

0 Bar

Valve to open
cylinder

Gas flow

Wing nut to
attach cylinder

Pressure regulation
valve

White

Oxygen
cylinder

Black

Side of anaesthetic
machine

Fig. 8.2

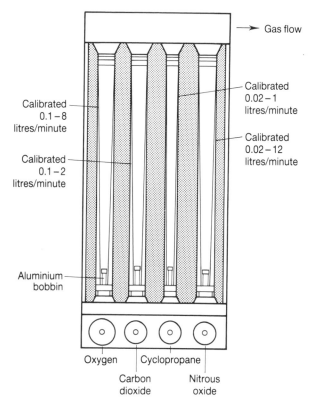

Gas flow

Calibrated
0.02 – 1
litres/minute

Calibrated
0.1 – 8
litres/minute

Calibrated
0.02 – 12
litres/minute

Calibrated
0.1 – 2
litres/minute

Aluminium
bobbin

Oxygen   Cyclopropane

Carbon   Nitrous
dioxide   oxide

Fig. 8.3

The gas mixture flowing out of the flowmeter bank is at a lower pressure and consists of an accurate mixture of oxygen and nitrous oxide.

Addition of volatile anaesthetics

The gas mixture flows on through a single manifold which passes through the back-bar conduit of the anaesthetic machine. Vaporizers containing liquid anaesthetics can be mounted on the back bar. Modern vaporizers are easily detached allowing different anaesthetic agents to be used. When the vaporizer is switched on, part of the gas mixture is diverted through it to become saturated by the vaporized liquid anaesthetic. The saturated vapour then rejoins the gas that has bypassed the vaporizer, to become diluted to clinically useful concentrations.

A glass-ether vaporizer, or Boyle's bottle, and a modern halothane vaporizer made of metal are depicted in Fig. 8.4. The principle of action of these two vaporizers is similar; they both contain liquid anaesthetic which will vaporize to an extent governed by their saturated vapour pressure at room temperature. In the case of the Boyle bottle the amount of gas entering the vaporizer (the splitting ratio) can be altered by moving the lever. The gas enters the vaporizer above the liquid anaesthetic; and its level above the anaesthetic can be altered by depressing the plunger. Vaporization requires latent heat of vaporization. In the case of the ether, large amounts of heat are required to vaporize the anaesthetic agent. Therefore, the concentration from the vaporizer will fall drastically as the temperature and the vapour pressure of ether falls. For this reason, the entire gas flow may be passed through the vaporizer and even bubbled through the liquid.

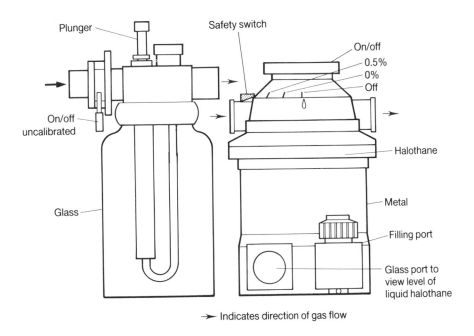

Fig. 8.4

The halothane vaporizer has a safety switch that must be depressed to allow the control on the top to be rotated. Counterclockwise rotation increases the fraction of the gas flow diverted through the vaporizer. The concentration of halothane can be varied from 0.5 per cent to 5 per cent. The modern halothane vaporizer is designed to maintain a constant output of volatile anaesthetic agent. It is made of metal which is a better heat conductor than glass. It also has a temperature-compensation device. The halothane vaporizer in Fig. 8.4 has a bimetallic strip inside to compensate for the cooling of the liquid halothane. As cooling takes place due to latent heat of vaporization, the strip, made of two different metals with different coefficients of expansion, bends to allow a greater fraction of the total flow to enter the vaporization chamber.

Safety features

The pipelines and cylinders supplied to the anaesthetic machine are colour coded. The pipelines are permanently fitted to the machine. The housings for the cylinders have a pin-index system. These are projections that fit into indentations on the cylinder neck. It should therefore be impossible to cross over the gas supply and so supply the 'wrong' gas. An alarm is fitted that will sound if the supply of oxygen fails and so results in a hypoxic supply of nitrous oxide leaving the machine. Some modern devices have the supply of oxygen and nitrous oxide linked. If the nitrous oxide supply is turned on oxygen automatically flows so that a hypoxic gas supply cannot be administered. The machine has a pressure-release valve so that the supply of gas cannot exceed a dangerous level. Suction apparatus is also mounted on the anaesthetic machine.

Anaesthetic breathing systems

The following terms are used:

Fresh gas supply
Gas of known composition supplied from the anaesthetic machine.

Rebreathing
The inhalation of previously exhaled, carbon dioxide-containing gas.

Alveolar minute ventilation
That part of the tidal volume that takes part in gas exchange in the lungs, multiplied by the respiratory rate.

Once the desired gas mixture has been generated in the anaesthetic machine, it is necessary to have a conduit to deliver it to the patient. An anaesthetic breathing system is a device that delivers gas from the anaesthetic machine to the patient. An example of an anaesthetic breathing system is the Magill attachment named after Sir Ivan Magill. The system is shown in Fig. 8.5. It consists of a length of large-bore tubing which is attached to the outlet of the anaesthetic machine. Anaesthetic gases pass down the tube to the patient. There is a reservoir bag to store gas delivered from the anaesthetic machine. The reservoir bag is needed because flow from the anaesthetic machine is constant, whereas patients breathe intermittently. At the patient end of the system is a spring-loaded expiration valve (Heidbrink) that will open when the pressure in the system rises to allow gas to be vented to the atmosphere.

The way in which the breathing system works during a single breath is shown in Fig. 8.5a, b, c. During inspiration the patient breathes in some of the gas passing down the wide-bore tubing and some of the gas stored in the reservoir bag which consequently diminishes in size. During expiration there is reversal of gas flow in the wide-bore tube, and exhaled gas flows towards the reservoir bag forcing fresh gas from the machine into the

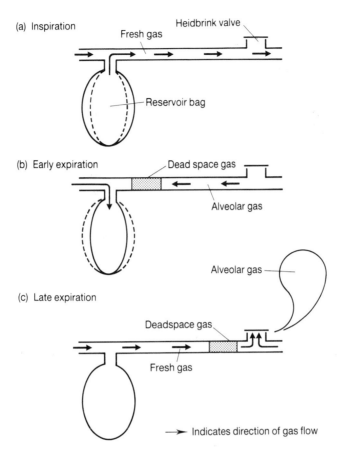

(a) Inspiration

Heidbrink valve

Fresh gas

Reservoir bag

(b) Early expiration

Dead space gas

Alveolar gas

Alveolar gas

(c) Late expiration

Deadspace gas

Fresh gas

Indicates direction of gas flow

Fig. 8.5

reservoir bag until the pressure within the breathing system reaches a critical value ($2\,cmH_2O$) sufficient to open the expiratory valve. The opening of this valve permits the flow to reverse so that gas escapes through the valve. For the purposes of explanation, it has been assumed that exhaled gas from the patient's lungs passes into the anaesthetic breathing system as distinct 'plugs' of gas and that mixing does not occur. The first part of exhaled gas comes from the anatomical dead space. This is gas that occupied the trachea and was not involved in gas exchange. It has the composition of fresh gas. The second part of the exhaled gas comes from the alveolar space and has been involved in gas exchange. This gas has a lower concentration of oxygen and anaesthetic gases, and also contains carbon dioxide. In the example, all of this gas is vented from the breathing system. If part of this gas is re-inspired, rebreathing is said to occur. The fresh gas flow from the anaesthetic machine must equal alveolar minute ventilation to prevent this.

There are several breathing systems that differ from the Magill system in the way in which the component parts are arranged. They are classified by the fresh-gas flow into the system that is required to prevent rebreathing of carbon dioxide previously exhaled by the patient. An example of another breathing system is shown in Fig. 8.6. This is the Bain breathing system. It differs from the Magill system in the way in which the component parts are arranged. The fresh gas is supplied to the patient by a small-bore inner tube, it is thus an example of a co-axial breathing system. In order to prevent rebreathing, three times the patient's alveolar minute ventilation is required. It is therefore less efficient in terms of fresh-gas economy than the Magill system.

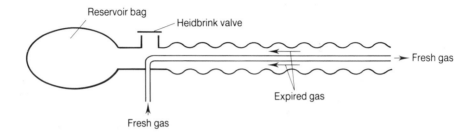

Fig. 8.6

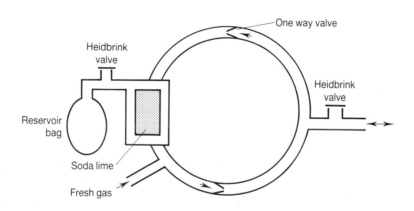

Fig. 8.7

In the two breathing systems described rebreathing can occur if the fresh-gas flow from the anaesthetic machine is reduced below a critical value that is specific to the breathing system. In the circle system (Fig. 8.7) the exhaled gas passes through a cannister of soda lime which absorbs carbon dioxide. The gas then continues to move in a circular direction determined by the two unidirectional valves and is added to the fresh gas entering the circle system. The proportion of exhaled gas added to the fresh gas will depend on the rate that fresh gas is added to the system. If the fresh-gas supply is high, most of the exhaled gas will be vented from the system through the spill valve. The virtue of the circle system is that the fresh-gas supply can be reduced to lower values than in the Magill or Bain systems. This is economical in terms of the fresh-gas flow needed and reduces atmospheric pollution. The fact that exhaled gas is recirculated and may form part of the inspired gas mixture is relatively unimportant because carbon dioxide is removed during its passage through the soda lime. Exhaled gas will have a lower concentration than fresh gas and will dilute fresh gas but this can be compensated for by increasing the concentration delivered from the anaesthetic machine.

Automatic ventilation

In the description of breathing systems it was assumed that the patient was breathing spontaneously. When patients are anaesthetized it is frequently necessary to ventilate the lungs, for example when neuromuscular blocking agents have been administered. This group of patients have normal lungs and relatively simple ventilators are all that is required. Patients in intensive care also frequently require artificial ventilation because they have respiratory failure. These patients have very abnormal lungs and require complex machines to ventilate them.

A lung ventilator functions by applying an intermittent positive pressure to the airway (IPPV). The ventilator must do work to overcome the elastic resistance of the lungs and chest wall, and the airway resistance. The power is supplied either from a pressurized gas supply or from electricity used to compress gas supplied to the ventilator. Expiration occurs due to the passive elastic recoil of the lungs and chest wall.

All ventilators produce a flow of gas into the lungs during the inspiratory period by developing a pressure gradient between the ventilator and the lungs. In one type, the constant-pressure generator, the pressure generated within the ventilator is relatively low and remains constant throughout the inspiratory period. The pattern of gas flow, and hence the tidal volume, is determined by the effect the generated pressure has on the lungs. If the lungs are stiff the pressure applied may not be sufficient to achieve the desired tidal volume.

In a second type, the constant-flow generator, the pressure available to drive the ventilator is very high. The gas-flow rate throughout the inspiratory period is constant, and unaffected by the effect that the flow has on the lungs. If the lungs are stiff the tidal volume set by the operator will be delivered at the cost of achieving high airway pressures.

The anaesthetic breathing systems previously described can all be used to provide ventilation of the lungs. This is achieved by closing the expiratory valve and compressing the reservoir bag. The Magill system is not reliable when used in this way, but the Bain system can be used with good effect. Rebreathing will occur, but alveolar ventilation can be increased to maintain arterial carbon dioxide concentration at normal levels. The circle system using soda lime to absorb carbon dioxide is eminently suitable. An alternative to manual compression of the reservoir bag is to connect a ventilator in place of the bag, this moves gas within the breathing system.

Penlon Nuffield series 200 (Fig. 8.8)

This ventilator is powered by compressed gas, usually oxygen. It is a constant-flow generator. The oxygen used to drive the ventilator passes through the machine and is the gas output from the machine. If the Penlon is connected to the reservoir-bag mounting on a Bain or circle system the output from the ventilator can be used to drive the anaesthetic gases within the breathing system into the patient. The ventilator has to be connected to the breathing system by a length of tubing so that the breathing system does not become contaminated by the oxygen delivered by the ventilator. During exhalation the gases will pass out of the breathing system down the hose connecting the ventilator to the system, rather than out of a pressure-release valve. The controls on the ventilator allow the operator to alter the inspiratory time, expiratory time and the inspiratory gas-flow rate. If the inspiratory time is set to 1 s, and the gas-flow rate to 500 ml/s, a tidal volume of 500 ml will result. The airway pressure generated by this tidal volume will be registered on the pressure gauge.

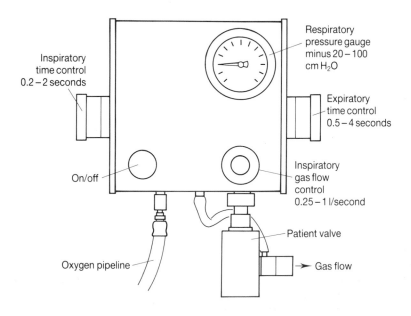

Fig. 8.8

Manley ventilator (Fig. 8.9)

The ventilator is a constant-pressure generator. The pressure to drive the gas contained in the bellows into the lungs is derived from the weight on top of the bellows. This ventilator is very commonly used in the operating theatre. It is connected to the gas outlet of the anaesthetic machine. The flow of oxygen and nitrous oxide from the anaesthetic machine provides the power to make the ventilator function. The total volume of oxygen and nitrous oxide set in the flowmeters will be delivered to the patient. The ventilator is therefore described as a minute-volume divider, because it splits the minute volume received from the anaesthetic machine into a preset tidal volume. Also, as it must deliver the total gas flow, the respiratory rate will be determined by the machine. However, the inspiratory flow rate can be adjusted by the control, and by moving the weight on top of the bellows.

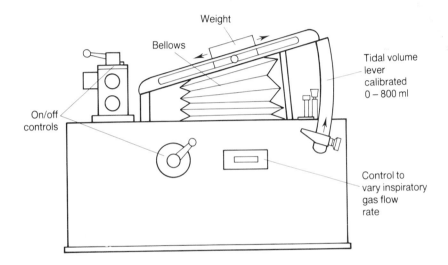

Fig. 8.9

Siemans Servo 900C (Fig. 8.10)

This ventilator requires a source of compressed gas as well as electricity for it to function. It is a constant-flow generator but can be adjusted to work as a constant-pressure generator if this is desired. It is typical of the sort of ventilator used in intensive care, where the ability to manipulate the respiratory pattern may improve oxygenation in patients with abnormal lungs. The ventilator has a number of alarms that allow the operator to be alerted if the limits set are violated. It also allows for a gradual transition from controlled to spontaneous respiration as lung function improves. A diagram of the ventilator is shown in Fig. 8.10 so that the number of variables in setting can be seen. The remainder of the description will be confined to the principle of function.

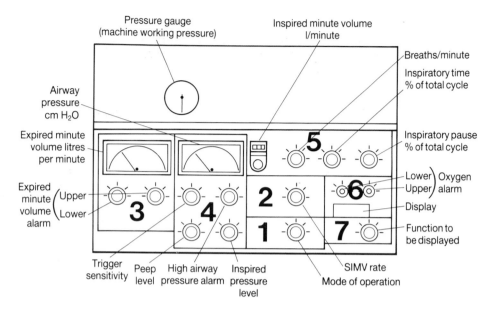

Fig. 8.10

Panel 1: mode selection

Ventilation can be totally or partially controlled. It may be desirable to allow the patient to ventilate themselves in a manner that progressively increases. In the synchronized intermittent mandatory ventilation mode (SIMV) the degree of mechanical ventilation per minute can be set but the patient can take a number of breaths for themselves in addition. Synchronization means that the controlled breaths will not clash with spontaneous efforts.

Panel 2: SIMV

This control allows the operator to set the number of mandatory breaths per minute. The lower the number of mandatory breaths the more the patient can breathe spontaneously.

Panel 3: expired minute volume

The expired minute volume is monitored and displayed. This panel has controls to set alarm limits for low or high levels of expired volume.

Panel 4: airway pressure

A meter indicates the airway pressure reading and an alarm can be set to warn when excessive pressure is reached. It is also possible to set a positive-end-excitatory-pressure (PEEP). This means that at the end of expiration, airway pressure does not fall to atmospheric pressure as normally. This facility may improve oxygenation by recruiting alveoli so that they continue to take part in gas exchange rather than closing. It is also possible to set the 'negative' pressure that the patient must generate to trigger a controlled breath from the ventilator.

Panel 5: respiratory pattern
The desired inspiratory minute volume can be preset. The number of breaths per minute can also be set and the time taken for the inspiratory period.

Panel 6: oxygen alarms
These controls allow the upper and lower limits of the concentration of oxygen to be determined.

Panel 7: monitoring
This control can be used to display a number of parameters of ventilation such as the oxygen concentration delivered by the ventilator, or the airway pressures developed in the course of controlled ventilation.

9

Preparation of the patient
R.F. Armstrong

- The preoperative visit
  general assessment
  cardiovascular assessment
  respiratory assessment
  renal assessment
  hepatic assessment
  assessment in specific conditions
- General anaesthesia or regional anaesthesia
- The preoperative check
- Premedication

Perioperative studies of morbidity and mortality reveal that surgery is still a procedure associated with significant risk. In a recent large survey 0.8–1.0 per cent of patients died within 30 days of surgery. Intraoperative hypotension due to unrecognized preoperative myocardial ischaemia may result in renal, cardiac or even cerebral damage. Airway contamination, due to regurgitation from a full stomach at the induction of anaesthesia, may set in motion a chain of events starting with hypoxaemia and ending in respiratory failure.

Dangerous preoperative conditions therefore need to be recognized before surgery begins and the risks of continuing the procedure measured against surgical postponement. Finally, those conditions which expose the patient to risk need to be excluded or neutralized. It is during the preoperative assessment that the important exercise of risk identification, quantification and neutralization occurs.

The preoperative visit

During the preoperative visit the anaesthetist will have several objectives in mind. Above all there will be the need to assess fitness for anaesthetic and surgery, but at the same time there is an opportunity to develop a relationship with the patient. This will involve a discussion of the events leading up to anaesthesia, the premedication and timing of the operation and an honest appraisal of the degree of postoperative discomfort and how this will be managed.

Any anxieties expressed by the patient need to be discussed and reassurance given in such a way that the patient can face the forthcoming ordeal with the knowledge that an experienced and competent person is going to be looking after them during the surgical procedure. There is an important concept here to introduce to the patient. The anaesthetist is not only giving the anaesthetic but is their doctor who will care for them throughout the operation.

General assessment

An early attempt to classify patients according to the degree of abnormal physiology present was made by the American Society of Anesthesiologists, and is known as the ASA physical status index. This classification has proved a useful way of objectively defining patient status (Table 9.1) and as such is still in widespread use.

Table 9.1 ASA physical status index

Class	Description
I	Normal healthy patient
II	Patient with mild to moderate systemic disease
III	Patient with severe systemic disease that is not incapacitating
IV	Patient with incapacitating systemic disease that presents a constant threat to life
V	Moribund patient not expected to survive 24 hours with or without operation.
	The suffix E is added if the procedure is an emergency

Cardiovascular assessment

Deep anaesthesia produces two fundamental changes in cardiovascular function, notably a fall in cardiac output and vasodilation (Chapter 2). The resulting reduction in blood pressure may threaten perfusion of the myocardium as well as other vital organs. Conversely light anaesthesia in the presence of intense surgical stimuli may produce tachycardia and hypertension, reducing available time for coronary perfusion during diastole and compressing blood vessels in the myocardium during systole. For these reasons any preoperative cardiovascular problem must be identified. In particular, ischaemic heart disease should be searched for. It is widespread and often asymptomatic. Risk factors such as family history, diabetes, smoking, high blood pressure and hyperlipidaemia may alert the anaesthetist to the possibility of ischaemia and this can be further evaluated by ECG, chest radiograph, echocardiography or ejection fraction determination. The presence of angina or heart failure is clearly important and if infarction has occurred then surgery should be deferred, if possible, for

6 months. For those patients wh~~ of myocardial infarction, rei described, with a 50 per cent ~

Goldman has constructed ~ years of age. As the score ~ increase (Table 9.2).

Table 9.2 Cardiac scoring

History	
age >70 years	
myocardial infarction (MI) ~	
Physical examination	
S3 gallop or jugular vein distension	
important aortic stenosis	
Electrocardiogram (ECG)	
rhythm other than sinus or PACs on last preoperative ECG ~	
>5 PVCs/min documented at any time preoperative	
General status, any one of:	
Po_2 <8kPa (60mmHg) or Pco_2 >6.7kPa (50mmHg)	3
K^+ <3.0 or HCO_3^- <20mmol/litre	
blood urea or creatinine elevated	
abnormal serum glutamine oxalotransferase (SGOT). Chronic liver disease or patient bedridden from non-cardiac causes	
Operation	
intraperitoneal, intrathoracic or aortic operation	3
emergency operation	4
Total possible	46

Goldman recommended that only truly life-saving procedures be performed on patients with risk index scores of 26 points or more (class IV). The mortality in this group was over 50 per cent. Patients with index scores of 13–25 points (class III) warrant preoperative medical consultation. Where potentially controllable factors exist operation should be delayed if possible until the patient is medically more stable.

Hypertension, though not considered a significant factor by Goldman, is nevertheless associated with intraoperative cardiovascular instability. The evidence suggests that a diastolic pressure over 110mmHg represents a hazard which needs treating and investigating before surgery.

Valvular disease may be a presenting feature or discovered by chance during the preoperative assessment. In all cases the advice of a cardiologist should be sought so that echocardiography may be carried out and the degree of cardiac compromise assessed. Atrial fibrillation will indicate the need for digitalization, and anticoagulation should be considered and

ent with mitral stenosis or prosthetic valves.
ill be needed to prevent endocarditis in patients
netic valves or ventricular septal defect (VSD) when
, GU, or colonic surgery.
bove all, an indication of underlying pathology (usually
sease) and this will modify the anaesthetist's choice of
dition, the pacemaker will need evaluation, including type,
n, battery strength and pacing effectiveness.

y assessment

ung disease is now extremely common and will therefore be a
type of pathology seen amongst patients presenting for surgery.
the clinical examination of these patients, two points need special
deration. These are sputum production and dyspnoea. The presence of
essive or purulent sputum is an indication that surgical postponement
ould be considered. This is because the postoperative patient may not be
able to expectorate properly due to pain and/or weakness. Dyspnoea is a
useful prediction of postoperative problems and grade IV dyspnoea shows
some correlation with the need for postoperative artificial ventilation.
Dyspnoea grading varies slightly between different centres but the one in
Table 9.3 has the virtue of simplicity.

Table 9.3 Respiratory grading system (Roizen)

Grade	Degree of dyspnoea
0	No dyspnoea while walking on the level at a normal pace
I	'I am able to walk as far as I like provided I take my time'
II	Specific street block limitation, 'I have to stop for a while after one or two blocks'
III	Dyspnoea on mild exertion, 'I have to stop and rest while going from the kitchen to the bathroom'
IV	Dyspnoea at rest

Whilst not necessarily contraindicating anaesthesia, grade IV dyspnoea
will demand a good team approach to the patient. Preoperative physiotherapy, microbiological advice, an experienced anaesthetist and surgeon
and facilities available for postoperative respiratory monitoring and support
are essential.

Finally, the presence of bronchospasm represents a significant hazard.
The anaesthetist will want to avoid certain drugs such as opiates, thiopentone and beta adrenoceptor antagonists due to their potential for
precipitating bronchoconstriction.

Once a thorough clinical examination is completed there is a galaxy of
pulmonary function tests available for more objective assessment. Of these,
the vital capacity (VC), the forced expiratory volume in the first second of
expiration (FEV_1) and the peak expiratory flow rate (PEFR) are commonly

used. Both VC and FEV_1 are conveniently measured with a Vitalograph and the PEFR by a Wright's Peak Flowmeter. Unfortunately, opinions differ about what levels constitute an unacceptable risk to the patient. In Table 9.4 a list of normal ranges are given with an adjoining column of values which anaesthetists would view with concern. The figures are a guide only and refer to a 70 kg male of average height.

Table 9.4 Common respiratory indices

	Normal	Abnormal
Vital capacity	5 litres	<1.5 litres
FEV_1	4 litres	<1.0 litres
PEFR	600 litres/min	<200 litres/min

Arterial blood gases Pa_{O_2}, Pa_{CO_2}

These measurements are the cornerstone of objective respiratory assessment. They are measured in units of pressure, i.e. mmHg or kPa. Normal values are shown in Table 9.5.

Table 9.5 Normal arterial blood gas values

	kPa	mmHg
PaO_2	10–13.3	75–100
$PaCO_2$	4.8–6.0	36–46

Pa_{O_2}
It is absolutely vital to understand that the Pa_{O_2} will increase as the inspired oxygen concentration goes up. This is readily understood with reference to the simplified alveolar air equation

$$\left[PA_{O_2} = F_iO_2 (PB - P_{H_2O}) - \frac{Pa_{CO_2}}{R} \right]$$

PA_{O_2} = alveolar partial pressure of oxygen
Pa_{CO_2} = arterial partial pressure of carbon dioxide
PB = barometric pressure (100 kPa or 760 mmHg)
P_{H_2O} = water vapour pressure (6 kPa or 47 mmHg)
F_iO_2 = fractional inspired oxygen concentration
R = respiratory quotient (assume 0.8)

If the alveolar partial pressure of oxygen (P_{AO_2}) is calculated then the arterial partial pressure (Pa_{O_2}) should be slightly lower. The relationship between inspired oxygen concentration and arterial P_{O_2} can be seen more easily from Table 9.6.

Table 9.6   Relationship between inspired and arterial oxygen

F_iO_2	Approximate predicted Pa_{O_2}
1.0 (100%)	90 kPa
0.9 (90%)	80 kPa
0.6 (60%)	50 kPa
0.4 (40%)	30 kPa
0.28 (28%)	18 kPa

Assuming the inspired oxygen concentration is known (i.e. high flow, fixed concentration, Ventimasks) then the patient's Pa_{O_2} in kPa should be approx. 10 kPa lower than the F_iO_2. If the Pa_{O_2} is less than one third of the predicted value then there is severe parenchymal lung disease and respiratory support may be necessary. For patients presenting for anaesthesia with a Pa_{O_2} of less than 6.0 kPa, breathing air there is some evidence that postoperative respiratory support will be needed.

Pa_{CO_2}
Preoperatively, a high Pa_{CO_2} is obviously of concern and predicts serious postoperative respiratory problems. During the aftermath of surgery, a high Pa_{CO_2} may also be worrying. Where renal compensation has taken place (high bicarbonate) the problem is clearly chronic and therefore less dangerous. However, once significant respiratory acidosis (pH of 7.2) develops in acute or chronic respiratory failure, IPPV should be seriously considered.

Renal assessment
Impairment of renal function may present preoperatively as oliguria (<400 ml urine/24 hours) or as a rising blood urea, creatinine or potassium. The problems may be acute (as a result of prerenal, renal or postrenal factors) or chronic, in which case the patient may be on dialysis or the recipient of a kidney transplant.

Renal failure

The preoperative management will depend upon which category of renal failure the patient occupies, though certain fundamental principles apply to all (Table 9.7). Fluid underload or overload should be corrected and any hypotension/hypertension reversed. Drug therapy should be used with caution, especially the nephrotoxic antibiotics and digoxin whose excretion will depend upon renal function. Blood transfusion in the anaemic patient may be necessary but can cause a high haematocrit and thus compromise renal blood flow.

Table 9.7 Categories of patients with renal failure

Acute

prerenal	renal	postrenal
hypovolaemia	acute G.N.	urinary
hypotension	sepsis	obstruction
hypoxia	nephrotoxins	

Chronic

conservative management	dialysis	transplant

Acute renal failure

There is often considerable difficulty in differentiating between prerenal and renal failure in the acutely ill and oliguric surgical patient. In these circumstances, blood and urine chemistry may be useful (Table 9.8).

Table 9.8 Urine and plasma values in renal failure

	Prerenal failure	Renal failure
osmolality mOsm/litre	>500	<350
urine sodium mmols/litre	< 20	> 40
U/P urea ratio	> 8	< 3
U/P creatinine ratio	> 40	< 20

In the preparation of the patient with acute renal failure for theatre, the anaesthetist will want a comprehensive work up of general and specific renal-function tests. Measurement of urea and electrolytes will give an indication of the severity of the disorder and may reveal dangerous hyperkalaemia. A potassium of >6 mmol/litre will contraindicate all but the most important surgery. A full blood count will detect any anaemia and may provide evidence of infection or blood dyscrasia. Blood gases will give a useful insight into acid-base status, as well as the ventilatory ability of the patient to compensate (by hyperventilation) for any metabolic acidosis. When severe metabolic acidosis exists (pH < 7.2), preoperative haemodialysis or haemofiltration may be necessary, and in decisions of this sort the advice of a renal physician is mandatory. In the fluid-overloaded patient, the difference between actual and predicted Pao_2 may provide a more sensitive measure of incipient pulmonary oedema than clinical examination or chest radiograph. Finally, measurement of central venous pressure (CVP) may resolve any lingering doubts about whether the renal failure is hypovolaemic in origin. A fluid challenge of 200 ml colloid given over 10 minutes will produce a temporary rise in CVP followed by a return to pre-challenge levels in the hypovolaemic patient. In the normally or overhydrated patient the rise in CVP provoked by a fluid challenge will be sustained.

A preoperative checklist (Table 9.9) can be helpful in preparing these patients for surgery.

Table 9.9 Preoperative checklist in renal failure

Test	Possible conclusion
full blood count	anaemic, septic
urea and electrolytes	uraemic, hyperkalaemic
clotting	coagulopathy
blood gases	hypoxic, acidotic
chest radiograph	overload
ECG	hyperkalaemic, tachycardia
CVP	hyper/hypovolaemic
drugs	nephrotoxic

Chronic renal failure (CRF)

In view of the part played by diseases such as diabetes and hypertension in the development of chronic renal failure, it is clearly important to treat hyperglycaemia or high blood pressure before surgery. These patients will merit close attention because of their sensitivity to fluid under or overload and in particular to the question of fluid balance. Many patients will have been treated with high-fluid intakes in order to maximize clearance by those nephrons still functioning. In these cases fluid restriction preoperatively may prove dangerous and precipitate sharp increases in blood urea and potassium, even to the extent of causing further and permanent deterioration in renal function. For this reason, judicious quantities of i.v. fluid should be given preoperatively under the supervision of an experienced clinician.

Low erythropoetin levels in CRF may lead to bone marrow suppression resulting in anaemia and coagulopathy. Preoperative blood transfusion however, by increasing haematocrit, may impair renal blood flow and thus needs careful thought and advice. The presence of heart failure adds to the difficulties and dangers inherent in this disease.

As a final complication, drug dosage needs careful monitoring, as reduced clearance may precipitate toxic drug levels. In particular, the use of digoxin, β adrenoceptor antagonists, antibiotics or muscle relaxants will all require caution. When dialysis or filtration is in use prior to surgery, it should be terminated at least 3 hours before starting and the full blood count, urea and electrolytes and clotting studies checked before theatre.

Hepatic assessment

Approximately 25 per cent of the cardiac output perfuses the liver, partly from the hepatic artery (500 ml/min) and partly from the portal vein

(1000 ml/min). Reductions in liver blood flow occur during the three common insults to regional blood supply namely hypotension, hypoxia and high catecholamine output. Whilst the normal liver seems capable of withstanding these insults, the damaged liver cannot. For this reason preoperative recognition of liver malfunction is important so that an appropriate anaesthetic can be designed.

In order to classify intraoperative risk Pugh has described a simple scoring system (Table 9.10).

Table 9.10 Hepatic scoring system

Points per abnormality	1	2	3
serum bilirubin mmol/litre	<25	25–40	>40
serum albumin g/litre	<35	28–35	>28
prothrombin time (normal 12) prolongation (secs)	<4	4–6	>6
Encephalopathy grade	none	1 or 2	3 or 4

Fewer than   6 points — good operative risk
7–9 points — moderate risk
>10 points — poor operative risk

An earlier classification by Childs includes, in addition, ascites and nutritional state. In order to improve the patient's chances of survival when decompensated liver disease is present (Childs class C, Pugh>10 points), attention should be given to the correction, where possible, of these problems. Because of poor vitamin K absorption in obstructive jaundice, vitamin K should be given intramuscularly in sufficient doses to lower the prolonged prothrombin time. Renal function should be closely monitored as renal failure may complicate the course of the jaundiced patient especially when serum bilirubin exceeds 140 mmol/litre or when endotoxaemia or hypovolaemia are present. To offset these added dangers, gentamicin or a cephalosporin should be started preoperatively if endotoxaemia is suspected and any dehydration treated aggressively to produce urine flows of approximately 1 ml/kg per hour.

Generally speaking in hepatic malfunction, drug doses should be lower than usual as cardiovascular and respiratory depression are more common and unpredictable. In theory, drugs affecting the Sphincter of Oddi (causing constriction) should be avoided in obstructive jaundice. In severe cirrhosis, morphine may provoke encephalopathy.

Assessment in specific conditions

The obstetric patient

The risks inherent in the delivery of a baby are made clear by a review of a recent confidential enquiry into maternal deaths. In the UK from 1979 to 1981 nine mothers died in the peripartum period per 100 000 births. Of these deaths 12.6 per cent were attributed to anaesthesia.

At term the pregnant patient has undergone several profound physiological changes. There is a decrease in the functional residual capacity of the lung with an increase in minute volume. Breathlessness is common and decreases in arterial oxygenation are seen as a result of airway closure brought about by the high diaphragm. Cardiac output increases by 40 per cent and there is a rise in plasma volume of approximately 45 per cent. Total haemoglobin rises by 20 per cent. Finally, there is increased secretion of gastric acid and a decreased gastric emptying time. The oesophageal sphincter relaxes.

For the anaesthetist several hazards exist which are peculiar to the obstetric situation. With the patient supine the weight of the gravid uterus can compress the inferior vena cava and aorta causing marked hypotension. Regurgitation and aspiration of gastric contents is a special risk due to high abdominal pressure and the changes in gastric physiology. Above all, there are two patients to deal with. It must be remembered in these circumstances, that practically all the anaesthetic analgesic and sedative drugs will cross the placenta and enter the fetal circulation. Muscle relaxants however do not cross the placenta in sufficient concentrations to affect the fetus.

Given these problems and the need for a mother to enjoy the experience of childbirth, epidural analgesia has become popular. For this technique, as well as general anaesthesia, specialist experts in this field are mandatory if the best results are to be obtained (Chapter 11).

Head injury

Preoperative management of the patient with head injury is a minefield for the untrained or unwary, especially in the multiple-trauma victim. As intracranial pressure rises so perfusion of the brain becomes impaired. Cerebral blood flow in these circumstances will depend on the difference between mean arterial pressure and mean intracranial pressure. This difference, the cerebral-perfusion pressure, becomes critical below about 60 mmHg when cerebral autoregulation starts to fail and cerebral ischaemia develops. It is of fundamental importance, therefore, to recognize rises in ICP and to meticulously avoid hypotension and hypoxia. By appropriate fluid resuscitation, correction of hypoxia with oxygen therapy and intubation of the patient who cannot protect the airway, secondary brain damage can be prevented. These measures should be carried out in all cases prior to transfer and/or CT scan.

For victims of multiple trauma, neck and chest radiographs need to be urgently considered before anaesthesia in case of cervical spine injury or pneumothorax. Clearly if life-threatening haemorrhage is present which cannot be controlled nor corrected by infusion, then surgical intervention will take an overriding priority (Chapter 15).

Muscle weakness

Occasionally patients present for anaesthesia with severe muscle weakness. In the Guillain-Barré syndrome this is due to a polyneuritis which produces a progressive peripheral nerve demyelination and the gradual onset of paralysis. In myasthenia gravis the site of the disease is at the neuromuscular junction. In both cases profound weakness may result with or without bulbar symptoms. A useful way of objectively charting the progress of these patients is to measure vital capacity (VC) with a respirometer or Vitalograph, twice daily. Normal VC will be approximately 50 ml/kg. When levels of 12–15 ml/kg are reached, intubation and ventilation should be urgently considered. In these situations careful assessment of coughing and swallowing ability is important so that aspiration of pharyngeal or gastric contents does not occur.

Patients receiving medication

No preoperative assessment is complete without taking a comprehensive drug history; in certain cases the type of medication being taken will be further evidence of any disease. Antihypertensive drugs, digoxin or amiodarone therapy will point to the presence of cardiovascular disease and the need to monitor this system with increased care. Beta adrenoceptor antagonists may cause severe bradycardia intraoperatively, whilst anticoagulants may need to be withdrawn. Other drugs, notably steroids and the hypoglycaemic agents, will indicate special precautions. Long-term corticosteroid therapy causes adrenal suppression so booster doses must be given with the premedication and tailed off gradually, postoperatively. When hypoglycaemic drugs, like insulin, are in use care must be taken to avoid a dangerous reduction in blood sugar during the fasting period before, during and after anaesthesia. Several regimens are popular and are based on the use of i.v. glucose with insulin given simultaneously by pump or infusion. In all patients, the longer-acting forms of insulin need substituting with short-acting insulin (soluble/Actrapid) at least 24 hours before surgery and in some cases (long-acting insulin and chloropamide) several days before. A simple system recommended by Alberti and Thomas is to omit the morning dose of insulin and to set up a 10 per cent dextrose infusion, 500 ml with 10 units soluble insulin and 10 mmol KCl to run in over 4–6 hours. Regular BM stix or blood glucose measurements can then be carried out and the insulin reduced or increased to keep the blood sugar within the range of 5–10 mmol/litre (Chapter 16).

General anaesthesia or regional anaesthesia

At the end of this period of patient assessment a decision will have to be made as to whether general anaesthesia or regional anaesthesia is more appropriate, given the patient's medical status and the operation planned. For many operations regional anaesthesia is impractical or impossible. Craniotomy, thoracotomy, faciomaxillary, and spinal surgery cannot, in most cases, be carried out under local or field block. However, limb surgery, abdominal surgery, including obstetric surgery, and pelvic surgery can be readily performed with a regional or local anaesthetic, if the patient finds this an acceptable option (Chapter 12).

In a regional block, a particular nerve or nerve bundle may be anaesthetized. Examples are a brachial plexus block in arm or hand surgery. For larger surgical fields introduction of local anaesthetic into the cerebrospinal fluid (spinal anaesthesia) or into the epidural space provides complete sensory blockade and muscle relaxation over a wide region. As in general anaesthesia there are pitfalls. Hypotension may occur as a consequence of sympathetic blockade. Dural puncture can cause severe headache or, rarely, neurological damage. Contraindications exist to these techniques such as pre-existing neurological disease, when any worsening postoperatively may be attributed to the anaesthetic. Anticoagulation may result in epidural haematoma and local skin infection can result in the introduction of bacteria to the CSF.

Nevertheless, a well-conducted regional block can provide a very high degree of patient and surgical satisfaction. The severe bronchitic can take deep breaths, cough and talk during the procedure. The obstetric patient may see and take part in the birth of her baby by caesarean section under epidural block.

There is one fundamental rule in the use of local anaesthetics; the administrator must know and understand the calculation of the maximum safe dose. In the case of lignocaine this is 3 mg/kg. Above this dose neurotoxicity occurs with the onset of convulsions. Labelling on vials of local anaesthetic may be unhelpful if the user does not understand what the various concentrations mean (Table 9.11).

Table 9.11

Concentration	mg/ml
0.5%	5
1.0%	10
2.0%	20
1: 1000	1
1: 10000	0.1

The preoperative check

Prior to administration of the premedication the nursing and junior medical staff need to check that the consent form for surgery has been signed and that the side of operation has been marked on the patient's skin. Any dentures should be removed and an identification tag attached to the patient's wrist. Before elective surgery, the patient will have been fasted overnight. In this way, stomach contents are kept to a minimum and the danger of regurgitation and inhalation at induction of anaesthesia is reduced. When emergency surgery is planned, the fasting period may be reduced to 4 hours. In these circumstances it should be remembered that pain, shock and drugs may reduce gastric emptying time and therefore that precautions to prevent airway contamination will have to be taken by the anaesthetist. Where loss of over 15 per cent of the blood volume (75 ml/kg) is expected, blood should be cross-matched and available.

Premedication

The objectives in patient premedication are threefold:
- to relieve anxiety
- to provide a degree of autonomic blockade
- to provide analgesia.

As a consequence of the reassurance and explanation which is such a vital part of the preoperative visit, the patient will to some extent feel less nervous about the forthcoming operation. Further anxiolysis is however necessary and this can be provided by *benzodiazepines* (diazepam, temazepam), *narcotics* (Omnopon, pethidine) or *phenothiazines* (promethazine). In all cases, over-sedation will result in respiratory and cardiovascular depression and it is important to prescribe the correct dosage taking into account body weight and concurrent illness. A particular advantage of the benzodiazepines is that anterograde amnesia is produced. This, and the lack of any dysphoric effects or nausea, make them an ideal group of drugs for premedication of minor to medium surgery. However, where major surgery is planned narcotics provide useful sedation with an analgesic effect which will last throughout anaesthesia and contribute to postoperative comfort.

Anticholinergics
These drugs produce their effects by competing with acetylcholine at parasympathetic muscarinic receptors. At the normal dose range, atropine (0.6 mg) causes marked drying of secretions and inhibition of salivation. This reduces the coughing and respiratory irritation provoked by inhalational anaesthetics. In addition, there is an element of protection against vagal overactivity produced, for example, by visceral traction, other anaesthetic drugs, or intubation. As a result, bradycardia and hypotension are less common. Scopolamine is an alternative anticholinergic with better drying effects but weaker vagolytic effects on the heart. Penetration of the blood–brain barrier by Scopolamine produces a mild sedative effect and can, on occasion, cause restlessness and disorientation, especially in the elderly. Glycopyrronium bromide is a new anticholinergic which does not cross the blood–brain barrier, thereby producing few of the central side-effects seen with Scopolamine. In addition, it has a good drying effect on secretions and causes less tachycardia than atropine when given intravenously.

Whilst omission of the anticholinergic part of the premedication has been advocated from time to time, most anaesthetists will prefer their use on the grounds of safety, even though a certain amount of patient discomfort (dry mouth) will be induced.

Certain categories of patients will need extra drugs with their premedication. Examples include asthmatics for whom bronchodilators can be used preoperatively, corticosteroid dependents who need booster doses, and certain cardiac cases with valvular damage in whom antibiotics are indicated. In all cases the premedication needs to be prescribed about 1 hour before surgery is due to start. Given the unpredictable length of surgical procedures, the correct timing of premedication needs a combination of obsessive care, skill, judgement and luck.

Further reading

Alberti K G M M, Thomas B J B. The management of diabetes during surgery. *British Journal of Anaesthesia* 1979; **51:** 693–716.

Buck N, Devlin H B, Lunn J N. *Report of a confidential enquiry into peri-operative deaths.* London: Nuffield Provincial Hospital Trust, 1987.

Childs C G. The liver and portal hypertension. *Major problems in clinical surgery.* Philadelphia: W B Saunders, 1966.

Goldman L, Caldera D L, Nussbaum S R *et al.* Multifactorial index of cardiac risk in non-cardiac surgical procedures. *New England Journal of Medicine* 1977; **297:** 845–9.

Morgan M. Report on confidential enquiry into maternal deaths. *Anaesthesia* 1986; **41:** 689–91.

Nunn J F, Milledge J S, Chen D, Dore C. Respiratory criteria of fitness for surgery and anaesthesia. *Anaesthesia* 1988; **43:** 543–51.

Pugh R N H, Murray-Lyon I M, Dawson J L, Pietroni M C, Williams R. Transection of the oesophagus for bleeding varices. *British Journal of Surgery,* 1973; **60:** 646–9.

Sykes M K, McNicol M W, Campbell E J M. *Respiratory failure* 2nd edn. Oxford: Blackwell, 1976: 112–24.

Consent to treatment. London: Medical Defence Union, 1989.

10

Practical procedures
R H Ellis

- Venepuncture and venous access
    indwelling intravenous needles
    techniques of intravenous cannulation
- Establishing and maintaining an airway
    the face mask
- Endotracheal intubation
    indications
    technique
- Cricoid pressure
    technique
- Arterial puncture and cannulation
    technique
- Central venous cannulation
    technique for cannulation of the internal jugular vein

Each of the procedures discussed in this chapter is a complex manoeuvre, and each is potentially harmful to the patient. An understanding of the principles on which the procedure is based, coupled with scrupulous attention to detail when performing it, offer the best chance of reducing the risk to a minimum.

When performing any of these invasive procedures a clean technique should be used, and care should be taken to avoid contamination of previously-sterilized items (tubes, cannulae, catheters, etc.) which are to be inserted into the patient. If the patient is especially at risk from infection (e.g. as a result of immunosuppression) a sterile technique should be used and the anaesthetist should wear a mask scrub up, and gown and glove. Such precautions should also be taken if the patient has an infective condition (such as hepatitis or AIDS) which may pose a threat to the anaesthetist.

Venepuncture and venous access

The simple needing of a vein should be used solely for withdrawal of a blood sample. The injection of any drug may occasionally be followed by an untoward reaction, and an already in-dwelling needle permits appropriate intravenous treatment to be given without delay.

In-dwelling intravenous needles
Simple in-dwelling needles allow repeated i.v. injections following a single venepuncture; they may also be suitable for repeated sampling of blood, or for fluid infusions over a limited period of time. There are various devices,

such as the 'Y-Can' apparatus (Fig. 10.1a) which, once in place, do not leave a sharp needle in the vein and therefore have less tendency to 'cut out' during use. A simple 'butterfly' needle (Fig. 10.1b) may also be satisfactory.

(a)

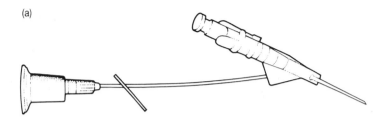

Fig. 10.1a   'Y-Can' apparatus.

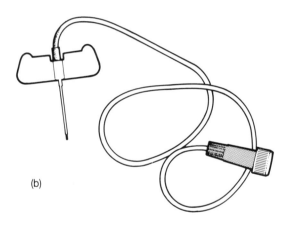

(b)

Fig. 10.1b   A 'butterfly' needle.

The preferred sites for in-dwelling needles are away from the wrist or elbow joints where movements of the limb may cause them to 'cut out' of the vein. The dorsum of the hand, the forearm and, less usually, the upper arm are ideal as the long bones tend to act as splints and prevent undue movement.

Technique of intravenous cannulation

Essential preliminaries

Examination of the patient
Specifically this is to select a suitable vein. The arm veins are usually used. A large vein on the forearm of the non-dominant arm should be chosen;

there should be no evidence of infection or skin disease nearby. The angle between the confluence of two veins is the best site as the veins are relatively fixed here and do not move away from the advancing needle.

Preparation of the apparatus
The specialized apparatus consists of
- A suitably-sized cannula (Fig. 10.2). The notion that it is easier to insert a small cannula rather than a larger one is mistaken. The size of the cannula should depend on the purpose for which the i.v. infusion is required. In adult practice a 16 French gauge cannula is satisfactory for the administration of clear fluids; a 14 gauge cannula should be used if blood or other viscous fluids are to be given.

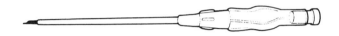

Fig. 10.2   A cannula.

- An infusion set (Fig. 10.3) should be made ready and attached to a bag of appropriate i.v. solution and the set should be primed with solution to remove all air bubbles.

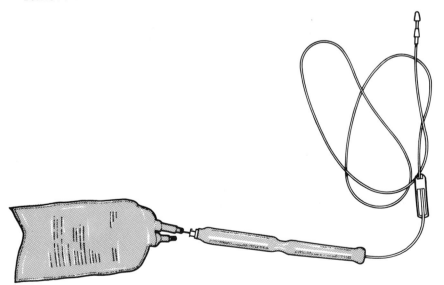

Fig. 10.3   An infusion set.

- A venous tourniquet will be needed, or an assistant can be asked to compress the arm.

The apparatus to be used should be checked beforehand. Make sure you know how it works, fits together, comes apart, etc. Anticipate and rehearse the sequence of manoeuvres to be performed.

Preparation of the injection site

The proposed site of injection should be cleaned with an antiseptic solution, and nearby unsterile areas covered with sterile towels. The venous tourniquet should be lightly applied to the arm in order to occlude the venous circulation and to distend the vein prior to cannulation. Care should be taken not to occlude the arterial supply as well so ensure the radial pulse can always be felt. If the patient is conscious an intradermal injection of local anaesthetic should be made at the site of puncture.

Insertion of the cannula

Palpate the distended vein in order to assess its size and the direction in which it travels up the arm. When you are certain that you have made these assessments, stretch the skin distal to the vein and perform the venepuncture by making two quite separate movements to enter the vein. Firstly, in one deliberate and brisk movement, insert the needle point through the skin at a point which lies just superficial and just to one side of the vein (if venepuncture is being made at the confluence of two veins, the needle point should be inserted a short distance distal to the confluence of the tributaries). Without advancing the needle any further at this stage, tilt the needle point upwards, so that it produces a dimple under the skin, and observe precisely how the point lies in relation to the distended vein (Fig. 10.4a).

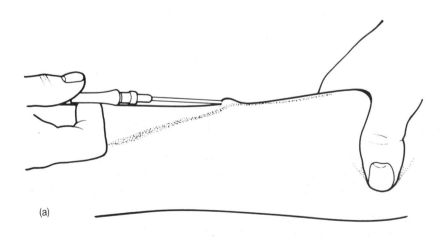

(a)

Fig. 10.4a Insertion of the cannula.

Then, making sure that the long axis of the needle coincides with that of the vein, advance the needle into the lumen of the vein. Successful entry is denoted by the appearance of blood in the small reservoir built into the hub of the needle. The hub should then be steadied and the cannula itself advanced gently into and along the lumen of the vein (Fig. 10.4b).

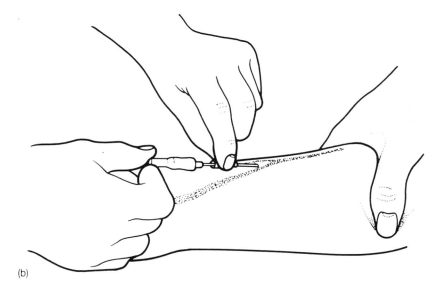

(b)

Fig. 10.4b

The infusion set should be connected and free flow of the fluid into the vein and not into the subcutaneous tissues nearby must be demonstrated before applying an antiseptic spray to the puncture site and securing the cannula with a sterile covering.

If the cannula is left in place for any length of time the puncture site, and also the vein along which the cannula and infusions course, should be inspected regularly. Any sign of redness or pain is an indication to remove the cannula and re-site it in a non-inflamed area.

Establishing and maintaining an airway

Every unconscious patient, or patient whose conscious level is impaired, is at risk from airway obstruction. Obstruction may occur

- due to blood, vomit, secretions and any variety of foreign bodies in the airway
- if the normal boundaries of the airways change position. They may do this because of gravity, because of local pathology such as cysts, tumours, etc., or because of oedema due either to localized conditions (such as infection or venous engorgement), or to some generalized states of fluid retention

- during anaesthesia in the supine patient. The commonest cause of obstruction in this case is the tongue falling backwards by gravity so that it meets the posterior pharyngeal wall and occludes the oropharynx. A floppy epiglottis may also pose a problem
- due to laryngeal spasm during anaesthesia. The larynx is the most reactive part of the airway, and responds to a variety of stimuli by involuntarily closing to a greater or lesser extent. Such stimuli may include
  - light anaesthesia
  - irritation by foreign bodies or secretions
  - irritation by pungent vapours

The **cardinal sign of airway obstruction** in a patient who is breathing spontaneously is a heaving chest. There is, virtually, no other cause of this in a patient lying, otherwise quietly, at rest. This laboured breathing occurs because the accessory muscles of ventilation act powerfully to try and overcome the obstruction. The muscles of the abdominal wall contract forcefully and pull the abdominal wall in. At the same time the intercostals attempt to expand the chest and a characteristic 'see-saw' pattern of respiratory movement is seen.

The **associated signs** are less reliable, and only appear later. These include
- sounds. A low-pitch, snoring noise is caused by the tongue or soft palate vibrating slowly in the stream of air which it is (partially) obstructing. A higher-pitch, crowing sound indicates laryngeal spasm and is caused by the more-or-less taut vocal cords and vestibular folds coming together and vibrating like the reeds of an oboe. If there is total obstruction no air flows, no vibration is possible and, ominously, there is silence.
- the reservoir bag of the anaesthetic circuit ceases to move fully. Obstruction may readily occur when the patient is not connected to an anaesthetic circuit, and so this sign is neither consistent nor reliable.
- cyanosis. This occurs only after the obstruction has been present for some time: it indicates either that the cardinal sign (see above) was unobserved or that the obstruction has not been managed efficiently (see below). Cyanosis cannot occur, even with total respiratory obstruction, in a severely anaemic patient.

Respiratory obstruction is a grave emergency. If unrelieved it will kill the patient. Its occurrence must be recognized as soon as it happens, and it must be relieved without delay.

There are several ways in which the airway can be kept unobstructed, or airway obstruction can be treated in the supine patient. Initially the presence in the airway of foreign material, secretions, etc. should be looked for and, if found, these should be removed by suction. Then one of the following can be used
- pull the mandible upwards and forwards. (The tongue moves passively with the mandible, since many of the extrinsic muscles of the tongue are attached to it.) It may be enough to pull firmly up on the point of the jaw (Fig. 10.5). If not then both angles of the mandible should be pulled or pushed upwards and forwards (Fig. 10.6). This is usually easy to accomplish but in muscular, short-necked patients may require a forceful effort.

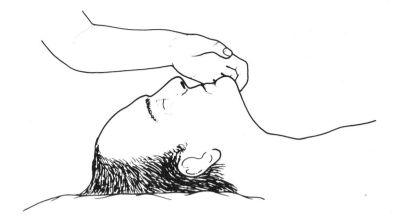

Fig. 10.5 Maintaining an airway by pulling up on the point of the jaw.

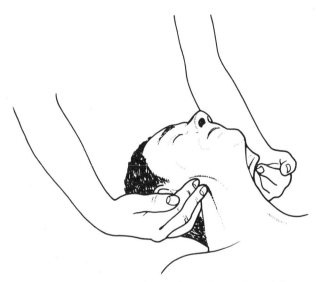

Fig. 10.6 Maintaining an airway by pulling the angles of the mandible up and forward.

- an oral airway may be used. The mouth is opened and the airway (Fig. 10.7a) inserted so that it comes to lie with its flange in front of the lips and its tip between the tongue and posterior pharyngeal wall. Caution should be exercised since, at light levels of anaesthesia, the airway may make the situation worse by stimulating pharyngeal reflexes and producing gagging, vomiting or coughing. Its careless insertion may damage teeth, lips and tongue.
- if the obstruction is accompanied by spasm of the masseter muscles, the teeth are clenched together and insertion of an airway is not possible.

Forcing the jaws apart by levering on the teeth is likely to make the situation worse. In these circumstances a *nasopharyngeal airway* (Fig. 10.7b) should be inserted through one nostril until it separates the tongue from the pharyngeal wall.

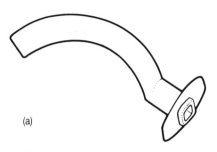

(a)

Fig. 10.7a   An oral airway.

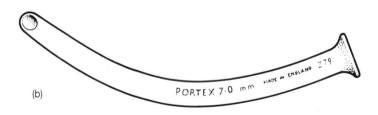

(b)

PORTEX 7·0 mm   MADE IN ENGLAND   279

Fig. 10.7b   A nasopharyngeal airway.

Respiratory obstruction which does not yield to the above measures is extremely dangerous. Further management is as follows
* if the patient is cyanosed, 100 per cent oxygen should be given with a close-fitting face mask, and the operation suspended until control of the patient's airway is regained.

- if the tongue causes resistant obstruction, the head (and if necessary the whole patient) should be turned onto one side so that the tongue falls towards the side of the mouth rather than towards the posterior pharyngeal wall.
- if *resistant laryngeal spasm* is the cause then the reservoir bag should be squeezed in order to try and force oxygen, under pressure, through the obstructed larynx.

As a last resort, the patient may be paralysed with a short-acting muscle relaxant and intubated. Performing such a manoeuvre in a hypoxic and hypercarbic patient is fraught with dangers but may be necessary to save life. Whenever an anaesthetic is being given, all the apparatus required for suction, intubation, and positive-pressure ventilation with oxygen must be to hand.

The face mask

Many straightforward general anaesthetics can be given using a suitable breathing system (Chapter 8) which is attached to a cushioned face mask (Fig. 10.8). This is applied closely to the patient's face in order to ensure a gas-tight seal between mask and face. Firm application is needed to ensure that there are no leaks between the edges of the mask and the face since such leaks permit air to enter the circuit during inspiration. This will lead to uncontrolled lightening of anaesthesia by diluting the anaesthetic mixture being breathed by the patient.

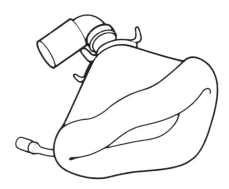

Fig. 10.8 A cushioned face mask.

This firm and backward pressure on the face tends to push the jaw and tongue towards the posterior pharyngeal wall and cause obstruction. Supporting the mandible (as described above) will compensate for this. It may be necessary to use one hand to keep the mask firmly pressed onto the face whilst the other supports the jaw (Fig. 10.9). Alternatively, the fingers can be used to support both angles of the mandible whilst the mask is kept in place with the thumbs with or without the help of the index fingers (Fig. 10.10).

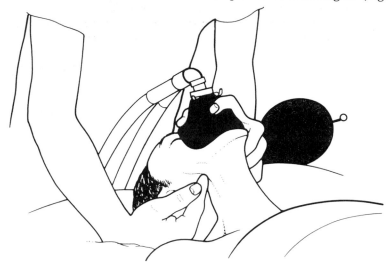

Fig. 10.9 Face mask held in place with one hand whilst the other hand is used to support one angle of the mandible.

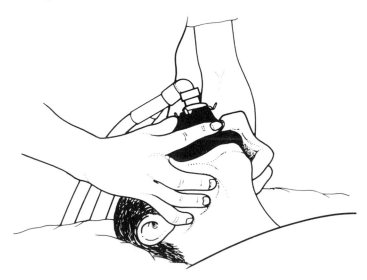

Fig. 10.10 Face masks held in place with the thumbs whilst the fingers support both angles of the mandible.

Artificial ventilation with a face mask

This is an essential skill in anaesthesia, but during its performance there is a risk that air will pass into the oesophagus as well as (or instead of) into the trachea and lungs. Should this happen stomach contents may spill into the oesophagus and pharynx, and thence into the unprotected lungs. This method of ventilation, therefore, is to be avoided if there is any possibility of a full stomach being present although the efficient application of cricoid pressure (p. 158) will prevent regurgitation. With this *proviso*, ventilation using a face mask may be used in the following circumstances

- prior to intubation
- as an alternative to intubation during brief procedures requiring full relaxation, e.g. electroconvulsive therapy
- in any circumstance when a patient is temporarily unable to breathe adequately — due to disease or to the continued effect of muscle relaxant or respiratory depressant drugs. Intubation should be performed if such respiratory inadequacy persists or if there is a full stomach.

One hand performs two tasks simultaneously – pressing the mask firmly onto the face to provide an air-tight seal and supporting the jaw to eliminate airway obstruction (Fig. 10.11). The other hand squeezes a reservoir or a self-inflating bag regularly to pressurize the airway and ventilate the lungs.

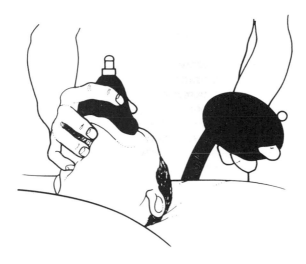

Fig. 10.11   One hand used to both hold the mask and support the jaw.

It is essential that a free rise and fall of the chest (not of the abdomen) occurs. If there is difficulty in producing this, both hands must be used to hold the mask and clear the airway whilst an assistant squeezes the bag.

Endotracheal intubation

This is one of the most commonly performed invasive procedures in anaesthetic practice and is used to ensure a patient's safety during anaesthesia. However, if performed without proper skill and care the procedure itself may be lethal.

Orotracheal intubation is usually preferred. During intraoral surgery the presence of a tube in the mouth may impede the operation, and nasotracheal intubation is indicated (see below).

Indications
- to enable prolonged IPPV
- to prevent contamination of the lungs — by separating the alimentary and respiratory tracts in the presence of a full stomach, intestinal obstruction, or when there is bleeding or secretion into or from the mouth and pharynx
- to deliver anaesthetics during head and neck surgery where a mask would impede surgical access
- to maintain an otherwise difficult airway
- to provide airway control during prolonged anaesthesia
- to secure the airway during resuscitation (Chapter 14)

Technique

Essential preliminaries

Examination of the patient
With intubation specifically in mind the presence of any deformities which might make intubation difficult must be detected. Large goitres, swellings within (or impinging on) the mouth, pharynx, larynx and trachea, skin contractures following burns of the neck, etc. are all likely to cause difficulties with intubation. Less obvious anatomical features must also be looked for since these, far more frequently, give rise to difficulties with intubation. Such features include:
- the inability to open the mouth fully
- the presence of a short fat neck
- the presence of protruding upper incisor teeth
- the presence of a small or receding chin and lower jaw
- reduced mobility of the neck, especially the inability to extend the skull at the atlanto-occipital joint

A trained and undistracted assistant is essential for the anaesthetist.

Preparation of the equipment
A source of oxygen under pressure, and suction should be available. All equipment should be checked beforehand to ensure that it is in working order, and that both anaesthetist and assistant are familiar with the ways in which the various components are used, joined together and come apart. Anticipate and rehearse the sequence of manoeuvres to be performed. The following special apparatus is necessary (Fig. 10.12).
- a laryngoscope (usually a Macintosh laryngoscope (1)) together with a second one in reserve

Fig. 10.12 Equipment for endotracheal intubation.

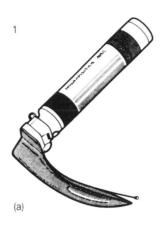

(a)

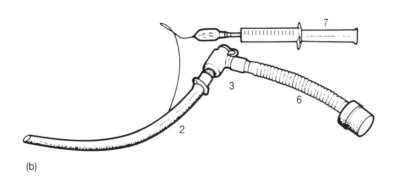

(b)

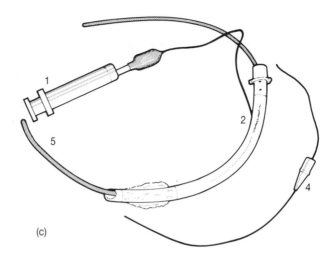

(c)

- a suitably-sized, usually cuffed, endotracheal tube (2) and connector (3). Normally an adult male will accept a 9.0 mm diameter tube, and an adult female an 8.0 mm. A tube 1 millimetre smaller than that predicted should also be available
- a stiffening introducer (4), and a long bougie (5) — in case of unexpected difficulty in visualizing the larynx
- a catheter mount (6) to join the connector of the endotracheal tube to
- a suitable breathing system or self-inflating bag (Chapter 8)
- a syringe (7) with which to inflate the cuff, and a clip to occlude the inflating channel
- an oropharyngeal airway

Rendering the larynx unreactive
The larynx is designed primarily to prevent foreign bodies entering the lungs and so its protective and sphincteric action must be overcome before a tube can be inserted safely through the vocal cords; virtually the only exceptions to this are in some neonates, in deeply unconscious patients, and in cases of cardiac arrest. The laryngeal reflexes can be attenuated or obtunded by
- local anaesthesia
- deep inhalation anaesthesia
- powerful respiratory depressants, e.g. opioids such as fentanyl, etc.
- muscle relaxants

Muscle relaxants and respiratory depressants will take away the patient's ability to breathe spontaneously, and should be administered only when efficient artificial ventilation has been demonstrated using a face mask and airway. Otherwise, a patient with some obstructing lesion which prevents artificial ventilation with a mask and airway, and which then gives rise to difficulty and delay in achieving endotracheal intubation, will be at serious risk from hypoxia.

Laryngoscopy

The way in which the laryngoscope is inserted is the key to successful laryngoscopy and intubation. An ill-considered, or forceful lunge at the patient's hypopharynx is unlikely to achieve its goal and may well cause serious damage to the lips, teeth, gums, tongue, pharynx and larynx. In contrast a deliberate and careful advance of the tip of the laryngoscope blade from the lips to the base of the tongue — following commonsense and obvious landmarks — should achieve its aim without undue hazard to the patient. The journey down to the larynx should be divided into the following stages, embarking on a subsequent stage only when the previous one has been successfully accomplished.

The technique will be described as for a right-handed operator.

- The patient should be supine. The head and neck should be placed in the position usually described as 'sniffing the morning air'. To achieve this a pillow (or two) under the head will ensure that the neck is correctly flexed (Fig. 10.13). The atlanto-occipital joint is then extended by either pushing gently on the vertex of the skull or by gently pulling upwards on the upper incisor teeth or gums.

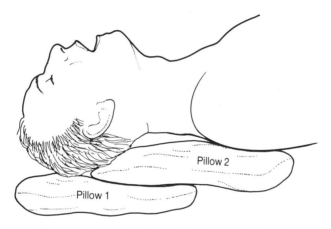

Fig. 10.13   Patient 'sniffing the morning air'.

- The laryngoscope should be taken in the **left** hand, and inserted into the **right** side of the patient's mouth, its tip being directed backwards until it lies just medial to the rearmost molar teeth (or gums in the edentulous) (Fig. 10.14).
- The handle of the instrument is then inclined medially so that the flange on the blade pushes the muscle mass of the tongue away to the left and brings the uvula into view (Fig. 10.15). The tongue must be displaced to the left, otherwise its incompressible bulk will, later, prevent the larynx from being easily seen. The uvula is important since it marks the mid-line. Having found the mid-line the tip of the blade should not deviate from it.

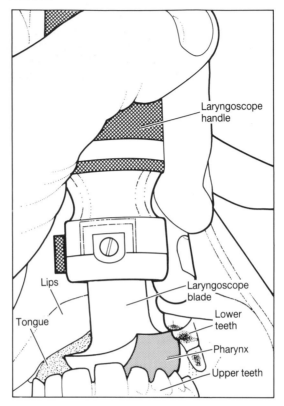

Fig. 10.14 Laryngoscope lying medial to rearmost molar teeth.

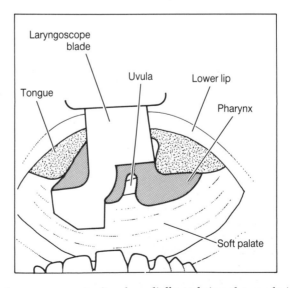

Fig. 10.15 Laryngoscope inclined medially to bring the uvula into view.

- With the tongue now displaced to the left, and the mid-line identified by the uvula, the tip of the blade should be advanced gently down over (but still applied to) the dorsum of the tongue, in the mid-line, until the tip of the epiglottis is seen. The tip of the blade is advanced until it lies in the valleculae between the front of the root of the epiglottis and the rear of the base of the tongue (Fig. 10.16).

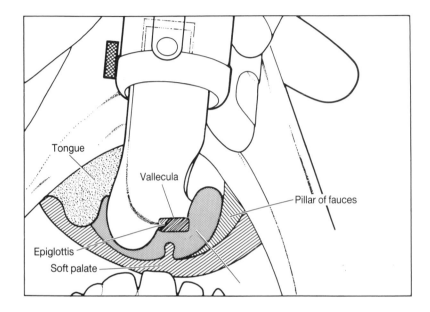

Fig. 10.16 Laryngoscope advanced until epiglottis is seen.

The tip of the laryngoscope is now in its correct position and should not be advanced further. All that is needed to reveal the larynx is to displace the epiglottis.
- This is achieved with the tip of the laryngoscope still in the valleculae. The laryngoscope should **not** be used as a lever and the incisor teeth or gums should **not** be used as a fulcrum. Instead moderate traction should be exerted both vertically and along the direction of the long axis of the handle of the laryngoscope (Fig. 10.17). This draws the epiglottis forwards and reveals the larynx below.
- It is not necessary to see the whole of the laryngeal opening. Quite often only the posterior (interarytenoid) region is seen (Fig. 10.18), but this is enough to identify the larynx and to permit a tube to be inserted into it, ensuring that the tube is seen to pass anterior to the arytenoid cartilages. If necessary, the assistant should be asked to push the thyroid cartilage firmly backwards and gently upwards (cephalad) in order to improve the view of the larynx.

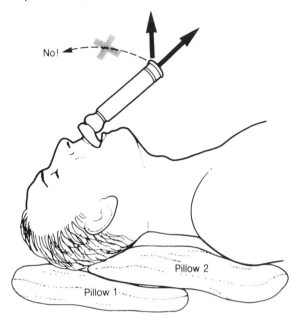

Fig. 10.17   Correct traction to be applied to laryngoscope once it is in position.

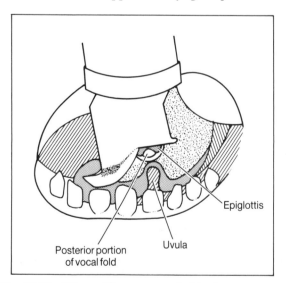

Fig. 10.18   View of larynx revealed by laryngoscope.

Insertion of the tube

The tube is then taken in the right hand and inserted through the right-hand side of the mouth, then — taking advantage of the curve of the tube itself — down to and through the laryngeal opening.

Occasionally, when some of the previously-mentioned anatomical features make intubation somewhat difficult, the curve of the tube should be accentuated with a stiffening introducer. Alternatively, a simple long flexible bougie should be passed through the vocal cords, and the tube can then be threaded over this guide and passed into the larynx.

The catheter mount and the rest of the breathing system should be connected and the cuff inflated with just enough air to provide an air-tight seal when the lungs are inflated by a modest, positive pressure applied to the tube.

Checking that the tube is in the trachea

It is far easier to pass the tube into the oesophagus than through the larynx. Therefore, having inserted the tube it is **absolutely essential** to check immediately that it is correctly positioned in the trachea, and that it has not inadvertently entered the oesophagus. Even if it is in the trachea, it may have gone beyond the carina and entered the right main bronchus.

The rise and fall of both sides of the chest as the bag is squeezed should be observed but this is not a reliable indication that the tube is in the trachea. A stethoscope **must** be used to make certain that air entry **can** be heard for certain throughout the lung fields (especially in both axillae) and that it **cannot** be heard in the epigastrium (i.e. over the stomach). If there is any doubt about these findings the tube should be removed and intubation attempted again when the patient has been adequately oxygenated.

As soon as the tube is known to be correctly placed it should be tied, or taped, securely in position, and — with an orotracheal tube — an airway inserted into the mouth to prevent the patient biting on the tube in light levels of anaesthesia.

A patient who is intubated is constantly at risk from lack of oxygen which is due commonly to obstruction of the tube or to its disconnection from the anaesthetic breathing system or ventilator tubing. It follows that such a patient should never be left unattended.

Nasotracheal intubation

Insertion of an endotracheal tube through the nose may be necessary during operations within the buccal cavity. The tube should be inserted along the floor of the nasal cavity into the nasopharynx and then pushed gently onwards into the oropharynx. A laryngoscope is inserted and the tube advanced through the larynx with the aid of a pair of intubating forceps.

Nasotracheal intubation may also be attempted when it is impossible to visualize the larynx directly with a laryngoscope: the tube should be directed towards and through the larynx using intubating forceps. If it is not possible to open the patient's mouth sufficiently to insert a laryngoscope a nasally-inserted tube may be directed towards the larynx solely by appropriate manipulations of the head and neck ('blind nasal intubation').

Intubation in children

Smaller apparatus is obviously required, but other important differences exist between children (up to the age of 8 years) and adults as far as intubation is concerned. The larynx in the child lies more anteriorly, and higher up in the neck than it does in the adult. In addition the epiglottis is larger and less rigid. Accordingly, having found the epiglottis (as described above) the tip of the laryngoscope blade is not advanced into the valleculae but, instead, is passed down over the dorsum of the epiglottis which is then lifted forwards to reveal the larynx. A straighter blade (such as the Seward blade) is normally used for paediatric intubation.

The narrowest part of a child's larynx is **not** between the cords (as in the adult) but is at the level of the cricoid ring; it is of circular cross-section. As a result a snug-fitting endotracheal tube does not require an inflatable cuff to seal the laryngeal opening.

Extubation

Adequate spontaneous ventilation must be ensured before removal of an endotracheal tube. It must be assumed that the larynx is relatively insensitive or incompetent and removal of the tube should always be preceded by efficient pharyngeal suction. In addition, unless some over-riding contraindication exists, the patient should be placed in the recovery position before extubation. Skilled supervision is essential as the patient may develop post-extubation laryngeal spasm and respiratory obstruction.

Cricoid pressure

No patient should ever be anaesthetized for an elective procedure within 4 hours of having taken food or drink (of any description or quantity). After 4 hours, although the stomach will still not be empty, it is usual to proceed on the assumption that vomiting or regurgitation of stomach contents into the pharynx — and then, possibly, into the lungs — is a manageable risk. However, no anaesthetic should be embarked upon without previously checking, *inter alia*, that an efficient sucker is to hand.

- *Vomiting* is an active muscular process, resulting in the powerful expulsion of gastric contents into the pharynx. It cannot occur in a paralysed patient, but such a patient is still at risk because regurgitation of stomach contents into the pharynx may easily occur.
- *Regurgitation* is a passive process and may occur in any patient receiving muscle relaxants if the intragastric pressure exceeds that in the oesophagus. The lower oesophageal sphincter is ineffective in preventing regurgitation.

In some emergencies anaesthesia may be required even though a full stomach is known, or assumed, to be present. Alternatives to general anaesthesia must be considered, but if general anaesthesia is decided upon there is a major risk of aspiration of gastric contents into the lungs. In these circumstances a nasogastric tube should be inserted preoperatively so that most of the gas, much of the liquid and some of the solid matter in the stomach can be removed by suction. This reduces the bulk of gastric contents and the intragastric pressure. However, the stomach cannot be emptied completely, and precautions must be taken against the aspiration of its contents into the lungs.

The vomiting risk at induction can best be circumvented by a rapid-sequence induction consisting of the administration of a quick-acting relaxant immediately after induction has produced a lightly-unconscious patient. Suxamethonium is the relaxant of choice as it enables an endo-tracheal tube to be passed as quickly as possible, and the inflated cuff of the tube then serves to protect the lungs from contamination. There is, however, an interval (which may be prolonged if intubation difficulties occur) between the onset of muscular paralysis and the successful place-ment of a cuffed tube in the trachea. During this interval the lungs may be completely unprotected and material regurgitated from the stomach can enter the airway. The correct application of pressure on the cricoid cartilage will protect the lungs in these circumstances.

The cricoid cartilage forms a complete and substantial ring around the airway at the lower end of the larynx. It consists of an arch, which can be felt subcutaneously in the neck, and a back-plate (or lamina) positioned immediately in front of the oesophagus. Firm pressure on the arch of the cricoid causes its back-plate to compress the oesophagus against the cervical vertebrae, obliterate the lumen of the oesophagus, and prevent the passage of regurgitant material upwards into the laryngopharynx.

Technique

Essential preliminaries

Examination of the patient
The presence or absence of those features which might make intubation difficult and prolonged should be noted. If severe difficulty is anticipated an alternative method of anaesthesia must be considered.

Preparation of equipment
In addition to that required for the intubation itself, an efficient sucker and a source of oxygen must be to hand. It must be possible to tip the patient into a steep head-down position at a moment's notice.

An assistant is essential
Prior to induction the anaesthetist and the assistant must anticipate and rehearse the series of manoeuvres to be performed. During the induction sequence the assistant must have no duty other than the application of cricoid pressure, and must be familiar with the relevant landmarks. The assistant should palpate the patient's neck and identify, with absolute certainty, the arch of the cricoid cartilage.

Application of cricoid pressure
As the induction sequence commences the assistant's fingers must be positioned accurately, but lightly, over the cricoid — the thumb and middle finger should be on either side of it and the index finger over the arch itself (Fig. 10.19). Firm pressure must not be applied before the onset of paralysis lest vomiting be provoked and the powerful expulsive effort, being obstructed by the cricoid pressure, lead to oesophageal rupture. As soon as paralysis occurs the assistant, taking great care not to displace the larynx to one side or the other, presses firmly backwards on the cricoid arch to obliterate the lumen of the oesophagus. It is helpful if the assistant places

his other hand behind the patient's neck to act as a counterpressure; this prevents the cricoid pressure displacing the neck (and larynx) too far posteriorly and thus pushing the larynx out of the anaesthetist's view.

The pressure on the cricoid must not be released until the endotracheal tube has been positioned, its accurate placement ascertained, and its inflatable cuff blown up to provide an effective seal.

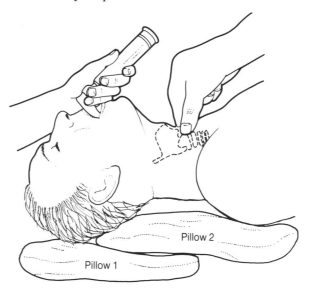

Fig. 10.19 Application of cricoid pressure. Cricoid pressure applied by the assistant is a bimanual procedure. For clarity the assistant's left hand, which is placed behind the neck to provide counter-pressure, is not shown.

Arterial puncture and cannulation

Arterial cannulation is usually performed in anaesthetic practice to enable
- continuous measurement of arterial blood pressure
- repeated sampling of arterial blood for the assessment of acid–base and blood–gas status (Chapter 6)

Any of the accessible, peripheral arteries may be cannulated, but the radial artery is most commonly selected; the dorsalis pedis and the femoral arteries are also suitable. The technique of radial artery cannulation will be described.

Technique

Essential preliminaries

Examination of the patient
Both radial and ulnar arteries should be examined. The radial artery should not be cannulated if the ulnar artery is absent, or if the ulnar collateral flow

to the hand is inadequate. On compression of the ulnar artery (temporarily, but sufficiently to occlude its flow) the thumb and fingers of the lateral side of the hand should remain pink and well perfused. If the radial pulses themselves are unequal, select the side on which the pulse is stronger.

Preparation of the equipment

Make sure you know how the apparatus you intend to use works, fits together, comes apart, etc. If the patient is conscious, an intradermal wheal of local anaesthetic should be raised at the site of puncture. Anticipate and rehearse the sequence of manoeuvres you will be performing. The following special items will be needed:

- a suitable cannula. The ideal cannula should be of the 'cannula over needle' type. It should be small (a 20FG cannula usually suffices), made of Teflon rather than plastic, and have parallel, rather than tapered sides. These features minimize the risk of occlusion and serious damage to the artery and the tissue which it supplies
- a 3-way tap with extension or manometer tubing for connection to the cannula. This is so that it may be flushed with an innocuous anticoagulant solution (500 units of heparin in 500 ml of 0.9 per cent saline) to prevent clotting in the system.
- the whole may be connected to a constant-flushing device, or to a transducer system (p. 163).

Determination of the local anatomy

The course of the radial artery varies from patient to patient and three aspects of the anatomy must be determined in each case immediately prior to cannulation in order to determine the precise site of puncture, and the direction in which the cannula should be inserted.

- firstly, the direction of the radial artery's course in the lower forearm, just proximal to the wrist, should be inspected from the anterior aspect of the wrist to determine the direction of its long axis
- secondly, the artery should be palpated at the wrist to identify the arched course it takes as it passes over the expanded lower end of the radius. The highest point of this arch should be identified, as should the angle (10°) at which the artery slopes upwards as it runs towards the wrist
- thirdly, the topmost point of the artery ('top, dead centre'), if viewed in cross-section, should be determined.

Insertion of the cannula

The assistant should abduct the patient's arm so that it is at a right-angle from the body. He should then support the forearm and hand with the wrist in a slight degree of extension which is just sufficient to move the muscles of the thenar eminence out of the way.

The cannula and its needle should be attached to a syringe barrel which acts as a reservoir to collect the blood which flows through the cannula during its insertion. The needle tip of the cannula is then inserted under the skin at a point which is:

- 0.5 cm distal to the highest point of the arch
- precisely above the topmost point of the lumen, and never to one side of the artery
- inclined at an angle of 10° to the horizontal plane.

Once the skin has been punctured with the cannula, pause and check that its orientation is as described above and then advance it until it pierces the anterior wall of the artery. If the point of puncture has been selected correctly, the needle point and cannula should pierce it at the apex of the arch of the artery. Blood appears in the syringe barrel. The hub of the needle must, then, be kept immobile whilst the cannula itself is advanced along the long axis of the artery: it will not impinge on either the posterior or the lateral walls of the vessel. Blood flowing slowly into the syringe barrel all the time indicates successful cannulation.

Once the cannula is in place it should be connected to the flushing system and secured with adhesive tapes. The puncture site must be kept clean, and a light splint should be used to immobilize the wrist and prevent kinking of the cannula and movement of its tip to-and-fro within the lumen of the artery.

The fingers should be inspected frequently for signs of circulatory occlusion. Should such signs appear, the cannula must be removed without delay. When an arterial cannula is removed the site of puncture should be compressed firmly with a sterile swab for 10 minutes and then — if no bleeding occurs and no haematoma forms — a sterile dressing should be applied. The circulation to the fingers should be inspected regularly over the next 4 hours.

Central venous cannulation

The pressure in a central vein accurately reflects the pressure in the right arium, and therefore — anatomically — a central vein is defined as one which is not separated from the right atrium by a venous valve. Central venous access may be effected either by cannulating the vein directly or by cannulating a more peripheral tributary and threading a long catheter towards the heart and into a central vein.

In practice only a few veins are suitable for cannulation. The femoral and other leg veins are unsatisfactory because their cannulation is associated with the risk of venous thrombosis and pulmonary embolus. The veins of the arm and the neck are preferred, and the basilic vein in the cubital fossa, the subclavian vein and the internal jugular veins may also be used.

The indications for insertion of a cannula or catheter into a central vein are:
- to measure the central venous pressure
- to permit the i.v. administration of irritant drugs
- to permit long-term venous access, e.g. parenteral nutrition
- to allow frequent blood sampling without multiple venepunctures
- to remove air from the right ventricle in case of venous air embolism

Technique for cannulation of the internal jugular vein

Essential preliminaries

Preparation of the patient
The right internal jugular vein is preferred since needling the left side may cause damage to the thoracic duct, and result in a chronic lymphatic fistula. A small support, placed between the shoulder blades, serves to extend the neck gently and accentuate the landmarks. It also causes the shoulders to fall away laterally. The usual preparations for sterile cannulation of a vessel should be made. Immediately prior to cannulation the patient should be tipped head down by 15° in order to distend the jugular vein. The head should be turned to the left in order to get the chin out of the way and to throw the sternomastoid muscle into relief.

Preparation of the equipment
You should familiarize yourself with the way in which the apparatus works, fits together and comes apart. If the patient is conscious, an intradermal wheal of local anaesthetic should be raised at the site of puncture. Anticipate and rehearse the sequence of manoeuvres to be performed. The following special items will be needed
- a suitable cannula. The ideal cannula should be of the 'cannula over needle' type. A 16 French gauge, parallel-sided, 'Teflon' cannula should be used. It is an advantage if the cannula is somewhat longer than an ordinary i.v. cannula, and those which are 3½ or 5¼ inches long are satisfactory. A complete 5 ml syringe should be attached to the cannula
- a 3-way tap and extension, or manometer tubing, for connection to the cannula so that it may be flushed with a heparin/saline solution to prevent clotting in the system
- The whole may be connected to a constantly flushing device or to a transducer system.

Determination of landmarks
There are several approaches to the internal jugular vein: the one to be described has easily palpable landmarks, which are
- the upper border of the medial half of the clavicle
- the lateral border of the sternal head of the sternomastoid muscle
- the medial border of the clavicular head of the same muscle

The triangular space formed by these boundaries should be delineated, and its apex — the point at which the two heads of the muscle diverge from each other — identified. The internal jugular vein runs beneath the skin, just medial to the lateral border of the triangle.

Insertion of the cannula

The needle and cannula are inserted under the skin at the apex of the triangle. They are then directed along the lateral border of the triangle, at an angle of 10° to the neck, whilst the plunger of the syringe is aspirated. As soon as venous blood enters it the syringe is steadied, in order to make sure that the needle tip does not slip out of the vein, and the cannula is threaded along the needle downwards into the vein (Fig. 10.20).

The needle itself should not be advanced since such movement may lacerate the vein and nearby structures. The cannula will be directed by the vein towards the superior vena cava and the heart. When it has been fully advanced the needle is withdrawn and the hub of the cannula is connected to an infusion or monitoring set. The head-down tilt is removed only after such connection is secure lest air be sucked into the vein and air embolism result. An antiseptic preparation should be applied to the puncture site which should then be kept clean with a sterile, occlusive dressing.

The patient must be observed carefully after insertion of the cannula lest unnoticed or inadvertent puncture of the pleura, or of a vessel within the thorax, leads to a pneumothorax, haemothorax or haemopericardium. If in doubt the chest should be examined and a chest radiograph performed.

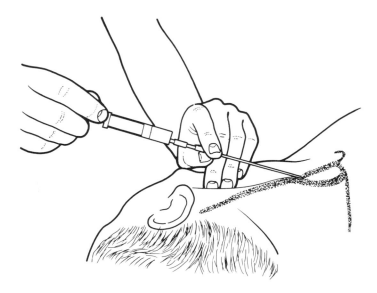

Fig. 10.20 Cannulation of the internal jugular vein.

11

Obstetric analgesia and anaesthesia
B. Morgan

- Obstetric analgesia
  - systemic analgesia
  - inhalational analgesia
  - electrical analgesia
  - conduction analgesia
- Obstetric anaesthesia
  - epidural anaesthesia
  - spinal anaesthesia
  - general anaesthesia
- Problems specific to obstetric anaesthesia
  - aorto-caval compression
  - neonatal resuscitation
- Cardiopulmonary resuscitation of the obstetric patient
- Preoperative assessment of the obstetric patient

Obstetric analgesia

The unique difficulties faced in obstetric analgesia are: firstly, the very wide range of pain states that need to be treated; secondly, the effects of such treatment on the fetus, the neonate and the labour process itself; finally, and most importantly, the side-effects of analgesia that increase maternal hazards. For instance the pregnant woman's inability to keep her gastric contents in her stomach is aggravated by systemic analgesics and so her risks during general anaesthesia are increased.

Although almost every childbirth is associated with pain, labour is not a single pain state but shows a wide variety in the severity and duration of pain. Labour ranges from the normal physiological process requiring little or no analgesic or other drugs but considerable psychological support, through to the pathological state of abnormal labour that requires conduction block for adequate analgesia and anaesthesia for some form of operative delivery.

There is considerable literature on non-pharmacological means of dealing with normal labour pain, this is often called psychoprophylaxis, but will not be dealt with in this chapter. Maternal attitudes to pain and the satisfactory experience of childbirth are crucial in the understanding of obstetric pain relief and its sensitive application. All medical staff involved in the care of pregnant women should be aware of the mother's psychological attitudes towards childbirth. Pain in labour is regarded differently to postoperative pain by mothers, as it is claimed to have long-term and far-reaching effects on her feelings of independence, self-confidence and through her the well-being of the family is influenced.

Systemic analgesia

Opiates have been widely used to treat labour pain. At the beginning of the century twilight sleep, a combination of Omnopon and Scopolamine, was used to provide analgesia and amnesia. The introduction of pethidine in 1939 was heralded as the ultimate analgesic. It was combined with the phenothiazines in the early 1960s and is still the commonest form of pain relief used in labour throughout the world.

The effectiveness of pethidine in producing pain relief in labour is poor. It has been shown to produce no better than satisfactory pain relief in 22 per cent of women. In another study pain relief was found to be poor and non-existent in over 60 per cent of women in labour.

Drug effects on the fetus and neonate are essentially no different from those on the mother. All drugs that cross the blood–brain barrier in the mother, as all analgesics must do, will also cross the placental barrier and then affect the fetal brain. The side-effects of opiates and other central-nervous-system depressants are respiratory depression, sedation or sleepiness resulting in poor muscle tone and reduction in the vigour of limb movements. Poor maintenance of body temperature, a special problem of the neonate, is aggravated. Drug metabolism is poor in the newborn therefore these effects last a much longer time than in the mother, days rather than hours. Neonatal effects of drugs can be minimized by using small doses of central sedative drugs. The fewer types of drugs used the better, however analgesics, anxiolytics, and antiemetics are often given in combination to women in labour. The effects on the neonate are of much greater concern in a sick or premature infant than they are in a healthy normal well-grown baby.

The sick fetus is usually chronically hypoxic. Further acute hypoxic episodes cause acidosis and an altered fetal circulatory pattern with compensatory increase in cerebral blood flow and reduction in flow in the descending aorta. The effect of these changes is for drugs to exert an even greater effect on such a neonate. Side-effects of systemic analgesics can be minimized in the fetus by keeping the dose small, but this reduces analgesic efficacy. It has been shown that prolonging the interval between drug administration and delivery for 2–3 hours produces more infants with cerebral depression. Drugs are given more than 4 hours before delivery to achieve minimal fetal effects but they also achieve minimal analgesia by that time. A rapid and widely used method of assessing the condition of the newborn is the Apgar score. At 1 and 5 minutes of life five aspects of the newborn are assessed: heart rate, muscle tone, respiration, responsiveness and colour; each receives a score of 0, 1 or 2, and an Apgar out of 10 (Fig. 11.1).

RESUSCITATION		Clinical scoring at 1 and 5 minutes after delivery		
TIME OF FIRST BREATH MINUTES AFTER DELIVERY		2	1	0
TIME OF FIRST CRY MINUTES AFTER DELIVERY				
MANAGEMENT (Include drugs and times)	Heart Rate	Over 100	Less than 100	Impalpable
	Respiratory Effort	Cry	Respiration alone	Absent
	Muscle Tone	Good Tone	Moderate Tone	Limp
	Reflex Irritability	Strong Withdrawal cry	Some Motion Grimace	No response
	Colour	Pink	Dark Blue	Pale
	Score at 1 min. _____ Score at 5 min. _____			

Fig. 11.1   Assessment of neonatal conditions at delivery.

Infants who are depressed by the influence of drugs will have a low Apgar score. This will not have serious consequences for the child, providing it does not subsequently become hypoxic during the early neonatal period. Apgar scores can also be reduced because of fetal hypoxia intrapartum. Therefore any infant whose mother receives systemic opiates may have two reasons for a low Apgar: central depressant drugs and hypoxia. The latter has much more serious long-term implications than the former.

Opioid effects can be antagonized by naloxone. However, the duration of action of this antagonist is much shorter than that of the opiates in the neonate. Phenothiazines have no known antagonist. Pethidine is used in preference to other opiates as it is believed to have less of a respiratory depressant effect on the infant than other opiates.

Maternal gastrointestinal side-effects of opiates are potentially the most serious. The report on confidential enquiries into maternal deaths in England and Wales 1982–84 states the 'almost universal use of opiates (pethidine) should be re-examined as its reduction would increase maternal safety'. Opioids are known to decrease the rate of gastric emptying. This has been shown indirectly by using the absorption of paracetamol as a marker. This drug taken by mouth is only absorbed into the plasma from the duodenum. Peak plasma levels in women in labour with no analgesia or with epidural analgesia occur at about 30 minutes, but following pethidine they occur at about 3 hours. This virtual cessation of gastric emptying leads to a large volume of stomach contents, from gastric secretions, which increases the danger of passive regurgitation and thus aspiration of this fluid into the lungs during general anaesthesia.

A further complication is that the lower-oesophageal sphincter tone is reduced anyway in pregnancy, leading to 70 per cent of women at or near term complaining of heartburn. Histological evidence of oesophagitis has been produced. Opiates and most anaesthetic drugs further reduce the poor lower-oesophageal tone. This further enhances the mother's inability to keep her gastric contents in her stomach and out of her oesophagus where such fluid can easily enter her lungs.

Inhalational analgesia

In the recent past a number of anaesthetic drugs that were volatile and analgesic in subanaesthetic doses were used for obstetric pain relief. The most successful of these was Trilene (trichloroethylene). However all these drugs have been abandoned as they produced considerable sedation in the mother.

Nitrous oxide and oxygen, premixed as a 50/50 combination, is at present the only inhalational analgesic in common use. It is administered by the woman herself and because the mask is self-held she cannot become unconscious. It has many advantages over pethidine; it is much more effective as an analgesic, it is more acceptable to mothers who feel they wish to be in control of their labour and analgesia, it is rapidly excreted in the expired air and has little effect on the neonate, especially as it is usually totally eliminated by the mother before the delivery. This is not the case when nitrous oxide is used during general anaesthesia for caesarean section where the possibility exists that the neonate may excrete nitrous oxide from the blood into its lungs and displace oxygen. Its major disadvantage is that many mothers dislike its central effects which come on rapidly. The technique of producing intermittent analgesia only during the contraction must be learned by the mother during labour and some seem unable to do this and thus declare the drug inefficient.

There is no time limit on the use of Entonox in labour, however it can be exhausting to use throughout a long labour and is usually started towards the latter part of the first stage. In the earlier part the woman is happy to walk about, finding the contractions easier when mobile and upright. It is especially of value in multiparous mothers whose labours are often shorter than in the primiparous.

Electrical analgesia

Transcutaneous electrical nerve stimulation (TENS) is also self-administered by the patient. It has been successfully used in many non-malignant chronic pain states. It is possible that its mechanism of action is by stimulating the large myelinated afferent fibres to reduce the nociceptive impulse conduction. Electrodes are attached to the mother's skin by adhesive tape and from a small battery-powered source, current is carried by electrical wires to electrode pads. The pads are placed over the dermatomes where pain is felt in labour; this is usually on either side of the vertebral column over the lower thoracic/lumbar area.

Success during labour is variable and depends partly on the mother's enthusiasm. It has been shown in small studies to provide good to satisfactory relief in over 80 per cent of mothers. Its role seems to be as an analgesic early in the first stage of primiparous labour; the mother can walk about while using TENS during a contraction. During normal multiparous labour it may be effective, but most drugs and techniques are declared satisfactory in these normal and usually fairly short labours.

Conduction analgesia

Epidural block via the lumbar approach is the most commonly used conduction block in obstetric patients and it has several advantages. It can produce complete analgesia and painless labour, although in practice this seldom occurs as the maintenance of the block throughout labour requires considerable attention. It is strikingly more effective than other commonly used analgesic techniques.

The details of epidural blockade are presented in Chapter 12. It is used in obstetrics to provide both analgesia during labour and anaesthesia for operative intervention. The presence of an epidural catheter means the need for general anaesthesia in a patient in labour can mostly be avoided. Epidural blockade can produce a range of blocks from the partial sensory block that is required to provide pain relief to the dense block of most sensory and motor modalities that is required for caesarean section.

Using epidural blockade for analgesia in labour requires a feeble block extending from T_{10} (dermatomal distribution at the level of the umbilicus) and later in labour down to S_5 (dermatomal distribution at the perineum and the lateral border of the foot). This type of block is best achieved with very dilute solutions of fairly large volumes of a local anaesthetic drug, most appropriately bupivacaine. The accompanying sympathetic block has the inevitable effect of causing vasodilation, so the mother usually experiences some fall in blood pressure. To minimize this fall an i.v. fluid preload of about 1000 ml of Hartmann's solution is given. The fetal heart rate is monitored as placental perfusion so fetal oxygenation is dependent on maternal blood pressure and changes may effect the fetus.

From 1972 midwives who have been instructed in the technique have been permitted to 'top-up' already existing epidural blocks to maintain analgesia for many hours. Between 1970 and 1984 there have been ten maternal deaths associated with epidurals, four of these occurred when the anaesthetist was not available, usually after a 'top-up' had been given by the midwife. In another four the patient also received a general anaesthetic or heavy sedation and died of complications of unconsciousness, although the epidural block was considered to be contributory. One patient died following what was assumed to be an i.v. injection of bupivacaine, and one sick mother with diabetes, pre-eclampsia and hydrothorax died in spite of the presence of the anaesthetist. The reports of 1973–75 and 1976–78 state that epidural analgesia is unsafe if the anaesthetist is not immediately available to attend to the patient. In the 1976–78 report the authors say that this is not the counsel of perfection; simply a recommendation to transfer the same level of care to the obstetric patient as that regarded as being essential for the surgical patient. It has been accepted by the College of Obstetricians and the College of Anaesthetists that 'a person proficient in the cardio-pulmonary resuscitation of a pregnant woman should be available within the maternity unit at all times if an epidural is in place.'

The reasons for these cautionary notes is that an epidural block may become much more extensive owing to the unwitting subarachnoid placement of the catheter, or convulsions and cardiac arrest may occur because of toxic levels of local anaesthetics.

The main disadvantage of epidural anaesthesia during labour is the effect of the block on the labour. There is insufficient evidence on this as no randomized study has ever been performed and there is little evidence that the block delays the first stage of labour but there is quite a lot of evidence that it causes delay in the second stage and is associated with a high rate of forceps delivery in primiparous women.

The effects of epidural blockade on the fetus are largely beneficial if hypotension is minimized or avoided. The fetus benefits from the reduction in maternal catecholamine levels and an epidural block can also eliminate uterine artery vasoconstriction and thus improve placental perfusion allowing the fetus to have a higher pH at delivery.

Obstetric anaesthesia

Epidural anaesthesia
Epidural blockade has become the anaesthetic of choice for caesarean section. Extending an already-existing analgesic block allows most emergency caesareans to be performed with this technique. Its advantages are numerous; the mother is awake to experience the birth of her child, her partner can be with her to give her emotional support, the risk of aspiration of gastric contents is almost eliminated, blood loss at operation is decreased, the incidence of postoperative morbidity is reduced and as has been shown in non-obstetric patients the risk of postoperative venous embolism is decreased. Pain at operation can best be avoided by ensuring a block from T_4 (nipple line) to S_5 (perineum) that is very dense with little or no sensation of cold or pinprick and dense motor blockade.

Disadvantages of the technique include the time taken to ensure an adequate block, hypotension, nausea and vomiting and pain at operation which must of course be treated.

Spinal anaesthesia
Injecting a small dose of local anaesthetic into the subarachnoid space results in an extensive and dense block that is a more effective surgical block than an epidural block. It is also of much quicker onset. However, it also causes more rapid and severe hypotension which must be anticipated and avoided by the early use of ephedrine.

The major problem of spinal anaesthesia in obstetrics is that the usual practice of having patients flat on their back to prevent too high a spread of spinal blockade must be avoided because of aorto-caval compression. This problem is usually solved by having the mother on a lateral-tilting wedge.

General anaesthesia
The hazards of general anaesthesia are increased during labour because of the mother's inability to keep her gastric contents in her stomach. In order to avoid gastric aspiration, or Mendelson's syndrome, the following technique is used: the mother is preoxygenated before induction with a sleep dose

of a rapidly-acting anaesthetic agent such as thiopentone. This is followed immediately by a full dose of suxamethonium. The application of cricoid pressure should occur as soon as possible and before the onset of unconsciousness. This manoeuvre is described in Chapter 10 and is used to compress the oesophagus thus preventing passively regurgitated material from passing up and into the lungs. Once the patient is paralysed with suxamethonium an endotracheal tube is passed, the cuff inflated and cricoid pressure released when the anaesthetist is satisfied that the trachea and not the oesophagus has been intubated. Long-acting muscle relaxants can then be given.

During the anaesthesia, unconsciousness must be ensured even though this may cause the baby to be sedated at delivery. Aorto-caval compression must be avoided by providing a 15° lateral tilt. Hyperventilation with resultant hypocarbia is undesirable. Lack of concern for these details reduces placental perfusion and thereby affects fetal oxygenation. The presence of a paediatrician is essential for delivery of an infant by caesarian section under general anaesthesia as these neonates often need resuscitation at a time when the anaesthetist must attend to the mother. The time interval from induction of anaesthesia to delivery and from uterine incision to delivery need to be kept to a minimum if the neonatal condition is to be optimal. Some reduction in the placental perfusion of healthy infants is probably inconsequential but may add to the hypoxia of the fetus already at risk. After the operation is complete the mother should be turned on to her side before she is extubated as inhalation may occur postoperatively before she has fully regained consciousness and before the trachea and larynx are restored to normal sensory levels.

The major use of general anaesthesia for caesarean section is when unexpected fetal distress occurs and delivery must be very speedy. It is not only the most rapid but also the most certain anaesthetic technique available. It is favoured when the mother has a systemic condition that makes her unlikely to cope with a major conduction block such as that required for caesarean section, and where massive blood loss is expected as for instance in placenta accreta. Overall the use of general anaesthesia in obstetrics is declining.

Problems specific to obstetric anaesthesia

Aorto-caval compression
A special problem in the obstetric patient is the compression of the mother's vena cava and aorta by the gravid uterus. This can occur from the 16th week of pregnancy and is an increasing problem until delivery. It is magnified in multiple pregnancy or with abnormal presentations such as a transverse lie. In the acute form of this syndrome the maternal venous return is obstructed causing the mother to complain of feeling faint and to show signs of hypotension. When conscious the mother cures the problem by moving her position. The syndrome has, however, some chronic element as most commonly during pregnancy the venous tone in the feet is raised and compensatory venodilation of the azygous system occurs.

The other aspect is aortic compression where, although there are no maternal symptoms and very few signs, the fetal placental flow can be seriously compromised. There are maternal signs of reduced urine output and altered blood pressure between arm and leg, i.e. above and below the block. Avoiding aorto-caval compression is very important during all forms of anaesthesia undertaken during pregnancy. Lateral tilting of the mother by placing a 15° wedge under her right hip can be an adequate prophylactic measure for a short period, such as at caesarean section or forceps delivery, but ideally at all times the mother should lie in the full left or right lateral position only being turned onto the lateral wedge at the last possible moment.

Neonatal resuscitation

The flow chart in Fig. 11.2 has been published by the Royal College of Obstetricians and Gynaecologists, to ensure that all those present at a delivery can immediately undertake basic resuscitative measures without waiting for a more experienced person to arrive. This chart is accompanied by handbooks on basic and advanced life-support techniques.

Essentially, cardiopulmonary resuscitation of the neonate is no different to that of an adult but the assessment of who to resuscitate, when, and what the extent of the resuscitation should be, requires skill. It is those infants that are unable to breathe and have a slow or no heartbeat that require immediate ventilation and cardiac massage. Other less-depressed infants may require added oxygen and nasopharyngeal suction to improve their oxygen saturations.

Cardiopulmonary resuscitation of the obstetric patient

The pregnant woman near term has a poor outcome with conventional cardiopulmonary resuscitation. The major reason for this is the possible caval compression that prevents venous return to the heart. Thus the principles of cardiopulmonary resuscitation as described in Chapter 14 must include the additional factor of avoidance of caval occlusion. This is best done by immediate delivery of the fetus, if possible. This may offer the additional benefit of saving the child's life even if the mother is not successfully resuscitated.

If immediate delivery is not possible the uterus must be lifted off the maternal great vessels either manually by placing both hands under the uterus and lifting it towards the ceiling, or by placing the mother on a 15° hard wedge under the right side of her body. This frees the vena cava from uterine pressure for a short period.

Midwives and medical personnel on the labour ward need constant updating to maintain cardiopulmonary resuscitation skills. As they are so seldom required in practice, teaching has to be done on simulators, about every 4–5 months (Chapter 14).

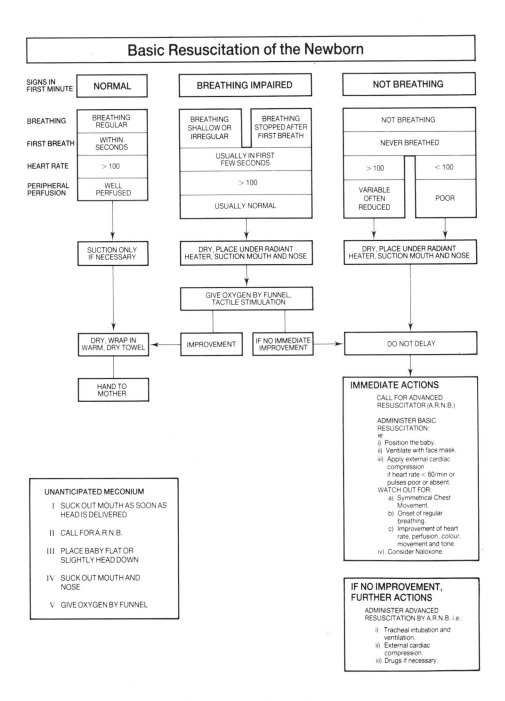

Fig. 11.2 Basic resuscitation of the newborn.
(ARNB = Advanced Resuscitation of the newborn)

Preoperative assessment of the obstetric patient

It is all too easy to neglect basic anaesthetic tenets in the busy active labour ward. However, there is some evidence that indicates that the pregnant woman, especially when in labour, is at greater risk of anaesthesia than the same young woman would be if not pregnant. Anaesthesia, being a greater hazard than usual, requires a more meticulous assessment of the mother preoperatively. This assessment includes her ability to flex and extend her neck, open her mouth and an assessment of the ease of intubation by looking into the back of her throat while she is extending her tongue without phonating. Sight of the faucial pillars, the soft palate and uvula indicates that endotracheal intubation will be possible but sight of the hard palate only indicates that intubation may be difficult or impossible.

One of the reasons for encouraging delivery in hospital is because of immediate access to anaesthesia and operative delivery in the event of fetal hypoxia. This, however, does not imply that every emergency caesarean section is unexpected and of great urgency. In the overwhelming number of cases there is ample time for the woman to be assessed by the anaesthetist, especially as these patients are often obese and are subject to the usual range of medical conditions, like any other patient having emergency surgery. Problems of a full stomach are common to all patients undergoing emergency surgery, but the problem is especially increased in pregnancy by the poor lower-oesophageal sphincter tone.

Premedication for caesarean section avoids the use of sedatives, tranquillizers or opiates and concentrates on improving the gastric condition. Ranitidine 150 mg orally with metoclopromide 10 mg will reduce the volume of gastric contents and increase the pH of the secretions. For planned procedures these can be given the night before and 2 hours preoperatively. For emergency surgery they should be given i.m. as soon as it seems likely that operative delivery may occur, or when blood is taken for cross-matching. This is the time when the anaesthetist should be called to see the woman as possibly requiring surgery.

Anaesthetic staffing of labour wards is often difficult to maintain to the desired standard of an immediately-available anaesthetist of more than one year's experience of anaesthesia. The reason why this stipulated minimum is unobtainable is the very large numbers of obstetric units delivering less than 2000 infants a year. This sort of obstetric provision is wasteful of anaesthetic manpower and can only be maintained with a substandard anaesthetic service in the majority of obstetric units.

Monitoring of mother and fetus during all anaesthetics is as important as monitoring patients having non-obstetric surgery. Whether general, epidural or spinal anaesthesia is being used a non-invasive automatic blood pressure monitor, an ECG and a pulse oximeter should be used during IPPV. An end-tidal CO_2 monitor is essential (Chapter 5). The fetus should be monitored during the whole anaesthetic procedure until the start of surgery. Fetal monitoring should be by continuous cardiotocograph or by heart-rate recording. When possible this should be by fetal-scalp electrode but if not with an external monitor placed on the mother's abdomen. Persistent fetal bradycardia requires an immediate response; turning the mother on her side, treating her hypotension, increasing her inspired oxygen and, if necessary, stopping hypertonic uterine contractions with i.v. salbutamol while preparing for delivery.

Postoperative care of the obstetric patient has exactly the same requirements as postoperative care for any surgical patient: a specific recovery ward, with a dedicated trained recovery nurse who is able to monitor the patient's vital signs and so exclude respiratory obstruction and blood loss and who can treat postoperative pain. All postpartum mothers must be watched for blood loss. The uterine blood flow is 500 ml/min and blood loss from the placental site can be very rapid if the postpartum uterus is insufficiently contracted. Blood loss when combined with an extensive conduction block is especially dangerous as the extensive sympathetic block eliminates all or most cardiovascular compensatory mechanisms, such as increasing pulse rate and vasoconstriction.

Anaesthetic care of the obstetric patient is demanding in terms of the hours and the increased risk that the patients present. However it is a rewarding aspect of anaesthesia both in terms of an acute pain-relief service and because of the successful outcome in most patients.

Further reading

Atlay R D, Gillison E W, Horton A C. A fresh look at pregnancy heartburn. *Journal of Obstetrics & Gynaecology British Commonwealth*, 1973; **80**: 63–6.

General professional training guide faculty of anaesthetists. *Royal College of Surgeons of England*, 1987.

Nimmo W A S, Wilson J, Prescott L F. Narcotic analgesics and delayed gastric emptying during labour. *Lancet* 1975; **1**: 890–3.

Report on confidential enquiries into maternal deaths in England and Wales 1970–72. London: HMSO, 1975.

Report on confidential enquiries into maternal deaths in England and Wales 1973–75. London: HMSO, 1979.

Report on confidential enquiries into maternal deaths in England and Wales 1976–78. London: HMSO, 1982.

Report on confidential enquiries into maternal deaths in England and Wales 1982–84. London: HMSO, 1989.

12

Local anaesthesia and analgesia
A.P. Rubin

- History
- Pharmacology
    - classification
- Anatomical sites
    - cutaneous anaesthesia
    - mucosal anaesthesia
    - injected local anaesthesia
- General principles
- Drugs and doses
    - the drug
    - concentration
    - volume
    - vasoconstrictors
- Complications and reactions to local anaesthetics
    - vasovagal
    - allergy
    - local toxicity
    - systemic toxicity
    - treatment of toxicity

History

The first local anaesthetic to be used clinically was cocaine, an alkaloid derived from the leaves of the *Erythroxylon coca* plant. The distinguished Viennese psychologist Sigmund Freud was aware of many of the properties of cocaine and used his friendship with a Viennese ophthalmologist, Carl Koller, to apply cocaine to the conjunctiva in 1884. Even though this was more than 100 years ago, experiments were conducted firstly on animals then on themselves and their colleagues before a clinical trial was set up. The first injection of local anaesthetic occurred in the same year and is usually credited to William Halsted, a New York surgeon. In the following years spinal and epidural anaesthesia were also discovered. The neurotoxicity, systemic toxicity and addiction potential of cocaine was recognized and a search for newer local anaesthetics began. Procaine was introduced in 1905 but had a short duration, caused systemic toxicity and occasional allergic reactions.

The breakthrough in local anaesthetic research occurred in Sweden between 1940 and 1960 with the discovery of the amino-amide drugs such as lignocaine, prilocaine and bupivacaine. These were more stable, had longer durations and had much less allergic potential. The toxicity problems remain and are a major limiting factor in the use of these agents.

Pharmacology

All local anaesthetics have the same three essential functional units: a hydrophilic chain joined to a lipophilic portion by an ester or amide linkage (Fig. 12.1).

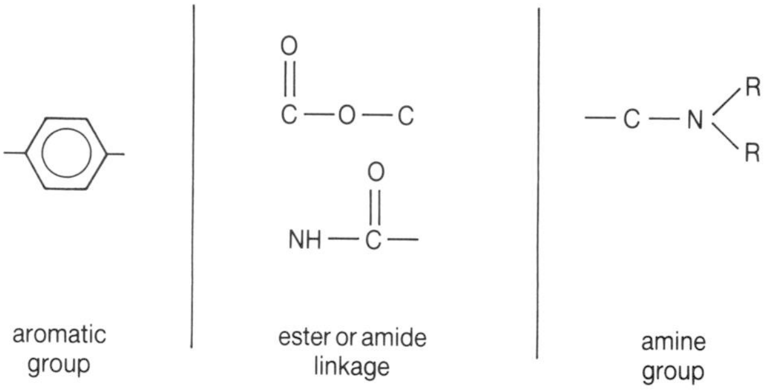

aromatic group	ester or amide linkage	amine group

Fig. 12.1   The three essential functional units of a local anaesthetic.

Local anaesthetics are usually in solution as the hydrochloride salts. They are weak bases and exist in equilibrium between a lipid-soluble, anionic uncharged form and a water-soluble cationic form. The pH of the commonly-used amide local anaesthetics is in the range 4.1–6.5.

The local anaesthetic has to penetrate the nerve fibre and the cationic form then blocks the sodium channels to prevent influx of sodium. This results in the blocking of membrane depolarization. The blockade is concentration-dependent and ends when the concentration falls below a critical minimal level. Thus local anaesthetics cause temporary blockade of nerve conduction and are applied locally close to the nerve.

Classification

Local anaesthetics may be classified in various ways:

Duration of action

Local anaesthetics may last less than 1 hour, 1 to 2 hours, or greater than 2 hours and typical drugs in each group would be procaine, lignocaine and bupivacaine respectively.

Chemical formula

They are either amino-esters or amino-amides. The amino-esters are easily destroyed in the body by pseudocholinesterase, whereas the amino-amides require complex metabolic pathways in the liver. Allergic reactions are relatively common to the amino-esters and almost unknown with the amino-amide group.

Effect on blood vessels

Most local anaesthetics are vasodilators with the exception of cocaine and to a small extent bupivacaine. Vasoconstrictor drugs, and in particular adrenaline, may be added to local anaesthetics to reduce absorption. This results in more effective and long-lasting anaesthesia and a reduction in the rate of rise and peak blood levels. Local anaesthetic agents are unusual in that they are placed at specific anatomical sites. Absorption into the blood stream removes them from the site of action, reduces local anaesthetic action and may cause systemic toxicity.

This can be compared with most other drugs such as aspirin, morphine or thiopentone which are given by standard routes of administration with the intention of absorption into the blood stream and carriage to distant sites of action.

Anatomical sites

Local anaesthetic administration may be divided into cutaneous, mucosal or by injection.

Cutaneous anaesthesia

There is a preparation called EMLA (eutectic mixture of local anaesthetics) cream which is a white cream containing a mixture of lignocaine and prilocaine in a eutectic mixture as an oil–water emulsion. A thick layer of cream is applied to the skin at least 60 minutes before the painful procedure and covered with an occlusive impermeable dressing. It is particularly useful in children prior to injection, blood sampling or the insertion of i.v. infusions.

Mucosal anaesthesia

Mucosal anaesthesia is also called surface or topical anaesthesia. A local anaesthetic may be instilled into the conjunctival sac to allow minor procedures on the surface of the eye such as the removal of foreign bodies or treatment of conjunctival lesions. The nose, mouth, pharynx, larynx and trachea are all amenable to the application of local anaesthetics, allowing procedures to be carried out on the nasal, oral, or pharyngeal mucosae, or allowing the painless passage of endotracheal tubes, bronchoscopes or oesophagogastroduodenoscopes. The agent may be instilled under direct vision using a nasal speculum, tongue depressor or laryngoscope. It also may be injected via the injection port of a fibreoptic laryngoscope or bronchoscope, or directly into the trachea through the cricothyroid membrane below the level of the larynx. The most commonly used solution for mucosal anaesthesia is 4 per cent lignocaine and the total dosage should be limited to 5 ml because local anaesthetic will be absorbed through the mucous membrane.

Injected local anaesthesia

Anatomical considerations are the limiting factor for injected local anaesthesia. Most patients do not like multiple injections and therefore sites are sought where a large number of nerves can be reached by a single injection. The subarachnoid and epidural spaces are the most central sites and a single injection can produce bilateral anaesthesia of large parts of the body.

Spinal anaesthesia

The spinal anaesthetic is an injection into the cerebrospinal fluid within the subarachnoid space, from here the local anaesthetic can fill the whole space and even, if in excess, enter the brain. A lumbar puncture is performed: the flow of cerebrospinal fluid indicates that the subarachnoid space has been entered and is thus a very definite end point. The nerve roots in the subarachnoid space are relatively bare having not acquired the dural or the myelin sheaths. They are thus easy to block and small volumes of local anaesthetic in the range of 2–4 ml are sufficient to produce profound sensory and motor block.

There is also block of the sympathetic outflow which causes vasodilatation and is likely to result in a fall in blood pressure. This may require i.v. fluids or vasopressor drugs such as ephedrine for its correction. The spinal solution may be made hyperbaric (heavier than the cerebrospinal fluid) by the addition of glucose. This allows for more accurate control of the level of anaesthesia by appropriately posturing the patient. The major disadvantage of spinal anaesthesia is the post-lumbar-puncture headache which is associated with leakage of cerebrospinal fluid, low pressure and dragging on the cranial meninges and venous sinuses. The headache is typical being occipital and made worse by sitting or standing and relieved by lying flat. It is a severe, incapacitating and very distressing headache which usually resolves spontaneously in a few days but may be cured more rapidly by the epidural injection of 10–15 ml of the patient's own blood. This acts as a patch, sealing off the dural hole and preventing further leakage of cerebrospinal fluid.

Epidural anaesthesia

In epidural anaesthesia the local anaesthetic is injected into the epidural (extradural) space which is the space between the dura and the bones of the vertebral canal. The epidural space is fat-filled and contains the paired nerve roots and the vertebral venous plexus. The epidural space is closed cranially so the local anaesthetic cannot directly enter the brain.

An epidural block is technically more difficult than a spinal block, the end point being the change in resistance to the passage of the needle from the ligamentum flavum to the epidural space. There are various methods of detecting this loss of resistance, either pressure on a syringe containing air or saline, or various gadgets which demonstrate the low pressure within the epidural space. A much larger needle is used but it is feasible to insert a fine catheter through the epidural needle which may remain in the epidural space for as long as necessary. Thus prolonged pain relief may be provided for the relief of labour pain, postoperative pain, posttraumatic pain and some forms of chronic pain.

While the spinal is almost always done in the lower lumbar region to avoid the risk of damage to the spinal cord which ends at the first lumbar vertebra, the epidural can be done at any level and segmental blocks can be achieved. A good example is the use of an epidural segmental block between the dermatomes of T_4–T_{12} to provide postoperative analgesia for an upper abdominal incision without causing leg weakness or interference with bladder function.

The dose of local anaesthetic required for an epidural is around ten times larger than for a spinal. This is due to several factors. Some of the local anaesthetic leaves the epidural space through the intervertebral foramina. Large amounts are absorbed by the vertebral venous plexus and the nerve roots in the epidural space have already acquired a thick dural covering. The exact site of action of epidural anaesthesia is not totally understood and it may be that the local anaesthetic has to penetrate through the dura into the subarachnoid space which would also cause a decrease in effectiveness.

Paravertebral and intercostal blocks

Local anaesthetic can be injected just outside the vertebral canal, as in the paravertebral block, or in an intercostal space where the intercostal nerve lies under the rib. Both these injections are effective but each injection can only be guaranteed to block a single nerve on one side so that multiple injections are required frequently. However, intercostal blocks with about 3–5 ml of local anaesthetic for each nerve are often used as a method of postoperative and posttraumatic pain relief.

Plexus blocks

In certain parts of the body, nerves are grouped together to form a plexus. If local anaesthetic can be applied to the plexus then several nerves can be blocked at the same time. The best example is the brachial plexus block but there are also techniques for blocking the lumbosacral plexus. With these techniques it should be possible to anaesthetize most of an extremity with a single injection of a large volume of agent.

The brachial plexus may be blocked at the level of the roots either as they emerge from the 5th cervical to 1st thoracic intervertebral foramina (interscalene approach), or as the plexus crosses the first rib (supraclavicular approach) or where the cords of the plexus are grouped together around the axillary artery (axillary approach). The lumbosacral plexus may be blocked in the psoas compartment by a posterior approach through the back or via the femoral nerve sheath in the groin. A sufficient volume will block the femoral, obturator and lateral cutaneous nerve of the thigh, but for full anaesthesia of the lower limb the sciatic nerve must be blocked separately. All these approaches require large volumes of local anaesthetic which are close to toxic doses.

Peripheral nerve blocks

In many areas single nerves may be blocked to produce anaesthesia in the area of their distribution. Good examples are the individual nerves at the elbow, wrist or ankle. The pudendal nerves may be blocked to produce anaesthesia of the perineum for operative vaginal delivery.

Digital nerve blocks
An injection on either side at the base of a finger or toe will anaesthetize the digit. The nerves are close to arteries which are effectively end-arteries, and vasoconstrictors should not be used as ischaemia might result.

Head and neck blocks
Head and neck blocks by injection are not very often used, with the exception of blocks of the eye and teeth. Many eye operations can be done by the injection of local anaesthetic around the globe into the orbit. This results in anaesthesia and immobility of the eyeball and is particularly appropriate for cataract surgery. Blocks are performed frequently for dental work and are mostly carried out by dentists.

Infiltration anaesthesia

Local anaesthetic may be injected subcutaneously to produce anaesthesia of small areas for the performance of painful procedures such as i.v. infusion, paracentesis of the pleural or peritoneal cavities, lumbar punctures or for the suturing of lacerations or tears.

Autonomic block

The autonomic nervous system also plays a part in pain, particularly that arising from visceral structures. Commonly used autonomic blocks include those of the stellate ganglion which innervates the vasculature of the head, neck and upper limb, the coeliac plexus which innervates the upper abdominal contents and the lumbar sympathetic chain which innervates the vasculature of the lower limb.

These blocks are often used for ischaemic conditions and in the management of cancer pain. Local anaesthetic block, when successful, may be followed by permanent destruction of these nervous tissues with neurolytic agents such as phenol or alcohol.

Intravenous regional anaesthesia (Bier's block)

In this unusual technique a limb with a cannulated vein is exsanguinated and isolated from the general circulation by a tourniquet cuff. Up to 40 ml of a dilute local anaesthetic, such as 0.5–1 per cent prilocaine, is injected intravenously and it spreads retrogradely into the tissues producing good anaesthesia of the limb. The safety of the technique depends on using a low-toxicity local anaesthetic, keeping within a safe dose, and ensuring that the tourniquet cuff remains inflated for at least 20 minutes so that large amounts of local anaesthetic do not suddenly enter the blood stream. Bupivacaine should **not** be used because of the risk of cardiac toxicity should the tourniquet become accidentally deflated.

General principles

Local anaesthetics should not be injected unless there are facilities for resuscitation of the patient in the event of systemic toxicity. The ability to ventilate the lungs with oxygen, to intubate the patient and to treat the potential central nervous system and cardiovascular system complications must be available.

Intravenous access must be ensured whenever more than minimal doses of local anaesthetic are administered and recommended doses must not be exceeded.

Injection must always be preceded by careful aspiration to detect an intravascular placement. It should also be slow with careful observation of the patient to detect symptoms or signs of reaction. Wherever possible a second doctor should administer the local anaesthetic and observe and monitor the patient from the point of view of both psychological well-being and physical state and to detect and treat any side-effects.

Drugs and doses

Various factors have to be taken into account when deciding on the choice of local anaesthetic to inject. These include
- the drug
- the concentration
- the volume
- the need to add a vasoconstrictor

The drug
There are a large number of agents available but the most commonly used are lignocaine, prilocaine and bupivacaine. Lignocaine or prilocaine are chosen when a short or moderate duration of block is required, while bupivacaine is preferred for longer duration as in the control of post-operative, post-traumatic or labour pain.

Cocaine

Cocaine is still used, not so much as a local anaesthetic but on account of its vasoconstrictor properties. It is applied as a 4 to 25 per cent preparation in the nose or nasopharynx. Not more than 200 mg should be administered.

Lignocaine

Lignocaine is the standard local anaesthetic and all others are compared with it. In common with other local anaesthetics there is a rather slow onset time and a slight unpredictability of anaesthetic effect. Unless adrenaline is added it also has a rather short duration of less than 1 hour. However, allergic reactions are very rare. It is available in a wide range of concentrations from 0.5 to 4 per cent, and not more than 3 mg/kg of lignocaine should be administered. If adrenaline is added, up to 8 mg/kg may be used (Table 12.1). Its toxicity is very well understood, particularly since it has been used as an antiarrhythmic by continuous i.v. infusion.

Table 12.1   Maximum doses of local anaesthetics (mg/kg)

	Plain	With adrenaline
Lignocaine	4	8
Prilocaine	7	—
Bupivacaine	2	2.5

Prilocaine

Prilocaine is an interesting amide which is the most rapidly metabolized of the agents used and thus has the lowest toxicity potential. It is therefore the safest local anaesthetic when large volumes are required or in i.v. regional anaesthesia. The recommended maximum dose is 7 mg/kg prilocaine (Table 12.1). Clinically it is very similar to lignocaine but the addition of a vasoconstrictor is unnecessary. It has one unique metabolite, orthotoluidine, and in large amounts this can lead to methaemoglobinaemia and hypoxia. This only occurs in high doses, e.g. 500–600 mg, and may rapidly be reversed with 1 mg/kg methylene blue intravenously.

Bupivacaine

Bupivacaine has increased lipid solubility and protein binding compared with lignocaine and this leads to increased duration of action. It has low placental transfer and tends to produce more sensory than motor block so it is very suitable for use in obstetrics. However it has a slower onset than lignocaine.

Adrenaline is sometimes added as it can decrease the absorption and increase the quality of blockade. However bupivacaine is a particularly toxic local anaesthetic and must be used with great caution. Not more than 2 mg/kg may be used (Table 12.1).

Concentration

The weakest concentration of drug that will reliably produce effective blockade should be used to reduce the risks of toxicity. Nerve fibres vary in diameter and the larger nerves need higher concentrations to be blocked than the smaller. The smallest nerves subserve pain and temperature and some autonomic functions; the intermediate subserve touch, pressure and vibration, and the largest nerves subserve motor function and proprioception (Table 12.2).

Thus the higher concentrations, such as 2 per cent lignocaine, are only required if full surgical anaesthesia and motor blockade are required. For most purposes an intermediate concentration, such as 1 per cent lignocaine, is sufficient to produce good sensory block.

Table 12.2   The function and diameter of the different nerve fibres

Fibre type	Diameter (μm)	Function
A α	12–20	motor, proprioception
β	5–12	touch, pressure
γ	3–6	motor to spindles
δ	2–5	pain, temperature, touch
B	<3	preganglionic autonomic
C	0.2–1.4	pain, postganglionic autonomic

Volume

The dose of local anaesthetic is made up of the concentration multiplied by the volume, and thus the smallest volume to produce effective anaesthesia should also be used. 10 ml of a 1 per cent solution is 100 mg of drug, and it is safest to think of the milligram dose to be administered. The volume required will obviously depend on the extent of anaesthesia sought, varying from less than 1 ml for the skin up to 50 ml for complex plexus and multiple peripheral-nerve blocks.

Vasoconstrictors

A vasoconstrictor such as adrenaline is very commonly added to lignocaine to improve the onset time, intensity and duration of anaesthesia. It will also retard the absorption of the local anaesthetic and thus help to reduce the risks of systemic toxicity. However, there are contraindications to the use of adrenaline particularly in situations where there are end arteries, as in the digits. If the peripheral circulation is compromised by disease and/or patients have cardiovascular problems, adrenaline should be used with caution.

Adrenaline may induce a tachycardia which will be dangerous in fixed cardiac-output states such as aortic stenosis, constrictive pericarditis and severe mitral stenosis. It should be used in the minimal concentration that will achieve local vasoconstriction and this concentration is 5 μg/ml commonly described as 'one in two hundred thousand'.

It may be made up from the 1 mg (contained in 1 ml, i.e. '1 in 1000') ampoule of adrenaline diluted 200 times with normal saline, but it is very much safer to use commercially available solutions where the adrenaline has been added by the manufacturer and where the label clearly states the concentration. As with local anaesthetics care must be taken to see that the solution is not injected intravenously. The total dose of adrenaline should be limited to 0.25 mg, i.e. 50 ml of solution.

Complications and reactions to local anaesthetics

Vasovagal

It is quite common for patients to suffer a vasovagal faint at the thought, sight or sensation of a local anaesthetic injection. Fainting is particularly common with injections in the head and neck region and when the patient is in the sitting position. Stopping the procedure and placing the patient supine with the legs elevated will rapidly resolve the problem.

Allergy

Allergy is mainly a problem with ester local anaesthetics although occasionally it may occur to the preservative methylparaben included in multi-dose vials of some amides. Patients claiming a history of allergy to local anaesthetics may be skin tested if a local anaesthetic is indicated.

Local toxicity

Local anaesthetic injections may cause direct trauma to nerves with temporary or even permanent damage. Great care must be taken to see that the local anaesthetic injection is not causing paraesthesia in the distribution of a nerve, or pain during the injection. If either of these occur the needle must be repositioned before continuing the injection.

Systemic toxicity

It must be stressed again that the intention is to place the anaesthetic locally and to minimize absorption into the blood stream. High blood concentrations of local anaesthetic or vasoconstrictor may occur due to accidental intravenous injection or due to an overdose of drug being placed in the tissues. Thus all local anaesthetic administrations should be of a safe calculated dose.

Aspiration must proceed injection and the rate of injection should be as slow as possible so that even if it is going intravascularly the rate of rise of blood levels of the drug will be slow. Toxicity to accidental intravascular injection will be very rapid whereas toxicity associated with an overdose injected into the tissues may well not occur for up to 20–30 minutes after injection.

Symptoms and signs

The toxic effects of a local anaesthetic include sedation, perioral and tongue numbness, lightheadedness, tinnitus and visual disturbances followed by anxiety, restlessness, muscular twitching and ultimately grand mal seizures and unconsciousness (Fig. 12.2). During this sequence progressive cardiovascular depression also occurs. At low blood concentrations lignocaine is an effective antiarrhythmic. However, it progressively depresses pulse rate and cardiac output, often hypoxia, acidosis or hyperkalaemia follow and serious arrythmias or cardiac arrest may occur.

Bupivacaine binds firmly to the myocardium, and may produce serious and prolonged ventricular arrhythmias such as extrasystoles, tachycardia and fibrillation. These may be very refractory to treatment.

Treatment of toxicity

The treatment of toxicity involves immediate cessation of the injection, administration of oxygen, maintenance of the airway and artificial ventilation. Twitching or grand mal convulsions may be terminated by the i.v. administration of diazepam 0.1mg/kg or thiopentone 1–3mg/kg. The

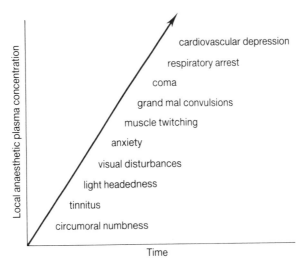

Fig. 12.2 Toxicity of local anaesthetics

presence of someone able to maintain the airway and ventilation is essential. The cardiovascular toxicity may require the use of specific inotropes or antiarrhythmic agents.

Local anaesthetics continue to be widely used and are of great benefit to patients in a large number of clinical situations. However they are dangerous drugs whose pharmacology and toxicity must be understood by all practitioners who use them so that serious or fatal consequences may be prevented.

Further reading

Scott D B. *Introduction to Regional Anaesthesia*. Appleton and Lange/medi globe, Connecticut, 1990.

Wildsmith J A W, Armitage E N. *Principles and practice of regional anaesthesia*. London: Churchill Livingstone, 1987.

13

Paediatric anaesthesia
K.J. Wark

- Psychological aspects
    age and personality of the child
    proposed operation
    parental response
    staff response
- Anatomy and physiology
    cardiorespiratory anatomy and physiology
    haematology
    central nervous system
    temperature regulation
    body fluids
- Preoperative visit
    premedication
- Apparatus
    facemasks
    laryngoscopes and endotracheal tubes
    intravenous cannulae
    anaesthetic breathing systems
    lung ventilators
- Monitoring during anaesthesia
- Anaesthetic management
    induction
    maintenance
- Fluid management
    preoperative dehydration
    maintenance requirements
    surgical losses
    body temperature
    postoperative
- Special problems with neonates
    surgical emergencies
- Postoperative analgesia
    choice of technique

Infants, particularly neonates and especially the premature, present special problems for the anaesthetist; they have physiological, anatomical and psychological problems which are quite different from adults. There are problems associated with their size and the immaturity of their systems and they cannot be considered as just small adults.

The paediatric anaesthetist must have the ability to understand and communicate with children of all ages; as well, meticulous attention to the smallest detail of anaesthetic technique is imperative.

Psychological aspects

The psychological impact of the anaesthetic, particularly the induction, may overshadow all other hospital experiences. Psychological preparation is probably more important for children than drug premedication before anaesthesia. The child needs to be given a careful explanation, not talked down to, in the presence of a parent. The anaesthetist needs to be particularly patient as many explanations need to be repeated if anxious parents 'block' prior information.

The child's reaction to hospital depends on:
- age and personality of the child
- operation to be performed
- parental response
- hospital and staff response.

Age and personality of the child

Depending on the child's age, hospitalization may have profound emotional consequences. Even in the first few weeks of life, the mother and baby 'bonding' may fail if they are separated for prolonged periods. Up to 4 years, children are particularly vulnerable to separation anxieties, believing that they are being punished. They can easily misunderstand the treatment and the reasons for it. Post-hospital regression in behaviour patterns is most common in this age group. The older child will have more understanding but may be more obviously anxious. An apparent air of bravado may cover some very basic fears. Children from unstable home situations are likely to be less able to cope. Also, children who have had many previous anaesthetics will need to be handled very carefully.

Proposed operation

The degree of anxiety is usually quite naturally related to the nature of the procedure. If it is an emergency procedure, then there will have been little time for preparation or discussion so child and family will be more stressed. Day-case surgery is likely to be less stressful as child and parent will be separated for only a short time.

Parental response

Hopefully, patients will have prepared their children for their stay in hospital. Unfortunately, quite often a child's fear and anxiety are a direct expression of the parents'. Parents are usually allowed to accompany their child to the anaesthetic room but it may be a frightening experience for them.

Staff response

Children are better treated in properly designated paediatric wards and theatres, where the staff are alert to their problems. A child can be prepared for the operation by preadmission visits, videos and picture books. A long trip to theatre, crowded lifts, a long wait outside theatres, personnel who are not 'child orientated' clattering round will all create further anxiety and tension. Familiarity and trust in the hospital are the main secret involved. The child should be allowed to bring to the theatre his favourite toy or other object that provides a sense of security.

Anatomy and physiology

The major differences between children and adults are greatest in the neonatal period. These differences are important for anaesthetists to understand.

Veins are much smaller and after 6 months are covered in a layer of subcutaneous fat. The common sites used are the dorsum of the hand or foot. Scalp veins or anterior-wrist veins are also used. The internal airway may be difficult to maintain and to intubate because of the following differences (Fig. 13.1).

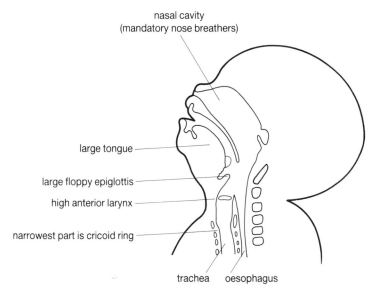

Fig. 13.1 Child's respiratory anatomy emphasizing the anatomical differences from adults.

- large floppy head and short neck
- small mouth with large tongue
- larynx is higher and more anterior (opposite C_3 rather than C_6 as in adults)

- epiglottis is large, floppy and 'V' shaped
- the narrowest part of the larynx is the cricoid ring
- trachea is short (4 cm in newborn and 8 cm at 18 months)
- infants of less than 6 months are mandatory nose breathers

Cardiorespiratory anatomy and physiology

- respiratory rate is much faster, 30–40 per min (compared to 12 per min for adults), but tidal volume at 7 ml/kg is relatively the same (Table 13.1)

Table 13.1   Normal ventilation

	Infant	Adult
respiratory frequency (breaths/min)	30–40	12
tidal volume (ml/kg)	7	7
O_2 consumption (ml/kg per min)	7	3.3

- neonatal respiration relies on diaphragmatic movement. Therefore, respiratory failure may develop easily with abdominal distension
- the small airways contribute a large proportion of the total airway resistance
- small-airway closure (closing volume) occurs within tidal volume range for children less than 6 years
- work of breathing is higher in neonates than adults relative to the O_2 consumption (Table 13.1)
- basal metabolic rate is twice that of adults, but the lung surface area/kg is almost the same, so a baby has less reserve to meet any increase in demand

   At birth the heart rate is 130–160/minute, and at the age of 5 the heart rate is 100/minute. Also neonates have a lower blood pressure than older children (Table 13.2).

Table 13.2   Normal values

Age	Heart rate (beats/min)	Blood pressure (systolic/diastolic) (mmHg)	Respiratory rate (breaths/min)	Blood volume (ml/kg)
newborn	120	70/45	30–40	85
2 years	110	80/60	20–30	80
6 years	100	90/60	15–20	80
12 years	80	110/65	12–15	70

The fetus has very little capacity to alter stroke volume because of the immature myocardium so relies on altering the rate. Changes in cardiac output reflect changes in the rate. Hypoxia will produce bradycardia or a fall in cardiac output, or both.

At birth, when ventilation starts, the pulmonary vascular resistance decreases markedly, with relaxation of the pulmonary vascular tone following the rise in arterial Po_2. The left atrial pressures rise above the right atrial pressures and close the atrial septum over the foramen ovale. Normally, the ductus arteriosis closes by 15 hours.

If a neonate becomes hypoxaemic the circulation will revert to a fetal pattern. An increase in pulmonary vascular resistance occurs, with reduced blood flow to the lungs creating further hypoxaemia so the duct may re-open. Transitional fetal circulation may occur with Respiratory Distress Syndrome (RDS) or congenital diaphragmatic hernia.

Haematology

Haemoglobin (Hb)

At birth the haemoglobin concentration is usually 17 gm/dl. Thereafter, it declines progressively — the physiological anaemia of infancy. The haemoglobin concentration will have fallen to 11 gm/dl by 6 weeks. This reduction is even more marked in premature infants and the average value at 6 weeks is 8 gm/dl, it is influenced by the nutritional status of the baby, especially levels of vitamin E, folic acid and iron.

Fetal haemoglobin (HbF) accounts for 60 per cent of all haemoglobin production at birth and is gradually replaced by adult haemoglobin so that by 3 months there is only 5 per cent HbF produced. Fetal haemoglobin confers protection for the baby under conditions of relative hypoxia. It promotes the transport of oxygen from the maternal to fetal circulation in the placenta. It shifts the oxygen dissociation curve to the left so that neonatal blood has an oxygen-carrying capacity at least 1.25 times that of the adult.

Blood volume

Normally 80–85 ml/kg body weight but may be 100 ml/kg in the premature baby (Table 13.2).

Coagulation

The infant is more at risk from bleeding compared to adults because
- platelet function is reduced
- reduced plasma coagulation factors. Vitamin K dependent factors (II, VII, IX and X) are deficient. All neonates are given vitamin K 1 mg parenterally routinely

Central nervous system (CNS)

Myelination of the nerve fibres is incomplete at birth. Also, the cerebral cortex and the blood–brain barrier are undeveloped. Therefore, the very young are more sensitive to opioids and general anaesthesia. Babies react non-specifically to pain but apparently cannot differentiate the origin of the pain. Neonates have higher circulating levels of β endorphine than adults and the immature blood–brain barrier may allow these to affect the CNS.

Analgesia for babies should be provided with the same care as for adult patients.

Temperature regulation

Infants lose heat rapidly in a cool environment because of their large surface area relative to weight and their lack of subcutaneous fat. Other responses such as shivering, vasoconstriction and nestling are only poorly developed.

The newborn's main thermoregulatory mechanism is chemical and involves metabolism of brown-fat stores. Cold exposure releases noradrenaline at sympathetic nerve endings and increases 3' 5' cyclic AMP.

The main danger of hypothermia is increased oxygen metabolism. It is important to attempt to maintain the baby in a *neutral thermal environment* when oxygen consumption is minimal.

Ninety per cent of heat loss is from conduction, convection and radiation. The rest is from evaporation (skin and lungs), inspired air and excreta. Therefore, the baby should be kept warm at all times.

Body fluids

The total body water content of a neonate is higher than an adult, because of a relative excess of extracellular fluid (Table 13.3). The infant kidney readily excretes dilute urine but its ability to concentrate or to conserve water is limited. There is also a limited ability to cope with excess water and sodium.

Table 13.3   Extracellular fluid, intracellular fluid and body water as percentages of body weight

	Extracellular fluid	Intracellular fluid	Body water
1 month	38%	32%	70%
1 year	26%	36%	60%
adult	27%	33%	60%

An infant's high metabolic rate and high oxygen consumption relate directly to a high water turnover (therefore, they rapidly become dehydrated). Fluid, sodium and potassium requirements must be monitored carefully and should be given over 24 hours in the neonatal period. Blood glucose should also be monitored carefully as hypoglycaemia may rapidly occur due to immature liver and glycogen stores and a high metabolic rate. Fluids should be given as 5 per cent or 10 per cent dextrose solution.

Preoperative visit

The preoperative visit by the anaesthetist is vitally important to allay the fears and to gain the confidence of the child and the parents. In fact, some anaesthetists believe that once trust and rapport are established then no premedication is needed. There is a wide range of techniques.

The child's physical state must be checked carefully by the anaesthetist. Table 13.4 details a routine check-list.

Table 13.4   Routine checklist for preoperative assessment

Name

Age ⎤   very important as drugs and equipment specific
Weight ⎦   to the child need to be prepared.

Consent by parents or guardian

Operation site and side marked if relevant

Previous anaesthetics

Medication

Temperature—if persistently raised this may mean an infection
     so the operation should be postponed if possible.

History   —including family history

Physical examination:
 general condition
 colour
 nutrition
 hydration
 respiratory system—if an upper respiratory tract infection (URTI) presents with
      purulent secretions and a raised temperature the operation
      should be postponed but this is not necessary if the child is
      afebrile with clear secretions. The danger of an URTI is an
      increased risk of laryngospasm, bleeding and bacteraemia.
 cardiovascular system—check for circulatory problems, murmurs or heart failure.
 veins—inspect for suitable venepuncture sites. Mark with a cross for
   EMLA cream to be applied (p. 197).
 teeth—any loose or damaged?

Investigations:
 Routine—haemoglobin and urinalyses
 Others—sickle test
    full blood count
    urea and electrolytes
    chest radiograph
    acid-base status
    liver function tests

Fasting state—usually 4–6 h. It is advisable to give children a drink of clear fluid
    4 hours preoperatively. It is very rare for children to become
    hypoglycaemic but if there is any delay then they must be monitored.

Premedication

This will depend on:
- the patient
- the anaesthetist's preference
- the operation to be performed

Methods of administration

- oral—well tolerated but unpredictable effect as it may be vomited or have unreliable absorption
- intramuscular—provides a reliable effect but child may have a 'needle phobia'
- intravenous—only for anticholinergics (not for narcotics unless closely supervised)
- rectal—not well tolerated in this country and unpredictable effect as unreliable absorption

Types of premedication

All premedication is prescribed on a dose for weight basis (Table 13.5).

Table 13.5   Useful drugs and dosages in paediatric premedication

---

Atropine
    dose: 0.02 mg/kg
    i.v. at induction
    i.m. 45 min preoperatively
    p.o. double dose 1–2 h preoperatively
    caution: reduce dose with pyrexia and tachycardia
Papaveretum and hyoscine mixture
    dose: papaveretum 0.4 mg/kg and hyoscine 0.009 mg/kg
    i.m. 1 h preoperatively
    maximum dose of papaveretum 15 mg
Pethidine compound injection
    dose: 0.08 ml/kg
    consists of pethidine 25 mg ⎫
                promethazine 12.5 mg ⎬ in 1 ml
                chlorpromazine 12.5 mg ⎭
    maximum dosage 1.5 ml
Diazepam
    dose: 0.4 mg/kg
    either as syrup, tablets or rectal sachets
Trimeprazine tartrate (Vallergan)
    dose: 2–4 mg/kg
    p.o. 2 h preoperatively
Routine premedication (as recommended by The Hospital for Sick Children, GOS)
- up to 8 months age or <8 kg body weight—atropine only
- small children >8 months or up to 15 kg body weight—atropine+sedation (e.g. pethidine compound injection)
- older children (>15 kg)—Omnopon and Scopolamine.

Nothing at all
Familiarity and trust are the main secret involved. This technique is most useful for day stay procedures.

EMLA cream
This is an eutectic ('melting readily') mixture of lignocaine and prilocaine. The cream should be applied about 1 hour before the operation under an occlusive dressing and after removal will provide effective topical dermal anaesthesia which should last for about 1 hour.

Analgesia
Preoperatively analgesics are prescribed for their euphoric and sedative effects and are useful as an adjunct to the anaesthetic. Drugs used include papaveretum and pethidine. Narcotics must not be prescribed to infants less than 6 months of age.

Sedatives
Mostly given orally, this group of drugs includes trimeprazine, diazepam and temazepam.

Anticholinergics
These drugs are necessary to reduce excessive secretions (often present in children) and to protect against the active vagal reflexes (stimulated by laryngoscopy). Drugs used include atropine, hyoscine and glycopyrrolate.

Apparatus

Paediatric lists demand that a full range of specialist equipment, suitable for the different sizes and shapes of infants, is available. Adult equipment is not suitable and a designated paediatric theatre and recovery area is the ideal. All equipment must be fully checked before use.

Facemasks
The Rendell-Baker-Soucek mask is commonly used and because of its face-fitting shape it has the lowest dead space. The MIE inflatable rim or Laerdal resuscitation mask both make a good air-tight seal on the baby's face.

Laryngoscopes and endotracheal tubes
Uncuffed tubes must be used in all children below puberty. The narrowest part of a child's larynx is the cricoid ring. Therefore, whenever a tube is inserted, a small *leak* should be heard. If the tube is too tight, it impinges on the cricoid mucosa causing oedema and possibly followed by fibrosis and stenosis. In a small baby, 1 mm of oedema at subglottic level will reduce the airway by 60 per cent and therefore markedly increase the work of breathing. Postoperatively, if oedema is present, stridor and signs of upper-airway obstruction will occur, these usually respond to the administration of humidified oxygen and dexamethasone. If symptoms persist racemic adrenaline given by nebulization usually results in a rapid resolution.

Several different types of polyvinylchloride (PVC) tubes are available and in common usage (Fig. 13.2).

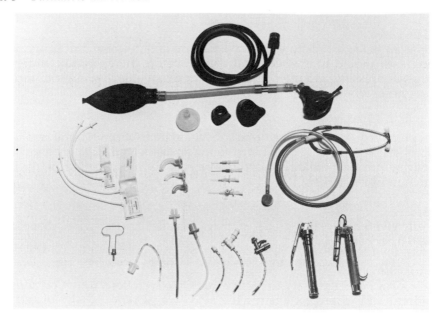

Fig. 13.2 Paediatric anaesthetic equipment. Clockwise from the lower-left corner. Various sizes of Guedel airway, various sizes of blood pressure cuffs, Jack Rees' modification of Ayre's T-piece with various sizes of Rendell-Baker-Soucek masks, end of precordial stethoscopes, Sheila Anderson-Magill and Robertshaw laryngoscopes, various sizes of endotracheal tubes with Portex Minilink connectors, Cole Pattern tube, flexometallic tube and RAE tube.

PVC Magill tubes

These are single-use tubes and were originally used only for long-term ventilation but have now largely superseded red-rubber tubes.

RAE tubes

A pre-formed disposable PVC tube with a bend at the mouth to prevent kinking and a connector at chin level to allow good access for work on the head and neck. It is especially useful for tonsillectomy. The length must be checked carefully.

Armoured tubes

Latex and silicone reinforced tubes are incompressible and unkinkable and are also useful when access is required to the head and neck. They are floppy so require an introducer for intubation and as they cannot be cut the position must be checked carefully.

Cole Pattern tubes

These have a wide proximal and a narrow distal part. They are useful for initial resuscitation as they are stiff tubes but they should *not* be used for maintenance of the airway as

- the shouldered part of the tube can cause laryngeal damage
- turbulence through the tube because of the narrowing increases the resistance and work of breathing

The size of the tube must always be chosen carefully to ensure a leak is present. It must be changed down a size if there is no leak. The following formula is widely used:

$$\left[\frac{Age}{4} + 4 = \text{internal diameter (mm)}\right]$$

There should always be a tube one size larger and one size smaller prepared in order to cover the wide variation for age and weight. Another aid is that devised from the guidelines of the Resuscitation Council which can be very useful in an emergency situation. It correlates weight with age, internal diameter and length of tube (Chapter 14, Fig. 14.9).

The *length* of the tube must also be carefully checked because of the small size of an infant's trachea and the dangers of intubating one lung. Useful formulae are:

$$\left[\begin{array}{l} \frac{Age}{2} + 12 = \text{length in cm for oral intubation} \\[2mm] \frac{Age}{2} + 15 = \text{length in cm for nasal intubation} \end{array}\right]$$

The tube should pass 2.5 cm past the vocal cords. It is important to then check that air enters both lungs (Chapter 5).

Fixation of the tube must be firm and secure to avoid kinking or displacement. There are a wide range of connectors available but for oral intubation the Cardiff or the Portex Minilink system are probably the most popular, while the Tunstall connector with forehead fixation is safest and easiest for nasal intubation (especially long-term). In the UK 8.5 mm connectors are widely used with 15 mm adaptors. It is important to check all parts of the system are compatible (Fig. 13.2).

The infant's anatomy requires a different design of laryngoscope.

- straight blade to visualize the high anterior larynx and to lift the floppy epiglottis
- small, light weight and easily handled
- design of blade to prevent the large bulky tongue obstructing

Intravenous cannulae

Intravenous access is mandatory for infants and children. Cannulae as small as 24 gauge are now in common usage and the choice from the many different brands and types of plastic is a matter of personal preference. It is important that they are properly fixed to the skin and in some cases plaster of paris is used for fixation to the scalp.

All fluids infused must be warmed and accurately calculated using either a syringe or a microburette. Syringe pumps or volumetric pumps provide accurate measurements.

Anaesthetic breathing systems

An Ayre's T-piece system with an expiratory limb and an open-ended 500 ml bag (Jackson Rees' modification) is used for children under 20 kg (Fig. 13.2 and Fig. 13.3).

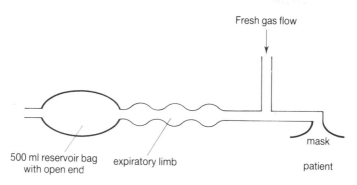

Fig. 13.3   Ayre's T-piece with Jackson Rees' modification (expiratory limb and open-ended reservoir bag).

Advantages
- simple and light weight
- no valves (no danger of sticking and no resistance)
- small dead space
- low resistance as fresh gas flow directed towards the patient, and minimal resistance only in expiration
- used for spontaneous respiration or intermittent positive pressure ventilation

Disadvantages
- a high flow of fresh gas is necessary
- humidification of the circuit is not easy
- scavenging can be difficult

The recommended fresh gas flow for spontaneous breathing is 2½ to 3 times the minute volume, but the minimal fresh gas flow to prevent rebreathing is 4 litres/min. When ventilated with the T-piece, the fresh gas flow will depend on the amount of leak around the endotracheal tube during controlled ventilation. The recommended minimal fresh gas flow is then 3 litres/min. The T-piece can either be used with manual compression of the reservoir bag or in conjunction with a ventilator. It is useful to be able to monitor the end-tidal CO_2.

For children over 20 kg any conventional adult breathing system may be used. The Bain system is a modification of the T-piece but the breathing bag and exhalation valve function as a Mapleson D. The components of the Bain system are of lightweight plastic so it is particularly useful.

Lung ventilators

Manual ventilation is recommended with neonatal anaesthesia, especially when the surgeon is operating near the trachea (e.g. tracheo-oesophageal fistula or diaphragmatic hernia). The anaesthetist is then able to detect early compression or interference with the airway.

Types of ventilator:

Main facilities required on a ventilator:
- accurate control of inspired oxygen (see hazards of oxygen therapy — Chapter 7)
- rate
- tidal volume
- inspiratory/expiratory ratio
- lightweight tubing
- humidification
- reliable alarms
- IMV (Intermittent Mandatory Ventilation)
- PEEP (Positive End Expiratory Pressure)/CPAP (Continuous Positive Airway Pressure)

PEEP is used to prevent airway closure within the normal range of tidal volume. The closing volume is usually greater than the functional residual capacity in small children. PEEP of 5 cm H_2O is usual.

CPAP is used for respiratory support when the child is breathing either spontaneously or with IMV and during weaning. It may be applied either by a nasotracheal tube, nasal prongs, facemask or head box with a tight seal around the neck.

Monitoring during anaesthesia

This must be maintained at all times (Chapter 5). Routinely this should include:
- ECG
- pulse oximeter—special paediatric probes for attachment to an ear, a finger or a hand are available
- blood pressure—the newer automatic monitors have a full range of paediatric and neonatal cuffs. It is important the right size of cuff is available (Fig. 13.2).
- end-tidal CO_2
- temperature probe. Oesophageal or rectal and surface measurements are used.
- precordial or oesophageal stethoscope. These allow the anaesthetist to listen to breath sounds and the heart rate.

    Other monitoring used for specific cases includes central venous pressure; urine output; direct intra-arterial pressure monitoring; trans-cutaneous O_2 and CO_2 monitors; pulmonary artery pressure and cardiac output.

Anaesthetic management

Prior to the induction, the anaesthetist will have carefully checked the equipment and the circuit. The drugs should be labelled and diluted as necessary. A skilled and dedicated assistant should be available.

Hopefully, the anaesthetic room has a quiet, non-frightening atmosphere. The child should be the centre of attention and the anaesthetist should explain all that is happening. Monitoring, especially a pulse oximeter, should be attached.

Induction

Methods of induction

- intravenous
- inhalational
- intramuscular
- rectally (rarely)

Intravenous
EMLA cream (local anaesthetic) applied to a preselected area (chosen by the anaesthetist), which is usually the dorsum of the hand, will aid insertion of a cannula. Coughing at the time of insertion will distend the veins and distract the older child. The agents used are

Thiopentone given as 2.5 mg/kg provides a smooth rapid induction. Care must be taken not to let the drug extravasate around the veins nor be injected intra-arterially. As with all paediatric drugs, the correct dosage for weight must be given.
Methohexitone, etomidate, propofol are all useful drugs but are not suitable for paediatric practice as they cause pain on injection.

Inhalational induction
This method may be chosen in the very small child, when venous access is difficult or unavailable or when the patient prefers it. It is best achieved by drifting the gases from the cupped hand across the nose and mouth of the child. This method, in skilled hands, is smooth and fast.

Halothane is now the most commonly used agent. It provides a smooth relatively fast induction. Nitrous oxide is used as a carrier gas. The rare risk of repeated exposure must be weighed against its smoothness.
Cyclopropane is explosive so its popularity has waned. It provides the fastest induction if given initially in a concentration of 50 per cent with oxygen. Atropine must always be given beforehand as it causes excessive secretions and spasm. Full antistatic precautions must be used.
Isoflurane can cause breath holding, coughing and spasm. In skilled hands, it can be very rapid.

Applying CPAP with a distended bag and tight-fitting mask can overcome problems with laryngospasm at induction. Once a deep plane of anaesthesia is achieved, venous access can be gained, and a relaxant given if required.

Intramuscular
Rarely, ketamine may be used by this method especially if venous access is difficult. Used in large doses it is associated with prolonged recovery.

Following induction the anaesthetist may elect to allow the patient to breathe spontaneously with a facemask or a laryngeal mask or may prefer to control ventilation.

Mask anaesthesia
The mask must fit the face and minimize dead space. An oropharyngeal airway may be required because of the bulky tongue. Adenoidal hypertrophy may cause obstruction in older children.

Intubation and ventilation
This depends upon:
- the anaesthetist's preference
- the size of the child (usually intubated if less than 10 kg as the airway can be difficult to maintain) or if they are less than 6 months of age
- any procedure lasting longer than 45 min
- for control of ventilation to prevent closing volume (small-airways closure) encroaching on tidal volume
- surgery around the head and neck or surgery requiring full paralysis e.g. neurosurgery, intra-abdominal procedures
- prone, sitting or abdominal postures
- to prevent aspiration of vomit
- airway problems e.g. a difficult airway to maintain
- ventilation problems e.g. hypoventilation

Intubation
This is different in the child because of the anatomical and physiological differences already described.
- preoxygenation is required because children rapidly become hypoxic
- in the smaller neonate an awake intubation may be used
- a straight-bladed laryngoscope is passed under to lift the large floppy epiglottis and expose the larynx
- a skilled assistant may apply gentle cricoid pressure (larynx is high and anterior)
- the endotracheal tube is passed 2.5 cm into the trachea. A leak must be present or the tube changed for a smaller size. The tube is secured firmly and checked to ensure both lungs are inflating (a radiograph is mandatory in an intensive care situation)

Dangers of intubation
- disconnection — a pressure-sensitive disconnect alarm is important
- tube malposition, e.g. bronchial intubation or extubation
- obstruction of the tube with secretions. Humidification and frequent suction are important especially when very small tubes are used
- post-extubation
  - sore throat and hoarse voice (usually transient)
  - stridor from subglottic oedema

Maintenance

Following induction, anaesthesia is usually maintained with a mixture of nitrous oxide and halothane, enflurane or isoflurane. Care must be taken when using adrenaline with halothane.

Analgesia or a regional technique must be added to this. Omnopon, morphine or fentanyl can all be used safely while the child is ventilated. Care must be taken with spontaneously-breathing patients and with small neonates. Codeine phosphate (i.m.) can be used in those children with airway problems.

Muscle relaxants

Suxamethonium. Infants appear to require a relatively larger dose than adults. It can be given i.m. (2 mg/kg) which can be useful in small children with difficult veins. Myoglobinuria can result from its use. Arrhythmias, particularly bradycardias, are common especially after a second dose. This can be avoided by using atropine either in the premedication or as an i.v. bolus.

Vecuronium. The major advantage is that it has no effect on the cardiovascular system. It is useful for short procedures but has a longer time of onset than suxamethonium. It can be used by an infusion technique with careful monitoring of the neuromuscular function as it is easily eliminated.

Atracurium. This drug releases histamine. It is useful for short procedures and for infusion techniques.

Pancuronium. This drug is more potent than curare but is longer acting. It has a slow onset time and produces a tachycardia.

Antagonism of muscle relaxants

Neostigmine in combination with atropine or glycopyrrolate is used to reverse non-depolarizing neuromuscular blockade. Children require smaller doses of neostigmine than adults, however, cold or acidosis may prolong the action of the muscle's relaxants and the infant must be anaesthetized carefully to avoid these factors. Adequate reversal is detected by the neuromuscular monitor and also clinically. A child crying loudly with good strong movements is 'safe'.

Fluid management

Calculation of the volume and type of fluid required must take into consideration:
- preoperative dehydration
  - normal fasting
  - abnormal losses, e.g. pyrolic stenosis, burns
- maintenance requirements
- surgical trauma
- body temperature

Preoperative dehydration

The patient must be carefully assessed preoperatively and surgery post-poned until dehydration is corrected. Sufficient fluid should be given to compensate for the preoperative fasting. The physical signs of dehydration are:

- 5 per cent loss — dry tongue
- 10 per cent loss — dry tongue, quiet, inactive child, flaccid skin, sunken fontanelle, tachycardia, tachypnoea, low blood pressure and urine output
- 15 per cent loss — unresponsive child with dry mouth, sunken eyes and fontanelle, thready fast pulse, hypotension, oliguria, respiratory distress.

Laboratory studies which may help with the diagnosis are haemoglobin concentration and haematocrit; electrolytes; urea and creatinine; osmolality (urine and blood). Replacement of losses will require monitoring of pulse, blood pressure, central venous pressure and urine output.

Fluids used depend on the type of loss, the preoperative haemoglobin concentration and the response of the patient. They include whole blood or plasma 5 per cent albumin at 10–20 ml/kg; physiological saline or dextrose/saline may also be indicated.

Maintenance requirements

Dextrose 4%/saline 0.18% is used normally except in the neonatal period.
    A useful guide is

$$\left[\begin{array}{l} \text{first} \quad 10 \text{ kg body weight} - 100 \text{ ml/kg/24 hrs} \\ \text{second} 10 \text{ kg} \quad ,, \quad ,, \quad\quad - \ 50 \text{ ml/kg/24 hrs} \\ \text{weight in excess } 20 \text{ kg} \quad - \ 20 \text{ ml/kg/24 hrs} \end{array} \right]$$

In addition, potassium 2 mmol/100 ml may be given provided urine output is adequate.

Surgical losses

Loss must be accurately assessed by weighing swabs, measuring suction and estimating loss on the drapes. Blood (usually replaced if greater than 10 per cent of the circulating blood volume is lost) must be accurately measured, warmed and filtered before infusion either by syringe or microburette. Fluid may also be lost by evaporation if overhead radiant heaters are used, from lack of humidification in the ventilator circuit, or from surgical cavities.

Body temperature

A rise of 1°C can increase fluid losses by 12 per cent.

Postoperative

A strict fluid-balance chart must be maintained and all losses recorded accurately. The appropriate fluids must be replaced hourly.
    The appropriate regimen will cover

- normal maintenance — usually dextrose 4 per cent/saline 0.18% with added potassium (dextrose 10 per cent in neonates)
- blood or serous losses
- insensible loss (from pyrexia or overhead radiant heaters)
- gastrointestinal losses (e.g. vomiting, ileus, etc.)

In addition, serum potassium concentrations should be measured often.

Special problems with neonates

- body temperature
  - always transfer in a heated incubator
  - always use a warming blanket and cover with gamgee, foil or plastic
  - warm all fluids to be used either intravenously or for skin preparation
  - humidify gases
  - operating theatre must be at 24°C
- haemorrhage — give vitamin K preoperatively
- apnoeic episodes — occur commonly in premature infants so must be monitored carefully after operation. Narcotics should only be prescribed if controlled ventilation is used
- hypoglycaemia — monitor blood sugar level frequently. Maintenance fluid should be 10 per cent dextrose. Postoperative twitching may be due to either hypoglycaemia or hypocalcaemia
- fluids — accurate measurement of all fluids, even those given with drugs, is important to avoid overload
- oxygenation — inspired concentration must be kept to a minimum. The risks to a premature infant of high inspired oxygen are
  - retrolental fibroplasia. In infants less than 36 weeks the Po_2 must be maintained between 6.6–10.6 kPa or there is a risk of retinal vasoconstriction
  - pulmonary O_2 toxicity
  - bronchopulmonary dysplasia — a high inspired oxygen and high inflation pressures will produce focal-air trapping, cyst formation and fibrosis
- intubation
  - always give atropine as the neonate has copious secretions and a very active vagus nerve
  - intubate awake if unskilled and if there is a tracheofistula present or if there is any difficulty with the airway
  - position endotracheal tube securely — ensure there is a leak around the tube and that both lungs are ventilated
- ventilation – usually manually with a T-piece
- analgesia — narcotics should only be prescribed if the patient is on a ventilator. Regional techniques or paracetamol may be all that is required

Surgical emergencies

Most surgery in the neonatal period is performed as an emergency. Antenatal ultrasound scanning has made early diagnosis possible and fetal surgery is developing. The mother can be transferred for delivery to a regional neonatal surgical unit.

Postoperative analgesia

Postoperative pain is physically and psychologically harmful to the child. Pain can also lead to hypertension and bleeding, and restlessness can interfere with dressings and surgical wounds. Intraoperative narcotics, local blocks or regional techniques can and should extend into the postoperative period.

Choice of technique

Intramuscular opiate

The intramuscular route is not ideal as it leads to peaks and troughs in the level of analgesia provided, but it may be the safest option when intensive care is not available. Narcotics are avoided in children less than 6 months of age because of the unpredictable response to opiates in this age group. Non-narcotic analgesia e.g. codeine phosphate 1 mg/kg i.m. 4–6 hourly should be given in all cases where airway problems may be present, it must not be given i.v. because of histamine release (Table 13.6).

Table 13.6 Common postoperative analgesic regimens

Papaveretum
    dose: 0.2 mg/kg
    i.m. 4–6 hourly
Morphine
    dose: 0.1–0.2 mg/kg
    i.m. 4–6 hourly
    (i.v. 10–50 µg/kg per h)
Pethidine
    dose: 1 mg/kg
    i.m. 4–6 hourly
Codeine phosphate
    dose: 1 mg/kg
    i.m. 4–6 hourly
    (not given i.v. as decreases cardiac output)
Paracetamol
    dose: 12 mg/kg
    p.o. or p.r. 6 hourly

Narcotics should not be prescribed to children less than 6 months unless ventilated.

Intravenous infusion of narcotics

This technique can safely be employed in unventilated infants provided liver function is not compromised and that very close surveillance of respiratory function is available in the postoperative intensive care ward.

Drugs must be infused by a syringe pump or volumetric pump via a single line, with no other access through that line and no other drugs given via that line.

Oral/rectal drugs

Paracetamol may be given orally or rectally 12 mg/kg 6 hourly and is useful in the very small child.

Local infiltration

This is performed by the surgeon during the closing of the wound. A long-acting local anaesthetic such as bupivacaine is useful. A dose of 3 mg/kg (0.25 per cent) must *not* be exceeded.

Caudal block

This is a simply performed and most useful block for all operations up to and including the umbilicus. It provides analgesia for some of the commonest paediatric operations e.g. herniotomy, orchidopexy, circumcision and orthopaedic procedures on the lower limbs. This block is often technically much more difficult in adults.

Technique
The child is placed in a left-lateral position and the needle is inserted into the caudal space at 40° to the skin. It is not advanced after it penetrates the sacrococcygeal membrane. The needle is aspirated to check for blood or CSF (Fig. 13.4).

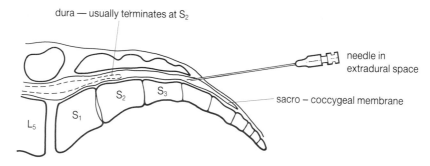

dura — usually terminates at S_2

needle in extradural space

sacro – coccygeal membrane

S_2 S_3

S_1

L_5

Fig. 13.4   Caudal anaesthesia. (Spinal cord terminates at L_3 at birth and L_{1-2} by 6 months).

Complications
- hypotension — rarely
- urinary retention (should be checked for before the child is allowed home if they are a day case)
- intravascular needle placement
- dural puncture — needle must not be advanced too far

Disadvantages
- motor block and paraesthesia can be frightening for the child but rarely occurs with 0.25% bupivacaine

- single shot technique — catheter cannot be left in because of proximity to anus

Ilio-inguinal block

Useful for unilateral inguinal herniotomy or orchidopexy but cannot be performed at the beginning of the procedure as it will often make the surgeon's task more difficult.

Epidural block

These are becoming more common and are useful for more major abdominal and thoracic procedures. A 19 gauge Tuohy needle with a 21 gauge epidural catheter is now available.

Penile block

Useful for circumcision and operations on the penis. Adrenalin must *not* be added to the local anaesthetic. Complications include haematoma formation.

Axillary block

For operations involving the deep tissues of the hand and forearm.

Further reading

Brown T C K, Fisk G C. *Anaesthesia for children*. Oxford: Blackwell, 1979.
Hatch D J, Sumner E. *Neonatal anaesthesia*. London: Edward Arnold, 1986.
Steward D J. *Manual of paediatric anaesthesia*. London: Churchill Livingstone, 1990.
Sumner E, Hatch D J. *Textbook of anaesthetic practice*. London: Baillière Tindall, 1989.

14

Life support and cardiopulmonary resuscitation

D.A. Zideman

- Basic cardiac life support
  - airway
  - breathing
  - circulation
  - infection
- Advanced cardiac life support
  - airway
  - breathing
  - circulation
- Prolonged resuscitation
- Post-resuscitation care
- Paediatric resuscitation
- Conclusion

Cardiopulmonary resuscitation is a simple psychomotor skill in which all members of the medical profession should be thoroughly proficient, frequently trained and formally and officially certified. It is a series of well-defined steps and protocols that should be followed following the collapse of a patient, whatever the cause.

Cardiopulmonary resuscitation (CPR) is divided into two stages

- basic cardiac life support (BCLS) — resuscitation carried out without the aid of equipment
- advanced cardiac life support (ACLS) — the use of advanced techniques (e.g. intubation) and equipment (e.g. defibrillator) in resuscitation

BCLS must be started immediately collapse occurs and continued until the equipment of ACLS arrives. BCLS in effect 'buys time' by providing an Airway, artificial Breathing by expired-air respiration and an artificial Circulation by external chest compressions. Thus a flow of oxygenated blood is maintained to the brain, heart and other vital organs by the rescuer until a spontaneous circulation can be restarted. In reality, BCLS is rarely successful on its own and ACLS is necessary to restart the heart. Nevertheless, it is important to remember that ACLS alone is not sufficient for a successful outcome, and that delays in commencing BCLS whilst awaiting the arrival of the ACLS team and equipment can seriously affect the eventual resuscitation result.

Basic cardiac life support

Current practice dictates that this follows the simple algorithm

    A — Airway
    B — Breathing
    C — Circulation

Before commencing the **ABC** sequence it is necessary to establish the conscious level of the casualty. He should be gently shaken by the shoulders and asked 'are you alright?' The rescuer should, of course, never place himself in any greater danger than absolutely necessary and must be constantly aware of potential hazards such as electricity, gas, traffic, or falling masonry, any of which could have caused the original incident.

Airway

An unconscious casualty will rapidly lose his airway as his tongue falls to the back of his pharynx. To open the airway and allow the unconscious casualty to breathe, tilt the head back and lift the chin forward (Fig. 14.1). Do not use the 'neck lift' method of opening the airway. The chin lift is of vital importance to the success of the technique. In cases of a suspected neck injury only tilt the head enough to obtain a clear airway. Foreign bodies can be removed from the mouth by a careful single-finger sweep.

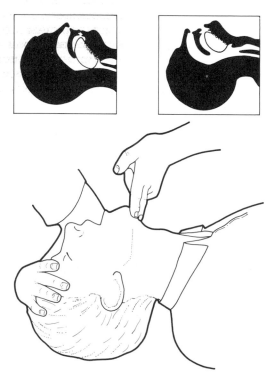

Fig. 14.1 Opening the airway.

Breathing

The rescuer now checks to see if the casualty is breathing (Fig. 14.2) by
- looking for chest movement
- listening for breath sounds
- feeling for breathing with the cheek

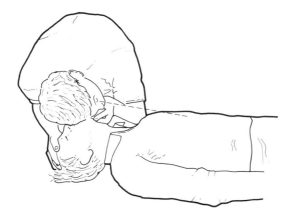

Fig. 14.2 Looking, listening and feeling for breathing.

If no effective breathing is detected then artificial ventilation is commenced by expired-air respiration.

'Mouth to mouth' ventilation describes the method of expired-air respiration to be used (Fig. 14.3). The casualty's mouth is covered by the mouth of the rescuer and the casualty's nostrils pinched closed. The rescuer blows his expired air into the casualty until the chest starts to rise. At this point he stops blowing, removes his mouth and allows the casualty to exhale. Two individual initial breaths are given. In infants and children the mouth and nose of the child are covered by the rescuer's mouth — 'mouth to mouth and nose respiration' — and the same technique is then followed.

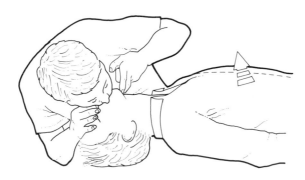

Fig. 14.3 'Mouth to mouth' resuscitation.

If breathing alone is required, as there is a carotid pulse present (see below), then respirations are continued at the rate of 12–15 breaths/min.

Circulation

The circulation is assessed by feeling for the carotid pulse in the neck (Fig. 14.4). This is the most relevant pulse as it checks that there is a pulsatile flow of blood from the heart to the brain. It is a common fault to rush this pulse assessment, but time must be taken to do it properly, especially if there is a bradycardia or abnormal cardiac rhythm.

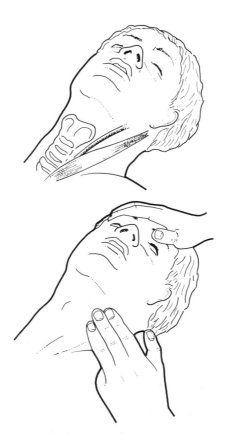

Fig. 14.4   Checking the carotid pulse.

If no pulse is felt then an artificial circulation must be created by external chest compressions. Chest compressions are carried out on the lower third of the sternum using the overlapping heels of both hands (Fig. 14.5). The sternum is depressed vertically 1½–2 inches (4–5 cm), 80 times/min. After 15 compressions, two mouth to mouth ventilations are performed. The 15 compressions and two ventilations are continued for 1 minute before the

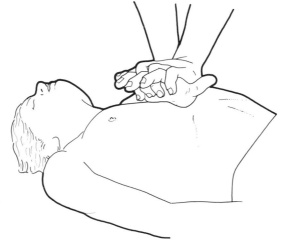

Note that the fingers are clear of the chest

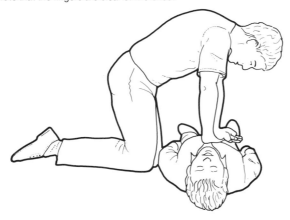

Fig. 14.5 External chest compressions.

breathing and ventilation are reassessed, they are then continued in 3-minute cycles before further reassessment. This resuscitation sequence should not be interrupted for more than 10 seconds for any reason.

If two rescuers are present, then the first should perform chest compressions at 60 compressions/min, whilst the second interposes an expired-air breath after every 5th compression.

External chest compressions were originally believed to work by direct compression of the heart between the sternum and the vertebral bodies. In the last decade an alternative physiology was formulated. Initially, it was found that if the cardiac-arrest patient was made to cough repeatedly his conscious level could be maintained until a more definitive therapy became available. Thus coughing, or raising the intrathoracic pressure, developed a cerebral flow of blood. Using two dimensional echocardiography and angiography it was further shown that in some humans the heart did not change in shape or size nor did the heart valves move during chest compressions. A new theory was formulated that by performing external chest compression, and thus raising the intrathoracic pressure, the whole of the chest cavity was acting as a pump. Each compression raised the intrathoracic pressure and this raised pressure was transmitted directly to the relatively thick-walled intrathoracic arteries. The raised pressure also caused collapse of the relatively thin-walled intrathoracic veins. Thus an arterial to venous pressure gradient was produced resulting in the forward flow of blood.

In children, chest compressions are also carried out on the lower third of the sternum, one finger's breadth below the internipple line, using either the tips of two fingers or the heel of one hand depending on the size of the child (Fig. 14.6). In the baby the compression:ventilation ratio is changed to five compressions to one ventilation. The compression depth is 1–1.5 cm and the compression rate is 100/min.

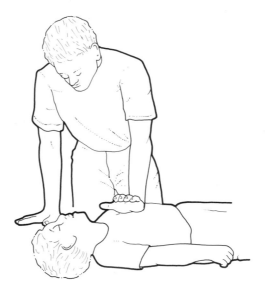

Keep your hand or fingers below the level of the nipple

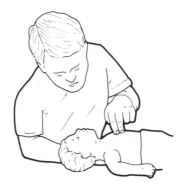

Fig. 14.6 Chest compressions on a child and baby.

In all cases where basic cardiac life support is started it must be continued until the advanced cardiac life support becomes available.

Infection
There has been much written on the risk of infection to the rescuer from 'mouth to mouth' resuscitation. Minor infection such as the common cold or, more recently, salmonella have been reported, but there have been no substantive reports in the world literature to date of any major infectious disease being transmitted in this manner. More specifically, in relation to the hepatitis virus and human immunodeficiency virus, statements have been issued saying that there is no risk of transmission of these viruses by 'mouth to mouth' resuscitation. An exception is made if there is visible blood in the saliva of the casualty.

With the above in mind a number of interpositional devices have been recommended in the past few years. Simplicity, efficiency and availability are of primary importance. At the time of writing, the best device seems to be the collapsible pocket mask with valve.

Advanced cardiac life support

The use of equipment and advanced techniques in cardiac resuscitation must come second to BCLS. Nevertheless the sooner ACLS is initiated the better the overall chance of a successful resuscitation. This section will deal with the techniques in an **A**irway, **B**reathing, **C**irculation, **D**rug sequence. It is important that all these procedures are carried out concurrently but that, for example, the treatment of ventricular fibrillation by early defibrillation takes priority and success may preclude any further progression of treatment.

Airway
The use of simple airway devices such as the Guedel airway, will help in controlling the tongue which is the most common cause of airway obstruction. The correct size must be selected; a size 3 is adequate for most adults. It must be carefully inserted to avoid damage to the lips, teeth or oral mucosa. Insertion is achieved by starting with the airway upside down (curved upwards) and inserting the airway into the mouth until the tip reaches the roof of the mouth. The airway is then turned 180° (curve downwards), gently advancing it until the bite block lies between the teeth of the casualty. Guedel airways do not always solve airway problems; they are only simple adjuncts and the airway must still be 'held open' by head tilt and jaw lift. Guedel airways may cause retching and vomiting if the pharyngeal reflexes are still present. The nasopharyngeal airway is an alternative and will often provide a simple controlled airway in the semiconscious subject.

The only guaranteed method of upper-airway control is by tracheal intubation with a cuffed tracheal tube. This is a practical technique which will not be discussed any further in this chapter. Suffice it to say, that a size 9 mm tracheal tube is used for an adult male and a size 8 mm tube for an adult female. Having intubated the trachea the tracheal cuff should be inflated to seal the airway and the tube firmly fixed in place to prevent accidental removal.

Breathing

The use of the self-inflating resuscitation bag has become the standard method of ventilation in ACLS. In its simplest form it is used as a bag–valve–mask system where the mask is held tightly onto the casualty's face to attain a seal and the bag squeezed with the other hand to achieve ventilation. The simplicity of the description belies the difficulty of the technique. This two-handed technique is difficult to achieve, especially for those unpractised in it. The chest must be seen to move with each inflation and if this is not easily achieved the rescuer should return to 'mouth to mouth'/expired-air ventilation.

An alternative method has been proposed for the two-man resuscitation sequence. The first rescuer seals the mask onto the face using two hands. Ventilation is then by the second rescuer reaching up to squeeze the bag after each set of five chest compressions.

It is important to add supplemental oxygen to the inspired gases of the resuscitation-bag system. Adding 4–6 litres/min of oxygen can raise the inspired oxygen to 40 per cent, but using an additional reservoir bag on the resuscitation circuit the inspired oxygen can be raised to 70 per cent.

Portable mechanical ventilators (resuscitators) are not recommended for resuscitation. This is especially so when the ventilator is pressure-cycled as this may lead to a premature triggering of the end of inspiration and result in inadequate ventilation. If such devices are to be used, they should be carefully selected, well maintained and used only when a properly-trained operator is available. If a portable ventilator is selected then an adequate cylinder-gas supply must be assured for the anticipated length of the resuscitation.

Circulation

Mechanical 'chest thumpers' are available but are not commonly seen in the UK at the present time. The support of the circulation during ACLS is mainly pharmacological. Thus in the first instance i.v. access must be established. The preferred route is central venous access and this can be attained via the internal jugular, external jugular, subclavian or femoral veins. Drugs administered by the central supradiaphragmatic route during resuscitation have been shown to reach the heart more rapidly and to be more efficacious than when administered by other routes. A large peripheral vein is a second choice. Other alternatives are the administration of drugs down the tracheal tube for absorption into the pulmonary vasculature, or by the intra-osseous route, via an intra-osseous needle inserted 1 cm below the tibial plateau. The direct injection of drugs into the heart is not recommended and should only be regarded as a final choice.

There are three main rhythm changes in cardiac arrest.
- ventricular fibrillation
- asystole
- electromechanical dissociation

Each has its own specific treatment algorithm.

Ventricular fibrillation

This is the most common cause of cardiac arrest (Fig. 14.7). It is described as electrical anarchy of the heart muscle, with a complete breakdown of organized electrical activity.

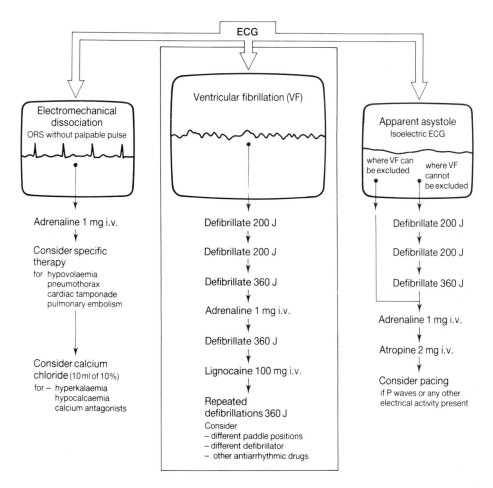

Fig. 14.7 Treatment algorithm for cardiac arrest.

The treatment of ventricular fibrillation is cardioversion by defibrillation. In a monitored or witnessed cardiac arrest, where the collapse is actually seen, then a single precordial thump is recommended as the quickest form of cardioversion. Defibrillation is the passage of an electrical current across the heart. Two paddles are positioned on the chest wall of the patient — one just below the right clavicle and the other a little outside the position of the normal apex beat (Fig. 14.8). The initial energy charge is 200 Joules (J). This is followed by a second 'shock' of 200J, then all further defibrillations are at 360J (maximum energy).

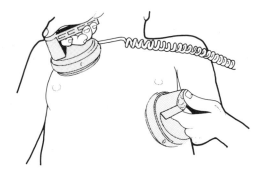

Fig. 14.8   Defibrillator paddles positioned on chest.

Adrenaline
1 mg (1 ml of a 1:1000 solution or 10 ml of a 1:10 000 solution) is administered after the first three defibrillations. Adrenaline, by its α-adrenergic action, raises the peripheral vascular resistance and improves coronary perfusion. The administration of adrenaline should be followed by 2 minutes of BCLS and if ventricular fibrillation persists then a further 360 J shock should be given.

Lignocaine
100 mg (10 ml of a 1 per cent solution) is the next recommended drug. This acts as a membrane stabilizer thus preventing refibrillation occurring following defibrillation.

Repeated defibrillation should be attempted at 360 J if fibrillation persists but consideration may be given to a different defibrillation-paddle position (anterior/posterior), a different defibrillator or the use of an alternative antiarrhythmic drug (e.g. bretylium tosylate).

Asystole

It is important to confirm the diagnosis of an isoelectric ECG as asystole (Fig. 14.7). The switches, connections and gain of the ECG monitor should be checked to see they are in the correct monitoring position. If there is any doubt, or if ventricular fibrillation cannot be excluded, then the defibrillation pathway should be followed. This is because asystole has an extremely poor prognosis when compared with ventricular fibrillation.

Adrenaline
1 mg (1 ml of 1:1000 solution, or 10 ml of a 1:10 000 solution) is the first drug of choice where ventricular fibrillation can be excluded. As in ventricular fibrillation, BCLS must continue following the administration of adrenaline. In addition to the α-adrenergic activity of adrenaline, its β-adrenergic effect will increase the rate of discharge of the myocardial nodes and improve the responsiveness of the heart muscle.

Atropine 2 mg
Atropine 2 mg is the next drug recommended. Autonomic chaos reigns during resuscitation and atropine, a parasympathetic blocking agent, will block the vagus nerve and its profound depressive effect on the sinus and atrioventricular nodes.

If the above fails, but there is still P wave activity on the ECG, then it is worth considering the possibility of electrical pacing of the myocardium. Many modern defibrillators will pace directly through large adhesive pads applied to the chest wall. Transoesophageal or transcutaneous pacing are other alternatives. Studies of pacing in resuscitation have so far provided disappointing results and many authors believe that this is because pacing is commenced too late in the resuscitation sequence to be effective.

Thus the recommendations try to reflect the need for early attempts at pacing the myocardium out of asystole.

Electromechanical dissociation

In electromechanical dissociation (EMD) there are QRS complexes on the electrocardiogram but no palpable pulse.

Adrenaline 1 mg
Adrenaline 1 mg is the first drug of choice, regardless of the cause. Further treatment of EMD depends on the cause.

Primary electromechanical dissociation
This occurs where there is a failure of the excitation–contraction–coupling mechanism. The major causes are:
- myocardial infarction (especially of the inferior wall)
- drugs (β-adrenergic blockers, calcium antagonists)
- toxins
- electrolyte abnormalities (hypocalcaemia, hyperkalaemia)
- apical thrombus or tumour (myxoma)

Calcium chloride
(10 ml of a 10 per cent solution) is recommended for the appropriate drug or electrolyte causes.

Secondary electromechanical dissociation
This occurs where there is mechanical embarrassment to cardiac output. It may be seen following trauma or may result from pericardial tamponade, cardiac rupture, pulmonary embolism, tension pneumothorax, hypovolaemia or prosthetic heart-valve malfunction. In these cases the underlying cause must be corrected if there is to be any hope of a return to normal myocardial function.

Prolonged resuscitation

Where resuscitation continues for a prolonged period of time, repeated doses of adrenaline, 1 mg at 5-minute intervals, may be considered appropriate.

Sodium bicarbonate as an alkali is sometimes used to treat the associated acidosis of resuscitation. The best treatment is efficient ventilation and proper chest compressions but sodium bicarbonate (50 mmol — i.e. 50 ml of a 8.4 per cent solution) may also be given provided that effective ventilation has been established. Sodium bicarbonate is best tritrated against arterial blood–gas results. Over-enthusiastic administration of sodium bicarbonate may result in alkalosis, hyperosmolality, and hypernatraemia and will eventually result in the failure of the resuscitation process.

Post-resuscitation care

Following successful resuscitation the patient should be carefully observed, monitored and treated in an intensive care area. Arterial blood gases, electrolytes and a chest radiograph are the minimum investigations. Any abnormality must be noted and treated. A proper and formal record of the resuscitation must be completed and should include the provisional cause of the event, the time course of the treatment (length of basic life support, time to first defibrillation), timed drug administration, timed physical intervention and the reasoned decision-making process. All must be carefully recorded as they may make a difference to the continued management of the patient.

Paediatric resuscitation

Brief mention has been made of the changes to the adult resuscitation sequence when applied to children. In the advanced cardiac–life-support sequence, allowances have to be made for the wide variety of equipment needed to resuscitate a wide range of sizes of children. The decision as to what to use must be considered a personal choice derived from training and experience. The administration of drugs to children is related to body weight. It is not possible to weigh a child in the emergency situation, but it has been found that the height/length of a child can provide a useful and simple measurement to judge the correct size and length of the tracheal tube and an appropriate dosage of resuscitation drug (Fig. 14.9).

Conclusion

The foregoing text provides a guide as to the recommended practice of basic and advanced life support. It is not sufficient to just read the text. Practical

Endotracheal tube

Length (cm)	Internal diameter (mm)
18 – 21	7.5 – 8.0
18	7.0
17	6.5
16	6.0
15	5.5
14	5.0
13	4.5
12	4.0
	3.5
10	3.0 – 3.5

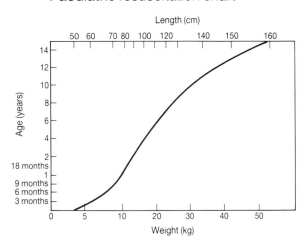

Paediatric resuscitation chart

Adrenaline (ml of 1/10 000) intravenous or endotracheal	0.5	1	2	3	4	5
Atropine (mg) intravenous or endotracheal	0.1	0.2	0.4	0.6	0.6	0.6
Bicarbonate (ml of 8.4%) intravenous	5	10	20	30	40	50
Calcium chloride (mmol)* intravenous	1	2	4	6	8	10
Diazepam intravenous per rectum	1.25 2.5	2.5 5	5 10	7.5	10	10
Glucose (ml of 50%) intravenous	10	20	40	60	80	100
Lignocaine (mg) intravenous or endotracheal	5	10	20	30	40	50
Salbutamol (mg) intravenous	25	50	100	150	200	250
Initial DC defibrillation (J)	10	20	40	60	80	100
Initial fluid infusion in hypovolaemic shock (ml)	50	100	200	300	400	500

* One millilitre calcium chloride 1 mmol/ml.   1.5 ml calcium chloride 10%   4.5 ml calcium gluconate 10%

Fig. 14.9   Paediatric resuscitation chart.

instruction in BCLS and frequent training and testing in the ACLS protocols are the only ways of establishing an effective and efficient resuscitation practice.

Further reading

Evans T R (ed). *ABC of resuscitation*. London: British Medical Journal, 1990.
Oakley P A. Paediatric resuscitation chart. *British Medical Journal*, 1988; **297:** 817–19.
Safar P, Bircher N S. *Cardiopulmonary cerebral resuscitation*. London: W B Saunders, 1988.
Standards and guidelines for cardiopulmonary resuscitation (CPR) and emergency cardiac care (ECC) American Heart Association, *JAMA* 1986; **255:** 2905–92.

15

Head injury and brainstem death
I. Calder

- Head injuries
  - first and second injury
- Types of head injury
- Consequences of head injury
  - loss of consciousness
  - hypoxaemia
  - deranged intracranial physiology
  - raised intracranial pressure
  - associated injuries
- Management of head-injured patients
  - transfer
  - anaesthetic technique
  - neurological intensive care
- Prognosis
- Brainstem death
  - incidence of brainstem death
  - causes of brainstem death
  - transplantation and brainstem death
  - diagnosis of brainstem death
  - who makes the diagnosis?
  - has there ever been a mistake?

Head injuries

First and second injury
The neurones of the central nervous system (CNS) do not regenerate. The neurones lost at the time of head injury (the first injury) are lost forever. Unfortunately many head-injured patients become hypotensive and hypoxaemic and lose more neurones as a result. Such loss of neurones is known as 'second injury'. Prevention of second injury is the aim of treatment. Second injury is common, its influence is shown in Table 15.1.

Table 15.1   Influence of systemic insults on poor outcome

	% dead/vegetative/severely disabled	
	no insult	insult
All	44%	76%
Operated haematoma	61%	86%
Diffuse injury	35%	73%
('insult' is hypoxaemia and hypotension)		

From Gentleman D, Jennett B (1990).

Types of head injury

Scalping is rare these days, but degloving scalp wounds do occur and are difficult injuries to treat. It seems that traditional scalping did not result in the immediate demise of the victim, but in a lingering dissolution due to the effects of blood loss and infection.

Closed injuries are the common type in this country. The skull is not penetrated, but damage to the brain and blood vessels inside the skull can occur and give rise to cerebral swelling or intracranial haematomas. The brain damage need not be at the impact site, a phenomenon known as contrecoup injury. There is an association with alcohol, which can lead to diagnostic difficulty. Readers will know that alcoholic stupor does not last more than a few hours.

Penetrating injuries are commoner in countries habituated to the use of firearms. The extent of cerebral damage depends principally on the velocity of the projectile, this is owing to the well-known relationship between energy, mass and velocity. Most rifle bullets and bomb fragments have high velocity and cause devastating injuries. An American authority once remarked that in some states there was little experience of penetrating head wounds due to the population's preference for 'Magnum' ammunition. The victims simply had no heads. Some handgun bullets have a sufficiently low velocity to permit survival, though severe neurological impairment is usual if both cerebral hemispheres are penetrated. Infection is likely with penetrating wounds.

Consequences of head injury

Loss of consciousness
This is the principal characteristic of brain injury. The severity of an injury is judged by the depth and duration of unconsciousness. 'What's the conscious level?', is always the first question to ask, or that you will be asked. A 'coma scale' emanating from Glasgow is in worldwide use; it is found on ITU charts everywhere. A stimulus is applied to the patient, verbal or painful (a pencil pressed into a nailbed is a standard), and the response is assessed under three headings, eye opening, verbal response and motor

response. These observations form the basis of neurological assessment and are repeated and recorded so that improvement or deterioration can be detected (Table 15.2). The Glasgow coma scale allows the conscious level to be described numerically.

Table 15.2 Glasgow coma scale

		Score
Eye opening	spontaneously	4
	to speech	3
	to pain	2
	none	1
Verbal response	orientated	5
	confused	4
	inappropriate words	3
	incomprehensible sounds	2
	none	1
Motor response	obeys commands	5
	localizes pain	4
	flexes to pain	3
	extends to pain	2
	none	1

Hypoxaemia

Even a minor depression of conscious level produces hypoxaemia. This is chiefly due to failure to maintain a *clear airway*. The airway is readily obstructed by the tongue; there is a colourful media expression 'swallowing the tongue' which describes this. The 'coma position', with the patient on his side, lower leg bent and upper leg straight, helps to avoid tongue obstruction. *Aspiration* due to glottic incompetence can also occur when the conscious level is depressed and will cause hypoxaemia, this is more severe if solids are involved. *Pulmonary oedema* occasionally occurs in head-injured patients. Obstruction of the airway is known to be a cause and this probably accounts for some cases, but it is believed that the condition of 'neurogenic' pulmonary oedema is an entity. Such patients may appear to 'froth at the mouth' and tend to have severe injuries.

Hypoxaemia is also caused by chest injuries, fat embolism and adult respiratory distress syndrome (ARDS). Always remember that the hypoxaemic effect of any ventilation/perfusion abnormality (all of the above) is aggravated by a *reduced cardiac output*, due to increased oxygen extraction in hypoperfused tissues.

All head-injured patients should receive additional oxygen, have their arterial haemoglobin saturation constantly monitored with an oximeter and have arterial hypotension promptly treated.

Deranged intracranial physiology

Intracranial pressure (ICP)
The dura mater is a tough membrane that contains blood, cerebrospinal fluid (CSF), brain and spinal cord. The dural sac in the spinal canal is distensible, so that CSF can be displaced into it from the head if an increase in volume of the blood or brain occurs. This displacement of CSF can prevent a rise in intracranial pressure, but ICP may rise *sharply* when the capacity of the system is exhausted. Thus a factor such as vasodilatation superimposed on cerebral swelling can cause large rises in ICP.

Cerebral blood flow (CBF)
The brain is a high-blood-flow, low-volume system. It contains about 200 ml of blood, but takes a fifth of the cardiac output. Brain cells are easily damaged by ischaemia. The cerebral blood flow is 'autoregulated' so that a reasonably constant flow is maintained despite variations in blood pressure (Fig. 15.1). It is believed that the ability to autoregulate is lost in damaged brain, so that flow becomes directly related to pressure. Hypotension is then more likely to produce cerebral ischaemia and hypertension to produce a hyperaemic brain.

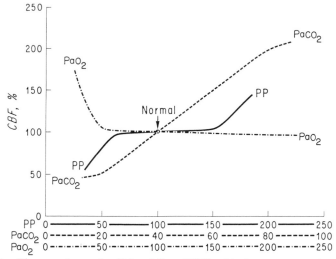

Fig. 15.1　Changes in cerebral blood flow (CBF) with changes in perfusion pressure (PP), the arterial CO_2 tension ($PaCO_2$) and the arterial O_2 tension (PaO_2). Reproduced with permission, from *Anaesthesia and the Brain*, Michenfelder J D. Churchill-Livingstone, New York 1988.

The *carbon dioxide* tension has profound effects on CBF in normal brain (Fig. 15.1). Cerebral vasoconstriction is the normal result of hyperventilation but the effect usually wears off in a matter of hours. The response is believed to be absent or even paradoxical in some cases of brain injury.

Raised intracranial pressure
The normal ICP is about zero, 25 mmHg is raised and 50 mmHg usually fatal (although ICP can be even higher if it rises slowly, as in 'benign' intracranial

hypertension). Rises in ICP after head injury are caused by *haematomas, 'swelling'* or *vasodilatation* in the face of exhausted compensatory mechanisms. Raised ICP may interfere with *cerebral perfusion* and expanding lesions can cause *internal herniation*.

The measurement of ICP would seem to be of obvious benefit to unconscious head-injured patients; in some centres it is routine, yet in others it is rarely practised. It is surprisingly difficult to demonstrate a clear benefit from an aggressive approach to ICP measurement and there is definite morbidity, principally infection, associated with the insertion of ICP-measuring systems. The most reliable readings are obtained from intraventricular catheters which have the worst infection risk and are the most difficult to place. The accuracy of subdural and extradural systems has often been criticized but technological advances, such as fibreoptic systems, have improved reliability so that ICP measurement is likely to be more widely practised.

Cerebral 'swelling'

This intentionally vague term is used to describe cerebral oedema on computerized tomography (CT) scans. Cerebral oedema is thought to be leakage from either blood vessels ('vasogenic') or brain cells ('cytotoxic') and both types may be present. Vasogenic oedema is the result of physical trauma or hyperaemia. Cytotoxic oedema can be caused by hypoxaemia and ischaemia.

Haematomas

These can be extradural, subdural or intracerebral and more than one type may be present. They reduce conscious level (disorientation is a reduction in conscious level) and are more likely in patients with skull fractures. The risk of haematoma can be estimated on the basis of the presence or absence of these two factors (Table 15.3).

Table 15.3 The risk of haematoma based on the presence of abnormal consciousness and/or fracture

Abnormal consciousness	Fracture	Risk
−	−	1:6000
+	−	1:120
−	+	1:32
+	+	1:4

Intracranial haematomas are diagnosed by CT scanning; it is currently recommended that all patients with a skull fracture or a persisting abnormality of consciousness should be scanned.

Vasodilatation

An increase in cerebral blood volume due to vasodilatation may produce a rise in ICP if compensatory shifts in CSF are impossible. Waves of raised

ICP are seen in patients with brain tumours or hydrocephalus, but are unusual in head injuries. The waves are believed to be due to vasodilatation of the cerebral vessels against a background of exhausted compensation (Fig. 15.2). More sustained rises or spikes are seen in head-injured patients.

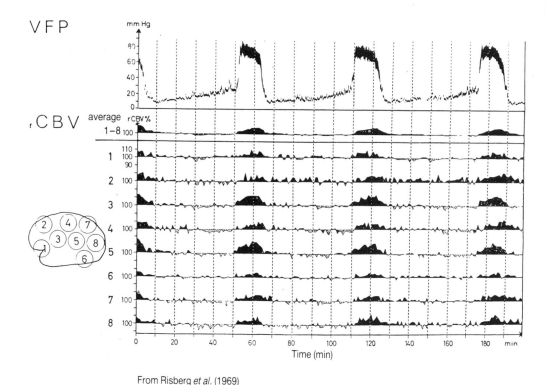

From Risberg *et al.* (1969)

Fig. 15.2   Coincident rises in cerebral blood volume (CBV) and intracranial (ventricular fluid) pressure (VFP). Reproduced, with permission, from Risberg et al. *Journal of Neurosurgery*, 1969; **31**: 303.

Cerebral perfusion

An adequate perfusion pressure is necessary to maintain cerebral function, particularly when autoregulation is obtunded. The *cerebral perfusion pressure* (CPP) is the mean arterial pressure minus the intracranial pressure. Poor perfusion leads to cerebral swelling, which leads to raised ICP, which leads to poor perfusion. Low blood pressures must be energetically treated. The CPP should never be less than 40 mmHg. An excessively high cerebral blood flow may also promote swelling by producing a *hyperaemic* brain, so that arterial hypertension must also be avoided. Jugular venous oxygenation has been used as a guide to cerebral perfusion. An oximetric catheter is placed in the internal jugular vein. The oxygen content of the jugular blood reflects cerebral hyperaemia or ischaemia.

Patients with raised ICP sometimes develop hypertension and occasionally a bradycardia (the 'Cushing response'), but it is not a constant sign. Chronically-raised ICP produces papilloedema and sixth nerve palsies, but deterioration in conscious level is the principal sign in acute rises.

Internal herniation

An expanding lesion in the cranial cavity may cause herniation of either the forebrain through the tentorium cerebelli, or of the brainstem through the foramen magnum. Both types of hernia cause paralysis of the vital centres. Tentorial herniation produces a third nerve palsy ('blown a pupil'), since the third nerve nucleus lies in the upper pons. Respiratory arrest will eventually occur. Internal herniation is often described as 'coning'.

Associated injuries

The head injury may be only one of the patient's problems. Limb fractures and abdominal injuries frequently occur simultaneously and will cause hypovolaemia. Hypovolaemic shock does not occur as a result of a closed head injury since extravasation of about 200 ml of blood inside the skull will kill the patient. Correction of hypovolaemia is the next imperative after the airway. General anaesthesia will often be required in the treatment of other injuries, such as the stabilization of fractures. There is the theoretical possibility that the signs of an intracranial haematoma (i.e. loss of consciousness) will therefore be masked. But in most cases the priorities are clear and a natural order of treatment is established. Intracranial haematomas can present several days after the trauma so that there is little point in delaying treatment of other injuries.

Cervical-spine injuries are said to occur in up to 10 per cent of head-injured patients. Fortunately, neurological damage is often avoided and may occur in as few as 15 per cent of cervical-spine fractures. Cervical-spine radiographs are notoriously difficult to interpret and it should be remembered that an unstable spine can appear normal on a plain radiograph. No harm is done by putting a surgical collar on all patients until things are sorted out.

Management of head-injured patients

Analgesia will be required for painful injuries and must not be denied to head-injured patients. Opiates or synthetics such as pethidine do have sedative effects, but naloxone will reverse them if necessary. Small i.v. doses are better than i.m. administration, except for *codeine* which must *not* be given i.v. Some non-steroidal anti-inflammatory agents, such as diclofenac, may interfere with platelet function and are probably best avoided until the risk of haematoma has diminished.

Transfer of head-injured patients

The transfer of patients between hospitals, or even between different areas of the same hospital, has been shown to be associated with frequent episodes of hypoxaemia and swings in blood pressure. It is better to *intubate* and *ventilate* patients whose level of consciousness is deteriorating, before sending them to a neurosurgical centre. The effects of modern anaesthetic drugs can be rapidly and completely reversed on arrival if need be. Direct laryngoscopy and tracheal intubation cause a reflex hypertensive response, which may provoke a rise in ICP. More-or-less normal doses of hypnotic, analgesic and muscle-relaxant drugs will be required to safely intubate all but the most moribund patient. Nasotracheal intubation should be avoided if there is epistaxis or CSF rhinorrhoea (intubation of the posterior fossa has been achieved through a base-of-skull fracture). A Ryle's tube should also be inserted.

It is poor practice to fail to *stabilize a patient's circulation* before transfer. A CVP line is useful if there are doubts about the extent of fluid loss and, since carotid damage and pneumothorax are both unhelpful in these patients, there is something to be said for cannulating the femoral vein using a 'Seldinger' technique. Glucose-containing fluids should be avoided in the replacement of losses (see below). Judicious use of a sympathomimetic drug (ephedrine is easiest to use) is often valuable in hypotensive patients.

The negative effect of hypoxaemic and hypotensive insults have been seen in Table 15.1. The same authors have proposed a checklist shown in Table 15.4.

Table 15.4   Checklist—before transfer of a head-injured patient

Respiration	Is the Po_2 at least 100 mmHg? Is the Pco_2 no more than 40 mmHg? Is the airway clear? Is it adequately protected for the journey? Does the patient need intubation or ventilation?
Circulation	Is the systolic BP at least 100 mmHg? Is the pulse rate no more than 100/min? Is there peripheral perfusion? Is there a reliable i.v. line?
Other injuries	Has a cervical spine/chest injury been excluded? Could there be a haemo-pneumothorax? Could there be an abdominal bleed? Are there pelvic or long bone fractures?
Escort	Are the escorting doctor and nurse adequately experienced? Have they had proper instructions? What equipment and drugs have they got? Are the casenotes and radiographs with them?

Anaesthetic technique

Anaesthesia can be local, regional (e.g. spinal) or general. Whatever is done to the head-injured patient must have regard to the considerations above. Thus the airway must be absolutely guaranteed and the circulation must be neither too full nor too empty. Local anaesthesia will only cope with relatively minor surgery, and spinals and epidurals are contraindicated if there is a possibility of raised ICP, since a lumbar CSF leak may precipitate coning.

General anaesthesia

Guaranteeing the airway will mean tracheal intubation in most cases. As previously mentioned, direct laryngoscopy and intubation can cause marked hypertension, which can be reduced by i.v. lignocaine given 3 minutes before the procedure (1.5 mg/kg). Cervical movement should be avoided if instability is suspected, for fear of precipitating cord damage. Flexible fibreoptic intubation may be safer than direct laryngoscopy in unstable patients.

The volatile anaesthetic agents produce cerebral vasodilatation, halothane the most and isoflurane the least. They all cause respiratory depression and hypercarbia if the patient breathes spontaneously and hypercarbia produces cerebral vasodilatation, which can result in raised ICP. In theory hypercarbia must be avoided by controlling respiration and any tendency to vasodilatation minimized by using isoflurane. It has been pointed out by Michenfelder of the Mayo Clinic, the doyen of neuroanaesthesia, that there is remarkably little evidence that much harm was done in the days when patients breathed halothane spontaneously.

Nitrous oxide increases the volume of air-spaces in the body (e.g. pneumothorax) and should be avoided if intracranial air is seen on radiographs.

Neurological intensive care

Many head-injured patients require intensive observation, nursing, physiotherapy and effort generally. The aim of intensive care is the efficient management of the problems previously mentioned. The best results are likely to be obtained in units dealing with reasonable numbers of patients. Simple physical points, such as promoting good cerebral venous drainage by head-up tilt and 'fore and aft' head orientation are important. Control of the respiratory and cardiovascular systems is often necessary to ensure adequate cerebral oxygenation and perfusion.

Control of intracranial pressure

Hypoxaemia, hypercarbia, hypotension, hypertension, mechanical obstruction to venous drainage, hydrocephalus and haematoma must all be excluded. The ideal neurointensive care unit would be built around a CT scanner and an operating theatre. After making these exclusions we are left with the control of cerebral swelling. *Mannitol* is the mainstay of treatment, in a dose of 0.5 g/kg over 20 minutes. If swelling is due to hyperaemia (often said to be the case in penetrating injuries), then cerebral vasoconstriction with i.v. anaesthetic agents such as *thiopentone* or *propofol* may be more appropriate. Both these drugs are prone to cause hypotension and must be used with care. Vasoconstriction caused by induced hypocarbia (i.e. patients on IPPV) may help, although such patients are usually already ventilated to ensure oxygenation.

'Cerebral protection'

A drug which would protect the brain from the effects of ischaemia and hypoxaemia would obviously be a good thing. The search for such a substance continues. There is no doubt that *hypothermia* does protect the brain, but there is a tendency to ventricular fibrillation at the temperatures at which substantial protection occurs (i.e. less than 30°C). Drugs that decrease cerebral oxygen consumption have been investigated. *Thiopentone* has been shown to have a protective effect if administered before the brain is injured, but this is rarely practical. Nevertheless it is a useful drug because of its vasoconstrictor effect on the cerebral vessels. *Isoflurane* has been recommended, since it drastically reduces cerebral metabolism without seriously decreasing cardiac output or producing cerebral vasodilatation. Low concentrations of isoflurane have been used for sedating ventilated patients.

Calcium-entry blockers such as *nimodipine* have been shown to improve the outcome after subarachnoid haemorrhage, but whether this expensive drug is beneficial after head injury is not known. It is believed that 'excitatory amino acids' (EAA) such as glutamine are responsible for tissue damage after ischaemia and drugs that are *EAA blockers* are being investigated. It is also believed that ischaemic brain suffers from the action of lactate ions produced from glucose by anaerobic metabolism. It has been shown that experimental animals suffer less cerebral damage if glucose is excluded from i.v. drips. Therefore it seems wise to *avoid glucose* drips where possible, especially if an episode of cerebral ischaemia is anticipated. Membrane-stabilizing drugs like *lignocaine* and *phenytoin* have been claimed to have some protective action, but steroids have been extensively studied and there is no evidence of any beneficial effect in head-injured patients.

It must be emphasized that adequate cerebral *perfusion* and *oxygenation* are the basis of all cerebral 'protection'.

Prognosis

It is not possible to prognosticate accurately in an individual case, however the work of Brian Jennett and his colleagues in Glasgow has provided broad indicators. *Age* is a major factor; pessimism about the outcome must increase with age. If a patient has *fixed pupils* or *absent eye movements* for 24 hours, then there is a 95 per cent expectation of death or serious disablement. If coma persists the chances of recovery decrease, so that after 4 weeks of coma one must expect 70 per cent of survivors to lead a vegetable existence.

Brainstem death (BSD)

What is death? The UK code for the diagnosis of brainstem death rests upon the belief that death of the brainstem means that the rest of the brain is as useless as if it had been cut off with an axe. This is because the *reticular activating system* (RAS) and the *respiratory centre* lie in the brainstem. The function of the RAS is to regulate consciousness; destruction of the RAS means permanent loss of consciousness. Destruction of the respiratory centre produces apnoea. Pallis has proposed a definition of death as the *'irreversible loss of the capacity for consciousness combined with irreversible loss of the capacity to breathe'*. In this country brainstem death is synonymous with death. The conference of the UK Medical Royal Colleges and their Faculties, entitled their publications on the diagnosis of brainstem death, 'Diagnosis of Death'.

Mechanical ventilation emerged as a treatment in the 1950s; patients who would otherwise have died from respiratory arrest could be maintained by a ventilator. It was soon appreciated that ventilator technology had produced a new clinical problem, termed 'coma depasse' in one of the first (1959) publications on the subject. The patient in this state 'beyond coma', provides an extremely distressing spectacle for relatives, nurses and all others concerned. The first brain death criteria were produced from Harvard in 1968. The UK code was published in 1976.

Incidence of brainstem death
A survey of English intensive care units in 1989 revealed that there had been 1200 confirmed cases of brainstem death. The survey also enquired into organ donations and found that half these cases became organ donors. Permission for organ donations was not sought in only 6 per cent of cases and 70 per cent of requests were granted. These figures suggest that making organ-donation requests compulsory would have little effect on supply.

Causes of brainstem death
The mechanism of brainstem death is usually internal herniation or severe intracranial hypertension preventing perfusion. Roughly half the cases are due to head injury and about a third of cases are due to intracranial haemorrhage which is often assocated with a ruptured aneurysm. Encephalitis, abscess, meningitis, hypoxic encephalopathy can all also cause brainstem death as a result of brain swelling. A cause no longer encountered in this country is judicial hanging, which may produce rupture of the brainstem.

Transplantation and brainstem death
An episode of BBC television's Panorama programme screened in 1980, claimed that patients were being declared brain dead and their organs used for transplantation, when they were not. There was a terrific row. Panorama's claims were based on a misunderstanding of the code and were refuted. It is important to understand that the concept of brainstem death was developed before transplantation was a regular part of surgical treatment. It would make no difference to the number of patients declared brainstem dead if transplants stopped.

The diagnosis of brainstem death
There are three stages in this diagnosis, which must be taken in this order:
- the preconditions
- the exclusions
- the tests

The preconditions

There can be absolutely no question of the diagnosis of BSD being entertained unless these are fulfilled. The preconditions are that the patient is *unconscious* and *apnoeic*, the *cause is known* and is *irreversible*.

The crucial point is that it must be clear **why** the patient is in his lamentable condition and that treatment is not possible. It is, as always, a matter of history, examination and investigation. The causes of BSD have been mentioned. The CT scan of a patient who fulfilled the preconditions is shown in Fig. 15.3. He complained of severe headache during sexual intercourse, became unconscious and after admission to hospital became apnoeic. The scan shows massive intracerebral and intraventricular haemorrhage.

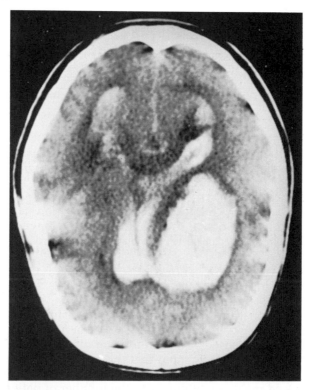

Fig. 15.3 CT scan showing massive intracerebral and intraventricular haemorrhage with blood in the fourth ventricle.

Exclusions

When a patient has fulfilled the preconditions, the UK code demands that reversible causes of depression of brainstem function are excluded. These are *hypothermia* (35°C or less), *drug intoxication* and *metabolic* or *endocrine* disturbance.

Drug intoxication may occasionally cause difficulty, which can always be resolved by allowing time to pass. Three days has been suggested as a safe period.

The tests

The tests demonstrate that brainstem functions have ceased.

Apnoea
The ventilator is disconnected but oxygen is insufflated through a catheter into the tracheal tube. The $PaCO_2$ must rise to 6.65 kPa (50 mmHg). A period of disconnection of about 15 minutes is usually necessary to achieve this. Oxygen insufflation is remarkably successful in preventing hypoxaemia. The record apnoeic survival on insufflation was reported from Sweden (3 hours 20 minutes).

Fixed pupils
The pupils are usually mid point, rather than large; but they must be fixed, despite a bright-light stimulus.

Absent corneal reflex
There must be no blink in response to the cornea being touched with a swab.

Absent vestibulo-ocular reflex
This reflex is also known as the 'caloric' test. Ice-cold water is injected onto the eardrum (at least 20 ml). Any movement of the eye in response indicates that the brainstem retains some function. The patency of the ear canal must be checked before testing.

Absent motor response
There is no motor response in the cranial nerve distribution to any stimulation. If a painful stimulus is applied to the toe of a BSD patient there may be reflex withdrawal of the leg but no grimacing. Withdrawal reflexes can sometimes be quite dramatic, a 'Lazarus' syndrome has been described with the patient appearing to rise from the bed. Such reflexes, due to spinal arcs, must be distinguished from fits or flexor and extensor posturing, which imply that there is traffic through the brainstem. If there is any doubt the diagnosis of BSD cannot be made.

Absent gag reflex
There is no response to stimulation of the glottis or bronchial tree. There should be no response to pushing the endotracheal tube in and out, or to a suction catheter pushed into the bronchus.

Oculocephalic reflex
The oculocephalic or doll's-head reflex is sometimes mentioned in connection with BSD but does not form part of the UK code. Many people find this reflex a bit confusing; remember that there are two sorts of doll, the china type with painted-on eyes and the 'lifelike' variety with swivelling eyes. The

test involves turning the patient's head from side to side and observing his eye movements.

- non-functioning brainstem—the eyes do not move (china doll)
- functioning brainstem—the eyes move (swivel-eyed doll)

Who makes the diagnosis?

The UK code stipulates that two doctors, one a consultant, the other a senior registrar or consultant, should make the diagnosis. They should have 'skill in this matter'. Neurologists, anaesthetists, neurosurgeons or ITU physicians are generally considered appropriate. It is difficult to imagine that there would be objection to any suitably-ranked doctor who had understood the procedure making the diagnosis. The doctors must *repeat* their diagnosis after an interval. No set or minimum interval is prescribed, most would regard about 3 hours as a minimum.

Has there ever been a 'mistake'?

Not that we know of. The majority of patients diagnosed BSD are disconnected from the ventilator and circulatory arrest ensues in about 20 minutes. It would be difficult to detect a mistake in such circumstances. However, not all patients have been disconnected, many have been ventilated to asystole and none have recovered. If ventilation is continued after the diagnosis of BSD, circulatory arrest will occur within a few days, rarely longer. The UK code is rigorous, observation of its practice is convincing.

Further reading

Andrews P J D, Piper I R, Dearden N M, Miller J D. Secondary insults during intrahospital transport of head injured patients. *Lancet* 1990; **335**: 327–30.

Campkin T V, Turner J M. *Neurosurgical Anaesthesia and Intensive Care*. London: Butterworths, 1986.

Gentleman D, Jennett B. Audit of unconscious head injured patients to a neurosurgical unit. *Lancet* 1990; **335**: 330–4.

Jennett B, Teasdale G, Davis F A. *Management of Head Injuries*. Philadelphia 1982.

Lindsay K W, Bone I, Callander R. *Neurology and Neurosurgery Illustrated*. Edinburgh: Churchill Livingstone, 1986.

Michenfelder J D. *Anesthesia and the Brain*. New York: Churchill Livingstone, 1988.

Pallis C. *ABC Of Brain Stem Death*. London: BMJ Publications, 1989.

Risberg *et al*. Coincident rises in cerebral blood volume and intracranial (ventricular fluid) pressure. *Journal of Neurosurgery* 31; **303**: 1969.

Teasdale G M, Murray G, Andersen E, *et al*. Risks of acute traumatic haematoma in children and adults: implications for managing head injuries. *British Medical Journal* 1990; **300**: 363–7.

16

Metabolism and endocrinology
J.A. Gil-Rodriguez

Pancreas

There are two different types of glandular tissue in the pancreas. The endocrine Islets of Langerhans which generate glucagon (alpha cells), insulin (beta cells) and somatostatin (delta cells); and the exocrine acini which secrete digestive juices into the duodenum.

Endocrine function

Diabetes mellitus

Diabetes is a chronic carbohydrate-metabolic disorder which results in abnormally high blood glucose levels. It can affect two different types of patients; the young who always require treatment with insulin to prevent ketoacidosis, and an older age group who, generally speaking, do not need insulin and can be controlled with oral hypoglycaemic drugs and/or diet.

In the young, if the insulin deficiency is severe amino acids are released from muscle and free fatty acids from adipose tissue. These are taken up by the liver which in turn releases glucose and ketone bodies. The level of glucose and ketone bodies in the blood rises and this leads to the well-known symptoms of diabetes; polyuria, dehydration and acidosis. In the older obese patient, there appears to be a degree of insulin resistance which is due to a decrease in receptors for insulin. Such patients show elevated blood levels of insulin and glucose.

A common complication of diabetes is retinopathy which affects about 75 per cent of diabetics with the passage of time. Laser photocoagulation and vitrectomy are useful in preserving and restoring vision. Renal failure presents in about half of all young diabetics, and myocardial infarction, hypertension and congestive heart failure are not uncommon, often associated with uraemia. On the other hand, diabetic neuropathy is not necessarily related to the level of blood glucose but possibly to the accumulation in the nerve cells of sorbitol, a byproduct of glucose metabolism. Vascular involvement appears at an early age in diabetics and frequently manifests itself in the extremities, particularly in the feet where ulceration is common. Secondary infection of these ulcers is a frequent reason for hospital admission.

Diagnosis

Symptoms suggestive of the diagnosis of diabetes are polyuria, thirst and eventually acidosis. Vision and peridontal problems and minor soft-tissue infections may also alert the doctor to the diagnosis. An elevated fasting blood glucose strongly supports the diagnosis of diabetes mellitus. However, even if this test is normal, a glucose-tolerance test may reveal diabetes. A normal glucose-tolerance test will exclude a diagnosis of diabetes.

Preoperative assessment and management

Approximately 25 per cent of all diabetic patients about to undergo surgery are undiagnosed on admission to hospital. Any patient presenting for surgery who is obese and over 60 years old should be investigated for diabetes.

Assessment of the diabetic prior to surgery and anaesthesia should include cardiovascular and renal-function tests, blood glucose and electrolyte determinations (particularly as hypokalaemia is a major factor in the development of severe cardiac arrhythmias during the induction of anaesthesia).

Serum creatinine should be preferred to blood urea nitrogen in the assessment of renal function. Urine analysis may demonstrate hyperglycaemia (glucose), poor control of the disease (ketones), renal complications (protein) and infection (bacteria).

A review of the medication may show that drugs which can produce or contribute to hyperglycaemia are being taken, e.g. thiazide and loop diuretics like frusemide. Immunosuppressive drugs are also known to produce mild hyperglycaemia and beta adrenoceptor antagonists, although not altering blood-glucose levels, can obscure the symptoms of acute hypoglycaemia.

Perioperative and postoperative management

Peri- and postoperative management of the diabetic has been greatly simplified with the introduction of continuous i.v. infusions of insulin. As little as 5 units of soluble insulin per hour, given as a continuous i.v. infusion, can prevent or reverse even quite severe ketoacidosis. Several treatment regimens are popular, all based on the use of i.v. glucose, with insulin given simultaneously by pump or infusion. In all patients the longer-acting forms of insulin need substituting with a short-acting insulin (soluble or actrapid) at least 24 hours before surgery.

For insulin-dependent patients who present for elective surgery, a continuous infusion of glucose and insulin should be set up preoperatively and continued during anaesthesia and into the postoperative period until the patient is able to resume normal oral intake. Potassium should be added to the infusion as insulin drives potassium into the cells and serum hypokalaemia may result. If the treatment is to continue for a long time, the infusion should be given through a central catheter to prevent thrombophlebitis. An Alberti infusion regimen of 10 per cent dextrose 500 ml plus 10 units soluble insulin and 10 mmol KCl 100 ml to run over 4–6 hours, has the advantage of simplicity. Blood glucose and serum potassium should be estimated before starting the infusion and thereafter every 2–3 hours. During surgery and anaesthesia blood glucose should be estimated every 30 minutes using the 'stix' method (BM stix or Dextrostix); using a reflectometer increases accuracy. This i.v. regimen should be continued as long as the blood glucose is between 5 and 10 mmol/litre. If the blood sugar falls to less than 5 mmol/litre, the insulin infusion should be reduced to 1 unit/h by decreasing the rate to 50 ml/h. Conversely, if blood glucose rises to between 10 and 20 mmol/litre, the infusion should be increased to 150 ml/h (3 units of insulin/h).

The advantage of this regimen over others is the flexibility of dosage and the inherent safety of giving the insulin and dextrose together. This lessens the chance of hypo- or hyperglycaemia if an accidental change in the rate occurs (the proportions remain the same).

An alternative to the i.v. infusion of insulin is the 'sliding-scale' technique. The urine is checked postoperatively every 4 hours and if the urine shows 1–2 per cent glucose, then an extra 5–10 units of soluble insulin is administered subcutaneously. If significant ketonuria is present an extra 5 units of soluble insulin are administered in addition to the amount required to cover the glycosuria. The sliding scale must be adjusted by occasionally correlating the urine glucose with the blood glucose level.

For the non-insulin dependent diabetic presenting for minor surgery, omission of the morning dose of the oral hypoglycaemic agent and preoperative starvation with regular perioperative blood-glucose estimations, is sufficient. Those patients on long-acting agents such as chlorpropramide are at risk from hypoglycaemia. The non-insulin dependent diabetic presenting for major surgery should be managed in the same way as the insulin-dependent diabetic.

Emergency surgery in the uncontrolled diabetic is a serious undertaking. Surgery should not be commenced until ketoacidosis is under control, usually within 8–12 hours of establishing i.v. insulin, electrolyte and acid-base therapy. A regimen combining the i.v. infusion of insulin (5–7 units/h) and repeated boluses of i.v. insulin every 2–3 hours (1–2 units/kg body weight), should be established under strict supervision. If after

3–4 hours the ketoacidosis has not been significantly reduced then the regimen will have to be altered by doubling the amount of the initial insulin bolus or by increasing the i.v. infusion rate of insulin from 5 units to 10 units/h.

The object of the preoperative management is not to try and correct all imbalances immediately because attempting to achieve this may produce dangerous swings in plasma osmolality, leading to possible cerebral oedema, and imbalances in plasma and CSF pH which will disturb the ventilatory compensation of acidosis. It should be sufficient to correct acute hypovolaemia and produce a falling blood sugar, indicating that glucose is entering muscle and adipose tissue. Acidosis should only be treated if it is potentially life-threatening (pH below 7.1). It is treated by administering bicarbonate 1 mmol/kg body weight over the first 1–2 hours. Potassium should be added to the i.v. infusion (Table 16.1).

Table 16.1   Treatment protocol for diabetic patients presenting for surgery

	Non-insulin dependent (NIDDM)	Insulin dependent (IDDM)
Elective surgery		
Minor	• omit tablets • preoperative fast • frequent blood-glucose estimations • 5% dextrose i.v. if patient on long-acting sulphonylurea drug	• omit insulin • preoperative fast • frequent blood-glucose estimations • *Alberti* regimen i.v. (10% dextrose + 10 mmol K^+ + 10 units insulin)
Major	as for IDDM	as for minor surgery
Emergency surgery	as for IDDM	as for minor surgery [plus] • correct ketoacidosis • correct volume deficit with 0.9% saline i.v. • correct severe metabolic acidosis with sodium bicarbonate

During anaesthesia IPPV is mandatory in all patients with ketoacidosis in order to control their $Paco_2$. Blood gases are checked immediately before induction of anaesthesia and this $Paco_2$ is regarded as the physiological optimum for the correction of the patient's metabolic acidosis. Ventilation to normocapnia may induce an acute and dangerous fall in the pH and to hypocapnia a serious reduction in cardiac output. Therefore, the infusion of bicarbonate and the reduction of ventilation to allow a rise in $Paco_2$, may prove to be the correct therapy. However, great care should be taken to to prevent swings in pH and serum potassium which can be extremely dangerous and sufficient to produce cardiac arrest.

Hyperinsulinism

This syndrome, characterized by fasting or postprandial hypoglycaemia, is generally due to an insulin-secreting tumour of the pancreas (insulinoma). These are rare tumours of the Islet cells which can be malignant (10 per cent of cases) but more commonly they are single benign adenomas, although occasionally they can be multiple or ectopic (liver). The diagnosis can be very difficult as can surgical removal since only about two-thirds of these tumours can be localized at surgery.

The main anaesthetic problem is the avoidance of hypoglycaemia during surgery, it must be corrected immediately by the rapid infusion of 5–15 per cent dextrose through a centrally-placed catheter. Blood glucose levels must be monitored throughout surgery, as handling of the tumour causes hypoglycaemia. The stix method of monitoring is rapid but can be quite inaccurate at low and high blood glucose levels. However, it can be very useful if combined with a spectrophotometer which can accurately read the purple colour of the dextrostix. This measurement will take less than 60 seconds to perform and will enable the anaesthetist to monitor accurately blood glucose levels throughout the surgical procedures. There may be a temporary postoperative hyperglycaemia resembling frank diabetes and requiring treatment with insulin. This state is transient unless more than 90 per cent of the pancreas has been removed.

Adrenal glands

Located at the superior pole of the kidneys, the adrenal glands are formed by two embryologically distinct parts, the medulla and the cortex.

Adrenal cortex

The adrenal cortex is a true endocrine gland, essential for life and secreting hydrocortisone, aldosterone and androgens, all of which derive from cholesterol.

Hydrocortisone and androgen production and release are controlled by the anterior pituitary adrenocorticotrophic hormone (ACTH). In turn ACTH is controlled by corticotrophin releasing factor (CRF) present in the hypothalamus. The serum level of hydrocortisone, through a closed negative-feedback loop, inhibits both ACTH and CRF. The principal role of hydrocortisone is in the control of anti-inflammatory and immune responses and the body reaction to stress. Thus in acute stress such as trauma, haemorrhage, infection, surgery, anaesthesia, etc., enormous surges of hydrocortisone production can take place. Hydrocortisone also has an important role in the maintenance of blood glucose levels as it stimulates glucose production by the liver and antagonizes insulin.

The main physiological function of aldosterone is the maintenance of blood pressure when the patient is in an upright position. It also has profound effects in the distal renal tubule, stimulating sodium reabsorption and renal loss of potassium, hydrogen ions and magnesium.

The control of aldosterone secretion is rather complex and related to the juxtaglomerular apparatus of the kidney. Low extracellular volume results in renin stimulation which in turn brings about the synthesis of angiotensin I. Angiotensin I is converted to angiotensin II in the lungs. Angiotensin II, an important peripheral vasoconstrictor, is also a potent stimulator of aldosterone production which in turn corrects the deficient extracellular volume.

Malfunction of the adrenal cortex is of importance to the anaesthetist because of over and underproduction of glucocorticoid, iatrogenic suppression of the adrenal cortex and overproduction of aldosterone.

Adrenocortical hyperfunction

Cushing's syndrome results from overproduction of glucocorticoids which, in about 80 per cent of the cases, is due to bilateral adrenal hyperplasia secondary to excessive secretion of ACTH by a tumour of the pituitary gland or from an ectopic site (carcinoma of lung, kidney, pancreas or thymus).

Patients with excess glucocorticoid production present with the classic constellation of signs and symptoms which are related to the degree and duration of the disease. Thus there may be potassium depletion and muscle weakness, poor healing and abnormal glucose tolerance. Protein catabolism reduces muscle bulk and osteoporosis is common. Immune response and fibroblastic activity are inhibited. The treatment is by surgical removal of the source of excess ACTH or glucocorticoids.

Patients with Cushing's syndrome are extremely fragile. Diabetes, hypertension, electrolyte abnormalities (hypokalaemia) and osteoporosis can all co-exist. Care should be taken when positioning the patient for surgery because of the danger of causing bone fractures or skin damage. Muscle weakness will necessitate IPPV for all but the shortest operations. Intravenous infusions of small quantities of insulin may be required to control elevation of blood glucose peri and postoperatively.

Hypertension, which is often related to significant blood volume increases associated with polycythaemia and sodium retention, may require perioperative treatment to control sudden surges of catecholamine released during handling of the adrenal glands.

Adrenocortical insufficiency

Addison's disease, or primary adrenocortical insufficiency, affects both sexes and all ages. It can be caused by granulomatous diseases such as histoplasmosis, tuberculosis and metastatic disease. Haemorrhage, amyloid and leukaemic infiltrations and autoimmune disorders are also common causes and in most cases both cortisol and aldosterone are lacking. When the adrenal insufficiency is secondary to a lack of pituitary ACTH, aldosterone secretion remains normal.

The onset of Addison's disease is often insidious. Patients feel generally unwell, weak and present with anorexia, nausea, vomiting, abdominal pains and weight loss. Hypotension is an important finding and is usually posture sensitive. There may be coexistent diabetes mellitus, hypothyroidism and hypoparathyroidism. Excessive skin pigmentation occurs, particularly in exposed parts of the body.

The diagnosis is made by a reduced plasma-cortisol response to ACTH. Therapy is with long-term cortisol administration (cortisone acetate or flurocortisone). The known chronic cases of adrenocortical insufficiency present few operative problems to the anaesthetist and should be treated as patients on long-term steroid therapy. However, problems may arise in patients with an acute illness who require surgery and are not previously known to have adrenocortical insufficiency. Preoperative blood glucose and electrolyte determination, and reversal of the intravascular volume depletion is an essential part of the treatment. Hyponatraemia and hypokalaemia require correction, and glucose administration to counteract hypoglycaemia should be instituted as soon as possible. Hydrocortisone given as an i.v. bolus followed by an infusion will be necessary and should be continued postoperatively on a regimen similar to that for patients with iatrogenic suppression of the adrenal cortex.

Management of patients receiving long-term corticosteroid replacement

Patients present for surgery on long-term steroid therapy mainly if they are being treated for asthma, rheumatoid arthritis, SLE, etc. The degree of adrenal suppression and cushingoid status will depend upon the maintenance dose and the length of corticosteroid treatment. These patients may be unable to increase their cortical output in response to surgery and will require replacement therapy starting before surgery with, for example, hydrocortisone 100 mg i.m. 6 hourly for about 3 days before major surgery or for 1 day before minor surgery. Alternatively, an infusion of 100 mg hydrocortisone over 24 hours, preceded by 25 mg given as an i.v. injection, will generally be sufficient for uncomplicated surgery. Another alternative preferred by some is the i.m. injection of a long-acting steroid preparation such as methyl prednisolone, 40 mg daily for 2–3 days before surgery. Postoperatively all causes of hypotension must be excluded before increasing steroid intake in response to apparent acute adrenal crisis.

Adrenal medulla

The adrenal medulla forms part of the sympathetic nervous system, secreting adrenaline and noradrenaline into the circulation. To the anaesthetist only catecholamine-secreting tumours of the medulla are of importance. These rare tumours, known as phaeochromocytomas because of their dark colour, cause a disease characterized by hypertension that may be sustained or paroxysmal. About 60 per cent of the tumours secrete noradrenaline (predominantly an alpha stimulant) producing an increase in peripheral resistance, thus increasing both systolic and diastolic blood pressures and reducing heart rate.

Only 5 per cent of the tumours secrete adrenaline alone (both alpha and beta effects but predominantly beta) with a net result of increased heart rate, cardiac output and systolic blood pressure.

The symptoms of phaeochromocytoma consist of attacks of headaches, palpitations, sweating, abdominal pain, nausea, irritability, visual disturbances, weight loss, angina and fainting spells related to posture. The diagnosis is confirmed by elevated catecholamine levels in urine and blood, and by high levels of vanillyl mandelic acid (VMA) in urine. The tumour can occasionally be localized by aortogram or pyelogram when it is seen as a posterior mass between the kidney and the diaphragm. Most cases are diagnosed preoperatively but sometimes the condition is first noted during unrelated abdominal surgery or during pregnancy.

Surgery is virtually the only cure for patients with phaeochromocytomas. Preparation for surgery should be started well in advance. The aim should be to produce a good adrenergic-receptor blockade preoperatively. Once the patient has been controlled with adequate alpha blockade, beta adrenoceptor antagonists may also be used, especially if tachyarrhythmias are a problem.

A good premedication will reduce catecholamine release. Anaesthetic agents to be avoided are halothane, because of its low threshold for catecholamine-induced dysrhythmias, and curare and alcuronium, because they may release histamine and thus aggravate catecholamine secretion.

Accurate and constant monitoring is absolutely necessary because of the rapid and sudden changes in circulation caused by the release of catecholamines. Pulmonary-artery-wedge pressure, intra-arterial blood pressure ECG, CVP and urinary output should all be monitored. Good, multiple venous accesses should be established in order to rapidly infuse the patient with blood and crystalloid fluids, and for the administration of drugs as necessary.

During surgery short-acting hypotensive agents, e.g. nitroprusside, can be used to deal with surges of catecholamine release and hypertensive crises as the surgeon handles the tumour. These surges can be minimized by early clamping of the venous drainage. Arrhythmias require treatment with the injection of beta adrenoceptor antagonists (propranolol).

Hypotension occurring after the tumour has been removed should be treated with fluid replacement rather than with catecholamine infusion.

Pituitary gland

The anterior pituitary is connected to the hypothalamus by a complex portal-vascular system. The posterior pituitary stores vasopressin and oxytocin synthesized by neurones in the hypothalamus. Together the pituitary and the hypothalamus control the release of hormones concerned with growth, lactation, thyroid, adrenal and gonadal functions (anterior pituitary), and the state of hydration (posterior pituitary).

Anterior pituitary

Hyperfunction

Hyperfunction generally due to hyperfunctioning tumours secreting excess prolactin, ACTH or growth hormone. Gonadotrophin and thyrotrophin-secreting pituitary tumours are extremely rare. All tumours of the pituitary gland may cause neurological symptoms and signs, particularly visual-field defects because of pressure on the optic chiasma.

Prolactin-secreting tumours, apart from any space-occupying effects they may have, present no problem to the anaesthetist. ACTH-secreting tumours are the cause of about 80 per cent of all the cases of the adrenocortical-hyperfunction syndrome known as Cushing's syndrome which has already been discussed in this chapter. Excessive growth hormone secretion, when prolonged, leads to acromegaly, a chronic disease of middle life character-ized by overgrowth of bone, connective tissue and viscera (heart, liver and thyroid). This disease is important to the anaesthetist because treatment, if there is visual impairment, is surgical removal of the pituitary. Airway management may be difficult in these patients due to the large lips, jaw, tongue and epiglottis. Face-mask ventilation prior to intubation may be impossible. The larynx and vocal cords are often visualized with difficulty and tracheal intubation can be so difficult as to warrant prophylactic tracheostomy. In addition to the airway-management problems, these patients commonly have hypertension and diabetes mellitus.

Hypofunction

This clinical condition in which all or several of the hormones of the anterior pituitary may be involved, usually results from the destruction of the gland by tumour (i.e. chromophobe adenoma). It is accompanied by secondary atrophy of the gonads, the thyroid gland and the adrenal cortex; the underproduction of thyroid hormone and ACTH (Addison's disease) have important anaesthetic implications.

Posterior pituitary

Hypofunction

Deficient or low levels of antidiuretic hormone (ADH) secretion result in the disease known as diabetes insipidus which is characterized by impaired renal conservation of water. The majority of cases are of unknown aetiology but usually follow pituitary gland or hypothalamic trauma or surgery.

Patients present with polyuria and polydipsia. Large volumes of urine (up to 25–30 litres/day in extreme cases) of low specific gravity (under 1010) are produced. Plasma osmolality rises and polydipsia closely matches polyuria so that, unless fluid is withheld, dehydration does not occur. The condition is usually treated with desmopressin (an analogue to vasopressin) 10–12 µg nasally once daily. It can also be given i.m. or i.v. and should be preferred to vasopressin which may cause hypertension.

It is important to monitor urine output and serum osmolality in patients with diabetes insipidus presenting for surgery. Serum osmolality can be calculated from the sum of serum glucose and urea concentrations plus twice that of serum sodium and potassium. If the osmolality exceeds 290 mmol/litre (normal 283–285 mmol/litre), hypotonic fluids and desmopressin should be given i.v.

Thyroid gland

The main function of the thyroid gland is the secretion of thyroid hormones which are important in the regulation of tissue metabolism. The hormone produced in the thyroid is made up of 90 per cent thyroxine (T4), the remainder being triiodothyroxine (T3) which is more potent and short acting than T4. Iodine is essential for the formation of thyroid hormones.

Four steps are involved in the biosynthesis of thyroid hormones
- iodine capture
- oxidation of iodine
- hormone storage in the colloid of the thyroid gland as part of the thyroglobulin molecule
- proteolysis and release of hormones

All these steps are controlled by pituitary thyrotrophin stimulating hormone (TSH) which is secreted by the anterior pituitary gland. Proteolysis of stored hormone in the colloid is inhibited by potassium iodide. This occurs in the normal gland but is greatly exaggerated in the thyroid gland of patients with Graves' disease.

Thyroid hormone secretion is regulated by a specific feedback mechanism. Thyrotrophin releasing hormone (TRH) from the hypothalamus increases the anterior pituitary gland production of thyroid stimulating hormone (TSH) which in turn increases the formation of T4 and T3.

The importance of this gland to the anaesthetist arises because of the effect of excessive or deficient hormone secretion (hyperthyroidism or hypothyroidism), and because of the physical enlargement of the thyroid which may, or may not, be associated with gland dysfunction.

Hyperthyroidism

Graves' disease is the most common cause of hyperthyroidism. Generally these patients have a relatively symmetrical and diffusely enlarged thyroid gland, and exophthalmos. The symptoms of hyperthyroidism are those associated with excessive catecholamine production, such as tachycardia, heat intolerance, increased perspiration, tremor and weight loss. Catecholamine production is not increased in hyperthyroidism but it is possible that the receptor sites for catecholamines are increased with the net result that many of the presenting symptoms are similar to those of a phaeochromocytoma.

Other causes of hyperthyroidism are subcutaneous thyroiditis and autonomous nodular goitres which can show both 'hot' and 'cold' nodules on radioactive scanning. Less commonly hyperthyroidism can be due to TSH secreting pituitary tumours.

Young patients are usually treated with antithyroid drugs (i.e. carbimazole, prophylthiouracil or potassium perchlorate). If within 2–3 years there is no remission, then subtotal thyroidectomy is often recommended. Older patients who have been treated with radioactive iodine are euthyroid and often do not present for surgery. Many hyperthyroid patients may present treated with beta adrenoceptor antagonists to suppress tachycardia, but the merit of this method of treatment has yet to be completely proven.

Preoperatively, antithyroid drugs should be changed to oral iodine (i.e. potassium iodide 60 mg three times daily) in order to reduce the vascularity of the gland. Patients with a nodular goitre who have both 'hot' and 'cold' nodules present on a radioactive scan, should never be given iodine as it can penetrate the cold nodules of the thyroid and convert a non-functioning nodule into a hot nodule and so accentuate the hyperthyroidism.

There is no contraindication to the usual anaesthetic agents and techniques, but drugs which stimulate the sympathetic nervous system should be avoided. There may be a problem with certain patients who present with large thyroids extending retrosternally into the thorax. In some of these patients there is also deviation of the trachea which could make intubation difficult. Tracheal damage during surgery or tracheal collapse due to eroded tracheal cartilages, may require tracheotomy in the postoperative period. At extubation the vocal cords should be visualized to ensure that both sides are moving fully, as recurrent laryngeal nerve damage may have occurred during surgery.

Hypothyroidism

Also referred to as myxoedema (non-pitting oedema due to subcutaneous-tissue accumulation of mucopolysaccharide), it can be caused by surgical ablation, administration of radioactive iodine, irradiation to the neck (i.e. in Hodgkins' disease), iodine deficiency, secondary to hypothalamic or anterior pituitary dysfunction, and, by far the most common cause, chronic lymphocytic thyroiditis or Hashimoto's thyroiditis.

Myxoedema patients present with a variety of symptoms including cold intolerance, apathy, hoarseness, constipation, slow movements, anaemia and bradycardia.

The prognosis is excellent provided thyroid-replacement therapy is maintained. Euthyroid patients present no problem to the anaesthetist and should be treated as normal. Untreated patients should not have surgery until their hypothyroidism has been controlled with replacement-hormone treatment (50 µg/day of thyroxine) because there is a high mortality associated with surgery and untreated hypothyroidism.

A rare complication due to profound hypothyroidism is myxoedema coma. It presents with extreme lethargy, severe hypothermia, bradycardia and alveolar hypoventilation with hypoxia and hypercarbia. Occasionally may be accompanied by pericardial effusion and congestive heart failure.

The anaesthetist should avoid the use of respiratory depressant drugs in premedication and should reduce the dosage of all induction agents, analgesics and volatile agents. Carbon dioxide, oxygen and temperature monitoring during surgery should be mandatory, and hydrocortisone administration should be carried out if unexplained hypotension occurs (adrenocortical insufficiency).

Parathyroid glands

Located behind the thyroid, these small glands secrete parathyroid hormone (PTH) which, together with vitamin D, acts to maintain a normal plasma concentration of calcium.

When the ionized calcium decreases, released PTH increases tubular reabsorption of phosphate which raises plasma calcium. Another hormone, calcitonin, produced in the C cells of the thyroid gland, antagonizes the effect of PTH when there is a high plasma ionized-calcium concentration.

Approximately 50 per cent of the plasma calcium is bound to plasma proteins (albumin), 40 per cent is ionized and the remainder 10 per cent is bound to citrate. If the plasma protein concentration decreases, the total plasma calcium will also decrease. Conversely, if the plasma proteins increase, as occurs in myeloma, then the total plasma calcium will increase. Acidosis tends to increase the ionized calcium, while alkalosis tends to decrease it.

The importance of these glands to the anaesthetist arises because of the changes in plasma calcium concentration that follow excessive or deficient parathyroid secretion (hypercalcaemia or hypocalcaemia).

Hypercalcaemia

Hypercalcaemia may not only be the result of hyperparathyroidism but can also be caused by sarcoidosis, myeloma, malignant tumours of breast, lung and kidney, immobilization (Paget's disease and paraplegia), adrenal gland insufficiency, vitamin D intoxication, renal failure, etc.

Common symptoms of hypercalcaemia are nausea, vomiting, thirst, polyuria, dehydration, muscle fatigue and hypotonicity. ECG changes include prolonged P–R and shortened Q–T intervals. Complications are renal calculi, chronic renal failure and hypertension.

Hypercalcaemia is treated with sodium phosphate, steroids and calcitonin. A plasma ionized calcium above 3.5 mmol/litre constitutes a medical emergency because there is imminent risk of cardiac arrest. Emergency treatment is by rehydration and loop diuresis; this increases renal excretion of calcium. Renal dialysis is also very effective.

Surgical treatment is indicated when the patient has recurrent kidney stones, neuromuscular symptoms, hypertension or renal failure. There is no specific anaesthetic technique for parathyroidectomy but the anaesthetist should prepare for a long and tedious exploration of the entire anterior part of the neck, and possibly the mediastinum, if the glands cannot be identified in the neck. Methylene blue is sometimes used by surgeons preoperatively because it is concentrated in parathyroid tissue and thus permits easy identification. The cyanotic appearance of the whole patient because of this dye causes severe problems for the anaesthetist.

Hypocalcaemia

Hypocalcaemia is mainly due to successful surgical parathyroidectomy. It can also be caused by vitamin D deficiency, chronic renal failure, hypoalbuminaemia, acute pancreatitis and hypomagnesaemia.

Usual symptoms of hypocalcaemia are paraesthesia, muscle cramps, tetany, laryngeal spasms and convulsions. The ECG shows a prolonged Q–T interval. These symptoms appear shortly after surgical parathyroidectomy, or thyroidectomy if all functioning parathyroid tissue has been removed. Emergency treatment should be by slow i.v. injection of 10–20 ml of calcium gluconate 10 per cent.

There is no particular anaesthetic technique recommended for patients with hypocalcaemia but low plasma ionized-calcium levels should always be corrected before surgery because of the increased risk of cardiac arrhythmias.

Malignant hyperthermia syndrome

Human malignant hyperthermia syndrome (MHS) is a pharmacogenetic myopathy transmitted by a dominant autosomal gene which, if unchallenged, produces no ill effects in the sufferer, but which is triggered by some drugs used in anaesthesia. MHS manifests itself as a life-threatening syndrome characterized by rigor and muscle hypercatabolism with a very rapid and, if untreated, progressive rise in body temperature leading invariably to death.

The MHS reaction is a sudden and sustained rise in myoplasmic free calcium. This in turn is due to a stress or drug-induced loss, by the sarcoplasmic reticulum, of its ability to resequester calcium which is needed for the muscle to return to the relaxed state. The lesion responsible is a genetic functional derangement in the excitation-contraction-coupling mechanism distal to the neuromuscular junction.

Clinical features

The MHS was first described in 1960. It is not such a rare condition, and occurs worldwide in approximately 1:5000 to 1:200000 of all patients, depending on the criteria of diagnosis. The syndrome affects all ages but is more common in the 20s, being almost unknown below the age of 3 and over the age of 50 years.

The usual presentation takes the form of increased sympathetic activity with tachycardia and unexplained tachyarrhythmias. Muscle hypertonicity or rigor is present in 80 per cent of the cases. Masseter-muscle spasm may occur following a triggering agent such as suxamethonium and may render tracheal intubation impossible. This sign is now recognized as reliable evidence of MHS in 60–70 per cent of all cases. Its presence should alert the anaesthetist to abort the anaesthetic.

At the same time as the development of muscle hypertonicity, the patient develops a progressive and often fulminant pyrexia. Core temperature can rise at 1°C every 5–10 minutes, and, without treatment, rises to 41°C or more and will eventually cause the patient's death.

Profound metabolic acidosis, hypoxia and hypercapnia are all present, resulting in cyanosis and hyperventilation in the spontaneously breathing patient. All electrolytes are elevated in plasma and hyperkalaemia is of great clinical importance because of the cardiac arrhythmias it may produce.

As MHS progresses, muscle damage and sarcolemma permeability are manifest by the rapid and progressive rise in plasma concentrations of muscle enzymes (creatinine phosphokinase, lactic dehydrogenase, alanine transaminase and aspartate transaminase), and the release into the circulation of myoglobin and thromboplastin. Myoglobinuria, renal failure and disseminated intravascular coagulopathy follow.

There are certain prerequisites needed for the precipitation of the MHS crisis. First, the patient must carry the MHS gene and must be exposed to a specific trigger agent for an adequate period of time. In addition, there are certain factors which will influence the sensitivity of the patient to the triggering agent, such as increased systemic catecholamine levels (pre-anaesthetic anxiety and stress), heavy muscular exercise before surgery, environmental heat stress, etc.

Almost all volatile anaesthetic agents can trigger MHS in susceptible patients, but it is more common with the potent halogenated agents such as halothane, enflurane and isoflurane. Nitrous oxide is not implicated as a MHS trigger agent; it has been used with impunity in countless MHS patients.

Of the i.v. anaesthetic agents, only ketamine and etomidate have been implicated and should therefore be avoided.

Suxamethonium is a specific trigger agent of MHS in the susceptible patient. Non-depolarizing relaxants do not trigger MHS and do not prevent initiation of the syndrome by the potent volatile inhalation anaesthetic agents.

Diagnosis

As transmission of the MH gene is dominant, those relatives of the patient who have a 50 per cent probability of possessing the gene (siblings, parents and children) should be screened, as preoperative identification of patient susceptibility to MH is a prerequisite for the prevention of the syndrome.

Invasive tests are based on the different responses to pharmacological challenges of normal muscle and muscle from MH patients. These tests are based on the measurement of the isometric-contracture tension of muscle fascicles in response to increased concentrations of caffeine and halothane.

Non-invasive tests lack specificity and are based on the assay of muscle enzymes. Of these, plasma creatine-phosphokinase activity has been the most widely used.

Treatment

The anaesthetist will need assistance in treating these patients as the complexity and urgency of the treatment is such that multiple involvement is always required.

When the onset of MHS is diagnosed early, all that may be needed is to discontinue the triggering agent. This may be sufficient to abort the syndrome. Failing this, the success of the treatment will depend upon the speed at which specific therapy is established and upon the supportive treatment of the concomitant symptoms (acidosis, arrhythmias, high temperature, etc.).

The specific agent in the treatment of MHS is dantrolene sodium, a hydantoin which binds to the sarcolemma and the T-tubular membrane reducing the rate and amount of calcium released. Thus, as triggering agents switch MH on, dantrolene switches it off.

For clinical use, dantrolene should be injected into a large vein or into a fast-running i.v. infusion as the pH is 9–10 and is very irritant to veins. The dose is 2.4 mg/kg body weight repeated at 15 minute intervals until relaxation of muscle rigor, control of temperature rise and cessation of arrhythmias has been achieved, or until a total dose of 10 mg/kg body weight has been given (average dose requirement is 4 mg/kg body weight).

Dantrolene has no adverse cardiovascular effect, is metabolized in the liver and excreted through the kidney. It has weak muscle-relaxant properties and patients may complain of muscle weakness following its administration. However, these effects are not strong enough to impair respiration or coughing.

It is possible for MH to recur after successful treatment. Prophylactic administration of dantrolene should be repeated in the postoperative period (2.5 mg/kg body weight).

If dantrolene therapy is instituted immediately after early diagnosis, supportive therapy may not be necessary. However, once the syndrome is fully established, supportive therapy is indicated to correct acidosis and hypoxia, to protect the kidney against myoglobinuria (by diuresis), and to arrest the development of disseminated intravascular coagulopathy (by giving fresh frozen plasma). In addition measures should be taken to decrease the patient's body temperature.

When therapy is instituted rapidly after early diagnosis, survival from MHS should be 100 per cent. However, because full awareness of the syndrome is not yet common, the present mortality is as high as 7–10 per cent.

Further reading

Barash P G, Cullen B F, Stoelting R K. *Clinical anaesthesia*. Lippincott, 1989.

Hutton P, Cooper G. *Guidelines in clinical anaesthesia*. London: Blackwell, 1985.

Katz J, Benumof J, Kadis L B. *Anaesthesia and uncommon disease*. Saunders, 1981.

Mason R A. *Anaesthesia databook*. Edinburgh: Churchill Livingstone, 1990.

Nunn J F, Utting J E, Brown B R. *General anaesthesia*. London: Butterworths, 1989.

Scurr C, Feldman S, Soni N. *Scientific foundations of anaesthesia*. Heinemann, 1990.

Smith G, Aitkenhead A R. *Textbook of anaesthesia*. Edinburgh: Churchill Livingstone, 1990.

17

Anaesthetic complications
T.H. Howells

- Preoperative complications
    existing patient pathology
    existing patient medication
    premedication
    preoperative starvation
- Intraoperative complications
    induction of anaesthesia
    maintenance of anaesthesia
- Postoperative complications
    early postoperative period
    late postoperative period

While this subject covers the vast area of the entire morbidity and mortality related to anaesthesia, it should be understood that although minor problems are not uncommon, serious complications are rare. So far as anaesthetic management is concerned the patient rightly expects that no significant problems will arise. Indeed, today's anaesthetist regards all anaesthetic complications as unacceptable and endeavours to manage the patient with that in mind. Nevertheless, the range of problems that may arise is so wide that some mishap is just waiting to occur and constant vigilance is required to ensure safe anaesthesia.

An idea of the range of anaesthetic complications is apparent when an attempt is made to classify the subject matter. For instance, problems related to existing patient medications and pathology, to pharmacological interactions, physiological disturbances, anatomical anomalies, technical aberrations, errors of judgement and technique can all be identified.

However, for the purposes of this chapter complications within the consideration of sequential anaesthetic management are presented. Classically we consider an anaesthetic as three fundamental components — the preoperative, intraoperative and postoperative management divisions. Each of these components may be further subdivided. Nevertheless, complications of a similar nature can occur throughout management. For instance, vomiting may complicate the premedication, the induction of anaesthesia and the postoperative phase, so that a complication chosen to be typical of one component of management should not be understood to be exclusive of any other.

Preoperative complications

Consideration of the preoperative phase includes
- existing patient pathology
- existing patient medication
- the prescription of preanaesthetic medication (the premedication or 'premed')
- preoperative starvation

Existing patient pathology

An otherwise fit patient may present with a single pathology requiring surgical correction, such as an inguinal hernia. On the other hand, an elderly patient needing a simple surgical operation may present with several health problems or pathology which extends to the brink of multiple organ failure. In these circumstances it is sometimes impossible to know, when complications occur, whether these are the result of surgical or anaesthetic intervention.

Hypertension is relatively clear-cut problem. A patient whose diastolic pressure is consistently above 110mmHg is liable to increased risk of a cardiovascular complication, especially when cardiac ischaemia is evident. Improvement in blood-pressure control is indicated before surgery is undertaken. A preoperative ECG, chest radiography and baseline biochemistry will assist management.

A pleural infusion will benefit from preoperative drainage; this will reduce the risk of compromising ventilation during anaesthesia and so the risk of pulmonary complications.

Fetal distress may indicate the need for an emergency caesarian section. The possible complication of acid aspiration during the induction of anaesthesia means that the mother requires protection by medication that reduces gastric acidity (Chapter 11).

Existing patient medication

Nowadays, many patients receive chronic medication and the anaesthetist must be familiar with each drug so as to avoid untoward interaction with anaesthetic agents.

Beta-adrenoceptor antagonist therapy will produce sensitivity to the hypotensive effects of anaesthetics.

Monamine-oxidase inhibitors preclude the use of pethidine and vasopressors. This avoids the possibility of cerebral haemorrhage.

Diabetic patients who are insulin dependent require careful management to avoid inadvertent hypo or hyperglycaemia (Chapter 16).

It is clear that the anaesthetist must be informed about each patient's medication, including drug sensitivities.

Premedication

Drugs used for premedication traditionally include a sedative and antisecretory component.

Narcotic analgesics should be used with caution in patients with respiratory disorders to avoid respiratory depression. When they are used an antiemetic is indicated to minimize nausea or vomiting.

Atropine is especially useful if an inhalational induction of anaesthesia is contemplated to avoid excessive salivary and bronchial secretions. Hyoscine should be avoided in the elderly because this drug may precipitate hallucination.

Hydrocortisone may be required if the patient has been receiving corticosteroid therapy to prevent cortisol deficiency during surgery (Chapter 16).

Bronchodilator drugs are indicated in asthmatics to prevent bronchospasm during anaesthesia.

Ranitidine and *metoclopramide* will diminish the risk of regurgitation of gastric acid as a complication of induction, for example in patients with hiatus hernia.

Antibiotics are used as part of the premedication for patients with heart-valve lesions to prevent infective endocarditis if the surgery creates a bacteraemia.

Preoperative starvation

This is a well-worn phrase indicating a need to withhold food and drink from patients in the period leading up to anaesthesia. During the instigation of general anaesthesia protective gastric, oesophageal and respiratory reflexes are depressed. One of the worst anaesthetic complications is the inadvertent inhalation of stomach contents. For this reason great emphasis is placed on ensuring that the patient's stomach is empty. Most nursing protocols insist on a period of total fasting for 6 hours before anaesthesia. This is almost certainly excessive in reality but concentrates the mind on the potential calamity.

When emergency surgery precludes starvation, or when gastrointestinal obstruction occurs, other methods are used to minimize the problem. The stomach may be emptied by intubation and aspiration or by administering metoclopramide, and gastric acidity can be reduced pharmacologically. Even so, it is never possible to be certain that the stomach is completely empty in an emergency situation.

It should be remembered that preoperative starvation can produce its own complications. Babies and small children can soon become ketotic if starved for an excessive period of time. It is sensible, therefore, to allow them milk feeds up to 6 hours before anaesthesia and to give them a sugar-containing drink 4 hours prior to surgery.

It is entirely possible that for normal adult patients there is no need to restrict water drinking in small amounts, but because this might lead to a misunderstanding, the strict rules of starvation should still prevail.

Intraoperative complications

The intraoperative (peroperative, operative) period of anaesthesia may be considered as
- the induction
- the maintenance
- the recovery (or emergence)

Induction of anaesthesia
This event is usually created by the i.v. administration of agents that induce the state of anaesthesia in one arm–brain circulation time. The alternative is the inhalation of anaesthetic gases or vapours. Each of the commonly used i.v. agents has its own characteristics and problems but they all share some similar induction complications.

Circulatory complications

An i.v. induction dose must be carefully titrated in the circumstances of slowed circulatory time, as in the elderly with cardiac failure, to avoid circulatory collapse. Patients with aortic stenosis or thoracic-inlet obstruction may take a long time to circulate drugs and the anaesthetist may be deceived into giving an inadvertent overdose. Patients vary in their susceptibility to i.v. induction for many reasons, and they may become apnoeic or suffer circulatory depression unless care is taken in dosage.

Hypotension in moderate degrees may accompany induction, but if anaphylactic reactions to induction agents occur hypotension can be severe.

Arrhythmias are common during normal intubation of the trachea but seldom give rise to problems.

Coughing and straining may raise the intraocular and intracranial pressure to a dangerous extent and care must be taken to avoid them when eye injury or brain damage is present.

Intra-arterial injection or extravasation of the agent may cause serious local problems particularly when thiopentone is used. It is important to avoid arterial sites when choosing a vein and to ensure that when a choice of vein has been made, nearby arteries can be palpated in a pulsing state and that the chosen vessel is indeed a non-pulsating vein. Should thiopentone enter an artery, intense vasospasm and thrombosis will occur. Vasodilators, anticoagulants and analgesics will be required to treat the complication.

Thrombosis, phlebitis and *haematoma* constitute minor complications. Haematoma is avoided by the application of gentle pressure over the injection site.

Respiratory complications

These are relatively common at the induction stage but are generally managed without difficulty.

Respiratory depression or temporary apnoea may be treated by controlled ventilation and increased inspired oxygen.

Reflex breath-holding, hiccup, coughing and laryngeal stridor are responses to irritation and may lead to a dangerous spasm. These problems are more common during induction with inhalational vapours and can be treated by withdrawing the irritant and ensuring adequate oxygenation. If the event does not regress, the solution may be found in expert hands giving an i.v. muscle relaxant and in resorting to wholly controlled ventilation. However, any precipitating cause of laryngospasm, such as foreign material impinging on the glottis, must be considered first.

Bronchospasm which is severe is rare and may be suggestive of an anaphylactic reaction. Bronchodilators such as aminophylline, salbutamol, adrenaline and hydrocortisone will usually release the spasm.

Alimentary complications

Regurgitation may complicate induction in patients with full stomachs and great care must be exercised to avoid the complication of inhalation by the use of a rapid-sequence system using cricoid pressure to occlude the upper oesophagus (Chapter 10).

Active vomiting is now rare with i.v. induction but it may complicate inhalation induction. The patient should be placed immediately into the lateral and head-down position.

Powerful suction must be available to the anaesthetist at all times and should have been properly connected and checked for instant use.

Anatomical complications

Damage may occur to the lips, tongue and teeth when facemasks are applied and when oral airways are inserted. Nasal bleeding can occur when nasal airways are used. During laryngoscopic and intubation manipulations, damage to the oropharyngeal and upper respiratory mucosa is not uncommon. The uvula and larynx may be considerably traumatized, especially during difficulty in intubation. The mucosa of the trachea is often compressed when tube cuffs are inflated and the presence of a tube lying between the vocal cords may give rise to cord defects following anaesthesia. The complaints of sore throat and hoarseness after anaesthesia are directly related to these traumas.

Maintenance of anaesthesia

Cardiovascular complications

Cardiac arrhythmias are common. Bradycardia may occur due to inhalational anaesthetics or when surgical traction affects the autonomic nerves. It responds to i.v. atropine, to reducing the dose of agent or to relieving the surgical stimulus.

Tachycardia may result from surgical stimulus and may be corrected by increasing the anaesthesia. It will occur in haemorrhage in association with hypotension.

Nodal rhythm is often seen when halothane is used and may be corrected by withdrawing the agent, or administering atropine or a beta-adrenoceptor antagonist.

Other arrhythmias are more sinister and may result in ventricular fibrillation requiring cardiopulmonary resuscitation.

Hypotension is a common feature during maintenance and the blood pressure needs monitoring continuously to ensure that no more than a moderate fall exists. It may be corrected by atropine when in association with slow heart rates, by restoration of blood volume when related to vasodilatation or blood loss, or by inotropes and vasoconstrictors. In emergencies the patient should be placed head down to improve essential organ perfusion.

Cardiac arrest can result from air, amniotic fluid or thrombotic embolism. These events can be fatal. The treatment of air embolism consists of placing the patient in the left-lateral position whilst also providing 100 per cent oxygen. It may be possible to aspirate air from the venous circulation through a large-bore central venous catheter and in extreme cases it may be necessary to aspirate air from the right ventricle directly.

Respiratory complications

The airway is always at risk in the unconscious patient. Without tracheal intubation the chin must be supported and artificial airway devices used whenever needed to correct airflow obstruction. Tracheal intubation offers the best airway protection but does not guarantee trouble-free maintenance. The tube may become obstructed, disconnected or slip out of position.

Lower airway problems may arise in the form of bronchial secretions or bronchospasm. Endobronchial suction may prevent or correct areas of lung collapse. Bronchospasm is a serious problem which may be relieved by aminophylline, adrenaline and hydrocortisone. Ventilation with high pressure may be essential and if the bronchospasm is intractable, the use of di-ethyl ether inhalation, which is a powerful bronchodilator, may be life saving.

Pneumothorax from lung-tissue rupture may occur during controlled ventilation or if expiration is obstructed, resulting in high airway pressure. If the pneumothorax becomes tensioned, dramatic lung compression can quickly endanger life and requires immediate pleural drainage.

Neurological complications

Awareness during surgery is much talked of and rightly feared. It generally occurs in unpremedicated patients under very light anaesthesia, typically during caesarian section. It stems from anaesthetists being overprotective about anaesthetic effects upon the patient or fetus. This is a misguided attitude, and awareness should be avoidable by ensuring that each patient is sufficiently anaesthetized.

Cranial nerve palsy has been described and peripheral nerve damage sometimes occurs under anaesthesia due to direct trauma. The brachial plexus may be traumatized when the arm is outstretched for venous access. It is important to ensure that tissue damage and nerve compression are avoided when caring for the unconscious patient.

When regional anaesthesia is employed, neurological complications may result from direct trauma. Rarely, subarachnoid and epidural blocks have resulted in infection, haematoma and frank paralysis. Some neurological disturbances, such as loss of bladder control and headache, may cause temporary problems. The current use of very thin needles has greatly reduced complications in subarachnoid techniques and serious sequelae from regional blocks are now uncommon.

Anatomical complications

As well as nerve damage any part of the unconscious body can suffer trauma unless care is taken to protect vulnerable tissues.

Conjunctival and corneal ulceration must be protected against by ensuring the eyes are closed and not compressed. Some anaesthetists also instil eye drops such as Lacri-Lube.

Diathermy burns can be caused by metallic contact with the skin, e.g. parts of the operating table.

Positioning of the patient for surgical access must be done with care to avoid joint strain especially in those who have existing skeletal problems.

Lifting patients on and off operating tables and trolleys is hazardous and may create severe trauma if performed carelessly.

Monitoring and its complications

Various monitoring systems are used from the time the patient arrives in the anaesthetic room until the patient leaves the recovery area. These help to minimize anaesthetic complications and non-invasive monitoring such as pulse oximetry and pulse-detection blood pressure measurements are virtually harmless. ECG monitoring is safe now that the danger of microelectrocution has been eradicated by the use of isolation transformers.

Invasive monitoring may create complications.

Central venous cannulation may produce pneumothorax, haemothorax and haematòma.

Intra-arterial cannulation may damage an artery as evidenced by the long-term absence of a pulse, although serious thrombosis and arterial occlusion are rare.

Postoperative complications

Early postoperative period

Emergence from anaesthesia is often associated with disturbances of orientation and some confusion may occur. At this early stage reassurance and gentle restraint may be required.

Pain from the operation site soon becomes apparent and needs management by an analgesic regimen. Systemic analgesics are commonly given to provide pain relief. These may be administered by mouth, sublingually or by parenteral injections. The powerful narcotic analgesics are generally given by intermittent i.m. injection and good analgesia may be achieved provided attention is given to dosage and frequency.

Intravenous infusions by continuous drip or by syringe pumps provide more satisfactory management but require closer attention. A patient-demand facility may be added to this system and offers the patient an involvement in pain control (Chapter 18).

Regional block by intermittent injections or by infusion techniques offers ideal pain control in many circumstances. Epidural or subarachnoid injections of narcotic analgesics are gaining much popularity. Pain relief is usually initiated and monitored by the anaesthetist although, of itself, pain is a complication of surgery. However, pain relief brings its own complications of respiratory depression, nausea and vomiting (Chapter 18).

Respiratory complications

Mild hypoxia often complicates recovery from anaesthesia for a variety of reasons and should be monitored by pulse oximetry in the recovery area. Controlled oxygen administration should be given to all major surgical cases, and any patients that show evidence of hypoxaemia, until satisfactory oxygenation is maintained by breathing room air.

Ventilatory depression may be caused by pain, by analgesic therapy, by the continued effects of muscle relaxants or by bronchopulmonary problems caused by secretions. Coughing and deep breathing should be encouraged by physiotherapy. Areas of lung collapse can be identified by careful auscultation and radiographs, and can be treated by the physiotherapist or the anaesthetist. Endotracheal or bronchial suction is very beneficial in these circumstances but occasionally direct bronchoscopic aspiration is indicated.

Gastrointestinal complications

Nausea and vomiting are considered by patients to be specific anaesthetic complications. Very few anaesthetic agents nowadays cause emesis but it is true that some patients are prone to suffer following anaesthesia. Powerful analgesics, however, do have emetic side-effects and need antiemetic treatment by such agents as phenothiazine, hyoscine or metoclopramide.

Minor complications

These are often manifest during the early recovery stages. Damage to eyes, lips, tongue; minor abrasions, sore throat, hiccups, swallowing difficulty, musculo-skeletal trauma. Headache, double vision and hypothermia are quite common. Shivering is often seen following inhalational anaesthetics, notably halothane.

Late postoperative period

By the time the patient has returned to the surgical ward most anaesthetic complications are over. However, until all the drug and the metabolic effects of anaesthesia are terminated, some complications may still arise.

Pulmonary embolism remains a dramatic event and derives from deep venous thrombosis. Attempts are made to prevent this by repeated small doses of subcutaneous heparin and the use of elastic stockings to cover the operative period. Early mobilization of the patient helps to minimize venous stagnation.

Lung tissue collapse remains as a potential complication and lung infection must be suspected whenever fever is present.

Long-term complications following anaesthesia are uncommon. However, a few patients take several months before regaining a full feeling of well being. The reason for this occasional persistent malaise is obscure. Reassurance is the most useful supportive measure.

18

Pain relief
D. M. Justins

What is pain?

Pain is defined as an unpleasant sensory or emotional experience associated with actual or potential tissue damage, or described in terms of such damage. This definition is important because it emphasizes that pain is not just a sensory phenomenon linked to tissue damage. The electrophysiological events that occur in the sensory nervous system following tissue damage are referred to as *nociception* and only become pain when conscious awareness occurs. A patient without peripheral tissue damage may still describe symptoms in terms of such damage. In most cases of acute pain there is a very obvious site of tissue damage but in many patients with chronic pain the origin of the pain may be obscure and psychological factors often make a significant contribution to the overall condition.

Classification
Pain is usually classified as acute or chronic but the boundaries between the two forms may be blurred. *Chronic pain* is regarded as pain which persists after all possible healing of any injury has occurred and long after pain could serve any useful or protective function. In many conditions, and most especially in cancer, there is continuing tissue damage which is superimposed upon the pain resulting from previous damage. Pain may also be described according to the presumed origin as:

- *nociceptive* — tissue damage
- *neuropathic* — nerve damage
- *psychogenic* — predominantly psychological

Measurement of pain
Since pain is a purely subjective experience it is difficult to make reliable measurements of pain intensity, but there are techniques that can be used to compare pain intensity at different times in the same patient and these techniques are useful in clinical practice and research. The most widely used measures are the visual-analogue scale and the verbal-rating scale. The *visual-analogue scale* is a 10 cm line which is marked at one end as 'no pain' and at the other end as 'worst pain imaginable' and the patient is asked to mark the point on the line that represents the intensity of their pain. This pain intensity can then be expressed as a number (the distance in cm on the line from 'no pain' to the mark made by the patient) and this gives a way of quantifying pain. The *verbal-rating scale* offers the patient a series of descriptions of pain intensity (such as 'no pain, slight, moderate, severe, very severe'), but it is important to note that these grades are not equally spaced in terms of pain intensity and therefore do not represent a means of quantifying pain.

The qualitative and emotional aspects of pain may be evaluated using a questionnaire such as the *McGill Pain Questionnaire*. The psychological impact of pain and the resulting behavioural responses of the patient and family can be assessed with a variety of questionnaires frequently used by clinical psychologists.

The degree of disability and physical impairment induced by pain can be gauged with *exercise tests* which are often best conducted by a physiotherapist. Thoracic and upper abdominal operations produce respiratory impairment and *respiratory function tests* can measure this.

The assessment of patients with complex chronic pain problems requires a multidisciplinary team using a wide range of assessment methods so that a complete picture of the patient and the pain can be established.

The assessment of pain-relieving techniques and pain research is bedevilled by the *placebo response*. Around 30 per cent of any group of patients suffering from pain will gain significant relief when given a treatment which is not specifically analgesic (although the treatment does not necessarily have to be inert). It appears that these placebo responders are obtaining pain relief through activation of endogenous analgesic mechanisms involving substances such as the endorphins and enkephalins. The placebo response demonstrates why double-blind controlled trial designs are essential in pain treatment research.

General principles of pain management

The formulation of a management plan for any specific patient can be based upon the general principles which are listed in this section and usually the most effective plan uses a number of therapies in a combined fashion rather than one single modality.

Remove the cause
Surgery for appendicitis and radiotherapy to shrink a tumour are obvious ways to remove the cause of pain. If movement of a fracture causes pain then splintage and rest will help to relieve the pain.

Prevent initial excitation of nociceptive nerves
Non-steroidal anti-inflammatory drugs such as aspirin inhibit prostaglandin activity in the periphery and reduce the excitability of nociceptive nerve endings. A simple ice pack can be very effective in treating an acute musculo-skeletal injury.

Interrupt peripheral nociceptive transmission
This is most commonly achieved with a local anaesthetic nerve block and is very useful in acute pain but often fails in chronic pain. This is because the neurophysiological basis of such pain is more complex and often the spinal cord and higher centres demonstrate neurophysiological changes which are not altered by peripheral neural blockade.

Alter spinal modulation of nociceptive transmission
The dorsal horn of the spinal cord is the site of very powerful control systems which can exert either an inhibitory or a facilitatory action upon the transmission of nociceptive stimuli. These control systems are modulated by local spinal influences and by descending pathways from the brain. Techniques such as transcutaneous electrical nerve stimulation (p. 168, 274) and acupuncture stimulate these inhibitory controls. The spinal (epidural or intrathecal) injection of opiate produces direct stimulation of the opiate receptors which play a key role in the inhibitory systems of the dorsal horn.

Interrupt spinal cord nociceptive transmission
The majority of nociceptive stimuli are transmitted to higher centres in the brain by the anterolateral spinothalamic tracts and these tracts can be destroyed or cut, although such a drastic technique is reserved for cancer patients.

Alter central processing of nociceptive information
A significant part of the analgesic activity of the opiate family of drugs is exerted at various sites in the brain, other analgesics such as nitrous oxide are also acting here.

Alter the emotional response to the pain
Both the anxiety of acute pain and the depression of chronic pain can be treated so that the patient becomes better able to cope with the pain.

Psychotropic drugs and antidepressant drugs have a role to play in some cases, as do various psychological strategies.

Alter the behavioural response to the pain
In many chronic pain patients the original pain complaint becomes submerged in a complex picture of disability and maladaptive behaviour which, though unrecognized by the patient, may actually represent the major problem.

In all cases of pain management a balance must be achieved between the methods of pain relief and associated side-effects on one side with pain and the patient's wishes on the other. A patient may settle for less than complete pain relief to avoid unwanted side-effects. A method of pain relief must be effective, safe and practical.

Acute pain

Some examples of acute pain
- postoperative
- obstetric
- traumatic
  - musculo-skeletal injuries
  - fractures
  - burns
- medical
  - myocardial infarction
  - acute pancreatitis
  - sickle crisis pain
- surgical
  - acute abdomen
  - acute peripheral vascular occlusion
  - ureteric colic
- orthopaedic
  - osteomyelitis
  - acute gout
  - prolapsed invertebral disc
- cancer
  - pathological fracture
  - raised intracranial pressure

This section will deal mainly with postoperative pain but the methods of pain relief can be applied with equal benefit to any form of acute pain.

Effects of unrelieved acute pain

Acute pain has psychological, physiological, and socioeconomic consequences. Unrelieved acute pain causes distress and suffering, falling morale and rising anxiety. Pain impairs breathing and coughing and leads to respiratory complications. Hypertension and tachycardia produced in response to pain may be harmful to a patient with cardiac disease and the increase in cerebral blood flow may cause further damage in a head-injury patient. Gastrointestinal motility is impaired. Mobility is restricted by pain and the risk of thromboembolism is increased. Patients with poor pain control are slower to convalesce and spend longer in hospital.

Problems of controlling acute pain

The big problem in acute pain management is unpredictable variability in:
- pain — incidence, intensity, time course
- patient — psychology, personality, placebo response
- pharmacology — drug, dose, delivery, pharmacokinetics, pharmacodynamics

The most important factor affecting the incidence and intensity of pain is undoubtedly the site of the operation. Thoracic and upper abdominal operations usually produce severe pain of at least 2–3 days' duration; minor peripheral operations produce slight pain of brief duration. Other things such as a drain site, a urinary catheter or a nasogastric tube can also be painful. Age, sex, race, and social background do not seem to be major consistent influences on the pain experience but personality is important and patients with trait anxiety, or with high neuroticism and extroversion scores on personality testing will report increased severity of pain and exhibit a lower pain tolerance. Some factors can be manipulated and these include ward design, comfort, sleep, distractions, state anxiety and feelings of fear or helplessness. A full understanding of the illness and proposed management is important. One critical factor which can be controlled is the attitude of the medical staff, particularly that of the nurses. The influence of pharmacological variables is discussed later.

Prevention of pain

Opiate premedication and nerve blocks performed before surgery commences may reduce the incidence of postoperative pain — *pre-emptive analgesia*. The idea that prevention is better than cure is not original!

Objectives of acute-pain management

The aims of management in acute pain are to minimize discomfort, facilitate recovery, and avoid treatment side-effects.

Methods of acute-pain management

Medication

Drugs available for acute pain control include:
- opioids including agonists (morphine, diamorphine, papaveretum, pethidine, fentanyl, alfentanyl, methadone) and partial agonists (pentazocine, buprenorphine, nefopam, meptazinol)
- prostaglandin synthetase inhibitors which include paracetamol and the non-steroidal anti-inflammatory drugs such as aspirin, indomethacin and diclofenac
- other drugs such as the i.v. induction agent ketamine which is also a potent analgesic
- inhalational agents such as nitrous oxide

- anxiolytic drugs such as the benzodiazepines enhance the effect of opioids

The prescription of a potent opiate is the most common method of postoperative analgesia yet pain control is often inadequate because medical staff ignore pharmacological influences. The most obvious influences apart from choice of drug are route, mode, time and frequency of administration. The individual response to treatment also varies because of pharmacokinetic and pharmacodynamic differences. Pharmacokinetics describes the uptake, distribution and elimination of the drug and there is wide variation between individuals (and sometimes in the same individual at different times). The patient characteristics which may influence pharmacokinetic variability include age (the elderly have a diminished volume of distribution for opiate drugs), hepatic disease, renal disease, acid-base balance, hypothermia, hypothyroidism and concurrent drug administration.

Even if all the pharmacokinetic variables are overcome so that a constant plasma concentration is maintained, individual patients will still vary in the degree of pain relief they experience. The concentration at which patients become pain free will also vary significantly. This means that analgesic administration must be individualized for each patient. The ideal is a steady plasma concentration that will maintain analgesia without causing toxicity.

The route of administration is one of the most important determinants of success. Irrespective of the route of administration, side-effects occur commonly with the opiates and include sedation, respiratory depression, nausea, vomiting, constipation, and dysphoria.

Available routes for opioid administration

Intramuscular Simplicity and economy are the only advantages. The injections are painful and there is wide variation in onset time, duration of analgesia and incidence of toxicity. Intramuscular injections are usually given 'on demand' but overworked nurses and strict drug regulations cause long delays between the request for analgesia and the actual onset of pain relief. The duration of action of the drug may be less than the prescribed interval so the patient is condemned to a period of pain before the next dose can be administered.

- Example: papaveretum (Omnopon) 20 mg 4-hourly for a 70 kg person.

Intravenous This route offers the advantage of immediate and reliable uptake of the drug by the systemic circulation with a rapid onset so that the dose can be titrated for each patient. The main disadvantage is the narrow safety margin between adequate analgesia and serious side-effects such as respiratory depression. Most i.v. techniques demand a high level of supervision and special equipment such as syringe pumps.

Modes of intravenous delivery
Intermittent bolus administration has the advantage of rapid onset allowing titration of dose against pain, but toxicity is common and the duration of analgesia is brief resulting in a pattern of peaks and troughs in pain control. This method is labour intensive.

- Example: papaveretum 5 to 10 mg for 70 kg person.

Continuous infusion avoids the peaks and troughs of intermittent administration and allows improved pain control but infusion pharmacokinetics are
complex and dose requirements change with time. The safety margin is
narrow and high levels of nursing surveillance are essential. Intravenous
infusions have proved to be very useful in infants and children, and even for
neonates after major surgery.
● Example: papaveretum 5 to 10 mg/h for a 70 kg person.

Combined   Continuous infusion plus intermittent bolus on-demand will,
in theory, allow control of background pain and acute exacerbations.

Control of intravenous administration

Medical staff generally control analgesic administration but pain is a
subjective experience and it is only the patient who can know the exact pain
intensity at any one time. *Patient controlled analgesia* (PCA) allows the patient
to control drug delivery according to his requirements. A PCA machine will
administer a preset dose of drug when the patient presses a button. The
machine contains a microprocessor which will prevent misuse or overdose.
Some machines also provide a background infusion.

PCA can produce very good analgesia with minimal side-effects and the
technique is popular with patients and nurses. Most patients benefit from
being in control but the technique is not suitable for every patient. Most
machines restrict patient mobility and are very expensive.

PCA machines have been used for i.m., subcutaneous and epidural
administration as well.

Subcutaneous
This is a simple and often effective method, particularly as an infusion,
although it is prone to wide variability because of unpredictable uptake from
the subcutaneous tissue.

Oral
The oral route is not ideal for acute pain control because first-pass
metabolism by the liver results in variable bioavailability of the drug and
leads to unpredictable results. Postoperative gastric stasis and inability to
swallow also limit the usefulness of this route.

Sublingual
This route avoids the problems of first-pass metabolism and inability to
swallow. Sublingual buprenorphine has been used with some success
although the slow onset time means that the drug is not ideal for severe
acute pain.

Other routes
These include buccal, nasal, rectal, and transdermal routes.

Epidural and intrathecal
A large proportion of any opioid which is deposited in the spinal canal will
act directly upon the opiate receptors which are densely concentrated in the

dorsal horn of the spinal cord. Small doses of opioid (e.g. morphine 1–2 mg) can produce high-quality analgesia of very long duration when given by this route. Significant side-effects are associated with the method and these include urinary retention, nausea, pruritis and, most dangerous of all, delayed respiratory depression.

Non-opioid analgesics
Paracetamol and the non-steroidal anti-inflammatory drugs are very useful in postoperative pain management. Drugs such as diclofenac can be given by injection.

Inhalation analgesia in acute pain management
Inhalation analgesia may be provided with a 50:50 mixture of oxygen and nitrous oxide (Entonox) and this can be used in ambulances, casualty, obstetrics and for wound dressings. Bone marrow toxicity limits the use of Entonox for long-term pain control.

Regional analgesia in acute pain management
Regional analgesia techniques (nerve blocks) simply aim to interrupt nociceptive transmission in the peripheral nervous system and are capable of producing complete pain relief without any central depressant effect on consciousness or respiration. Unfortunately there are disadvantages as well. Performance of the blocks requires a high degree of skill and is time consuming. Repeated administration may be impractical. Side-effects of the blocks are also significant and include immediate complications such as toxicity following intravascular injection of local anaesthetic, and delayed effects such as muscle weakness and urinary retention which occur when motor and autonomic nerves are blocked by the local anaesthetic.

Methods of regional analgesia
Regional blocks require meticulous attention to detail. One of the greatest dangers lies in exceeding the dose limits of the local anaesthetic and thus causing toxicity (Chapter 12). The maximum safe dose of bupivacaine is 2 mg/kg.

Topical and wound infiltration   Regional techniques do not have to be complex and topical application of local anaesthetic as a spray or ointment, or local wound infiltration (performed by the surgeon during the operation) are very simple and often remarkably effective.

Nerve blocks   Blocks such as digital, wrist, ankle, intercostal, ilioinguinal, penile, and femoral are simple to perform and are very useful especially in children. Intercostal blocks produce very effective analgesia following unilateral abdominal incisions but the risk of pneumothorax is a major disadvantage.

Intrapleural block   In this relatively new technique local anaesthetic is infused via a catheter inserted into the intrapleural space. Potential side-effects are a major disadvantage.

Plexus block   A catheter can be inserted near the brachial plexus and an infusion of local anaesthetic used to provide continuous analgesia following arm surgery.

Epidural analgesia This displays all the advantages and disadvantages of regional analgesia in postoperative pain control. These blocks can provide complete pain relief, improve respiratory function, suppress the endocrine-metabolic response to surgery, reduce the incidence of thromboembolic episodes, improve gastrointestinal function and speed recovery; but the reverse side of the coin reveals a high incidence of significant side-effects, mainly a consequence of the blockade of sympathetic nerves which results in hypotension. Urinary retention and muscular weakness are also common. The lumbar and thoracic routes are most commonly used but caudal injections can provide superb pain relief in adults and children following anogenital operations.

The available techniques of epidural injection use either intermittent bolus doses ('top-ups') or a continuous infusion of either local anaesthetic alone or a mixture of dilute local anaesthetic and opiate.

Cryotherapy This freezes nerves and has been used to produce very prolonged analgesia, most particularly after thoracotomy when the surgeon can apply the cryoprobe to the intercostal nerves under direct vision.

Stimulation-induced analgesia

Transcutaneous electrical nerve stimulation (TENS) and *acupuncture* are useful in some individuals but these methods do not recommend themselves as being universally effective.

Choice of postoperative pain control

Choice of the most appropriate method will be governed by:

- the nature of the surgery and the intensity of the pain
- the availability of drugs and expertise
- the efficacy and side-effects of the available methods
- patient factors such as pre-existing illness, age and psychological state

Combination techniques, for example using a local anaesthetic block, a non-steroidal anti-inflammatory drug (NSAID) and an opioid, may provide better analgesia with fewer side-effects than reliance upon a single method.

Special problems in postoperative pain management may arise with babies, young children, the elderly and in patients with severe respiratory disease, obesity, head injury, or opioid addiction.

In many hospitals the management of postoperative and other acute pain problems is supervised by a special acute pain team.

Chronic pain

Some examples of chronic non-cancer pain

- medical
  - chronic pancreatitis
  - intractable angina
  - irritable bowel syndrome

- surgical
  - chronic peripheral vascular disease
  - post-amputation pain
  - post-thoracotomy pain
  - abdominal-wall nerve entrapment
- musculo-skeletal
  - rheumatoid arthritis
  - cervical spondylosis
  - chronic low-back pain
  - vertebral collapse
  - reflex sympathetic dystrophy
- neurological
  - multiple sclerosis
  - trigeminal neuralgia
  - post-herpetic neuralgia
  - spinal cord injury
  - post-stroke pain syndrome
  - migraine
- psychological
  - tension headache
  - hysterical pain

Effects of unrelieved chronic pain

Chronic pain becomes like a disease in itself and produces effects that are different to acute pain. Depression, demoralization, disability, dependence upon others, and excessive drug consumption dominate the lives of these patients. The socioeconomic consequences are devastating.

Assessment of chronic pain

A high proportion of patients who present to pain relief clinics have been in pain for a considerable period of time and may already have tried a wide range of therapies, including multiple operations. The unrelenting pain and repeated therapeutic failures drag the patient down even further into a state of utter hopelessness so that it is essential to disentangle the various organic and psychosocial components in each case. Assessment should include a history of the present pain complaint, past pain complaints, general health, family history, past treatment including full details of medication, a physical examination, a psychological assessment, a social, family and work assessment (the importance of the family assessment cannot be overstated) and then any appropriate investigations. Some patients become involved in a constant search for a diagnosis and 'cure' and in these patients it is important to concentrate on pain management rather than additional investigations.

This total assessment is best carried out using a team which can focus a wide range of skills onto any particular problem; this *multidisciplinary approach* is central to the successful management of chronic pain.

Problems of chronic pain management

Assessment and management are difficult because of the complex nature of chronic pain, the potent influence of psychological, social and behavioural influences, and because these patients almost by definition will already have tried and failed with a wide range of therapies.

Objectives of chronic pain management

Elimination of pain is occasionally possible, but in many cases the pain is resistant to treatment and management has to be aimed at minimizing the distress and disability that the patient experiences as a result of the pain and treatment.

Methods of chronic pain management

The pain relief clinic

The multidisciplinary approach that was used in assessment is even more important in the management of chronic pain where a range of therapies is offered to each patient. A multidisciplinary pain-relief service will employ, or have access to, the following specialities: anaesthetist, neurologist, orthopaedic surgeon, rheumatologist, oncologist, psychiatrist, psychologist, physiotherapist, acupuncturist, nurse specialist, and social worker.

Medication

Analgesics are ineffective in a large proportion of chronic pain complaints although many musculo-skeletal pains respond to NSAIDs. These less potent analgesics should always be tried before resorting to stronger drugs. Patients with chronic non-malignant pain who do respond to opiate drugs pose a management dilemma because of the risk of dependence with long-term use. The adverse effects of these potent drugs may aggravate the disability suffered by the patient.

Psychotropic drugs are commonly used in chronic pain and in particular the tricyclic antidepressant, amitriptyline, is often very helpful. Part of this benefit may stem from the relief of any underlying depression but there is some evidence that the drugs have specific pain-relieving activity. The benzodiazepine group of drugs generally have no place in chronic pain management and patients who are already taking these drugs frequently exhibit a marked dependence syndrome which can be very difficult to treat.

Anticonvulsant drugs such as carbamazepine, phenytoin and sodium valproate are helpful in certain neuropathic pains. Trigeminal neuralgia responds to carbamazepine in a high percentage of cases.

Other drugs such as steroids and muscle relaxants (e.g. baclofen) find use in specific circumstances such as painful neuroma or muscle spasm.

Drug delivery systems

In some cases of chronic pain, and in cancer pain, the effect of a particular drug is enhanced by continuous delivery which may be epidural, intrathecal, or subcutaneous. External pumps may be linked to a catheter or small pumps may be implanted beneath the skin so that the patient's mobility is unimpeded by external paraphernalia.

Medication reduction

Patients benefit from eliminating unnecessary medication and special drug reduction regimens are available.

Neural blockade

The aims of neural blockade in chronic pain are:

- diagnostic — selective blocks can aid in pinpointing the origin of a pain
- prognostic — local anaesthetic injection can produce a reversible block so that the patient can judge the effect of a permanent block
- therapeutic — blocks may be used as an active part of the treatment

The solutions that are injected include local anaesthetics such as bupivacaine, steroids such as methylprednisolone, and neurolytic agents such as phenol or alcohol. Nerves are also destroyed using heat (radiofrequency lesion generator) or cold (cryoprobe).

Meticulous attention to detail is essential when nerve blocks are performed in chronic pain therapy. The patient must understand fully the aims and risks of the procedure. Sterile technique is mandatory and a nerve stimulator or image intensifier should be used to confirm needle position.

Examples of nerve blocks:

- trigger point injections
- somatic nerve blocks for a trapped or damaged nerve e.g. intercostal
- cranial nerve blocks e.g. for trigeminal neuralgia
- epidural injections e.g. for low-back pain
- blocks of the sympathetic nervous system
  - stellate ganglion e.g. for reflex sympathetic dystrophy of arm
  - coeliac plexus e.g. for chronic pancreatitis
  - lumbar sympathetic trunk e.g. for peripheral vascular disease
  - intravenous regional guanethidine block

The sympathetic nervous system and pain   The sympathetic nervous system is involved in a number of chronic pain states where patients complain of a typically burning pain in a limb which is associated with swelling, skin discolouration, temperature changes, alterations in sweating, skin atrophy and joint stiffness or osteoporosis. The causes and manifestations of these abnormalities are diverse but the term *reflex sympathetic dystrophy* is used as a general description. Common causes include major nerve injury, Colles's fracture, ligamentous ankle injuries and the shoulder–hand syndrome following a cerebrovascular accident.

Neurosurgery

The cutting of nerves which innervate painful areas has enjoyed an unjustified popularity but fails to take account of the more central neurological changes which occur in chronic pain. In fact peripheral nerve section sometimes creates a severe new pain.

Stimulation-produced analgesia

The use of stimulation to induce analgesia is certainly as old as ancient Greek and Chinese civilizations. Recent advances in neurophysiology have demonstrated that these techniques produce analgesia by stimulation of the inhibitory control systems located in the dorsal horn of the spinal cord and that endogenous opiates are involved in some cases.

Transcutaneous electrical nerve stimulation (TENS) uses a small battery-powered machine to deliver a small alternating current to a pair of electrodes positioned on the skin. The frequency and the intensity of the stimulus can be controlled by the patient and these machines are helpful in a wide range of conditions.

Electrodes may be implanted in the spinal canal (spinal-cord stimulation) or in the brain (deep-brain stimulation) but these techniques are not without risk and should only be used in specialist centres.

Acupuncture using either the ancient Chinese method or in more modern styles is capable of producing outstanding results in certain patients.

Physical therapies

Immobility creates a vicious circle of weak muscles, stiff joints and poor fitness and leads to even more pain. Physical therapy can produce marked improvements in the overall condition of the patient and is the key to success in specific conditions such as reflex sympathetic dystrophy.

Psychological methods

Clinical psychologists can play a major role in helping chronic pain patients learn to cope with pain, to think rationally about pain and associated disability, and to eliminate inappropriate or unhelpful behaviour in response to the pain. The methods used range from outpatient relaxation sessions to long-term inpatient programmes aimed at producing major changes in behaviour and attitude. The help of a psychiatrist may be needed to deal with severe depression, hysteria, or with personality disorders.

Cancer pain

Causes of pain in cancer patient

Pain in a patient with cancer may be due to many possible causes and in over 80 per cent of cases there are multiple causes.
- directly caused by the cancer
  - bone involvement
  - nerve compression or infiltration
  - visceral infiltration, obstruction or swelling
  - raised intracranial pressure
  - muscle spasm
- resulting from cancer therapy
  - surgical scars
  - chemotherapy
  - radiotherapy
- resulting from debility
  - pressure sores
  - constipation
- unrelated to cancer
  - patients with cancer are not spared the other pains of mankind
- total pain
  - overwhelming physical and emotional pain associated with fear of impending death and a sense of helplessness

Effects of unrelieved cancer pain

Pain in cancer is often unrelenting and increasing in severity so that the patients become depressed, demoralized and fearful, with major restriction of activity.

Problems of cancer-pain management

The multiple possible causes of pain and the progressive nature of the disease may make assessment very difficult. Emotional factors are extremely important. Many patients and medical staff are burdened down by wildly inaccurate misinformation about analgesic drugs and the risk of addiction (dependence) and this leads to woefully inadequate pain management. The patients deserve optimal pain management and analgesics should never be withheld because of a theoretical risk of addiction or because of a short anticipated life span. The need for analgesia should be dictated by the severity of the pain and nothing else.

Tolerance, which means that an increased dose of opioid is required to achieve the same degree of analgesia, may develop but this should not be confused with dependence. *Physical dependence* is the physiological condition that results in withdrawal symptoms when the opiate is stopped and this is a normal response to long-term opiate administration. *Psychological dependence* is the behavioural pattern of drug abuse which produces a craving for the drug and an overwhelming involvement in obtaining the drug and using it for psychological effects. This is the form of addiction that is feared by the ill informed but it is never a problem in cancer-pain patients.

Objectives of cancer-pain management

Complete pain relief may be impossible because of the multiple and often widespread nature of the pains so it is essential to discuss this with the patient and his family. The prime aim is to make the patient pain free at night so that sleep is possible. The next aim is to make the patient pain free at rest during the day. The final aim of making the patient pain free even when active is the most difficult to achieve.

Methods of cancer-pain management

Specific antitumour therapy

Surgery, radiotherapy and chemotherapy can be vitally effective in helping to control pain.

Medication

Analgesics   Oral analgesics form the mainstay of pain treatment in the vast majority of cancer patients and some very simple guidelines for rational use have been established. The fundamental points are:
- simplicity
- analgesic ladder. Start with a non-opioid (e.g. aspirin), if this fails then use a weak opioid (e.g. dihydrocodeine), if this fails go straight to a strong opioid (e.g. morphine). Do not try different drugs of the same class; always go to the next rung on the ladder if analgesia is inadequate.

Add non-analgesic drugs such as steroids and muscle relaxants when necessary.
- regular administration on a fixed-time basis and not only when the pain is severe. Once again prevention is better than cure.
- oral administration
- treat side-effects such as constipation and nausea
- treat insomnia
- monitor closely

Morphine and diamorphine are the opiates used in most cases and morphine can be conveniently given twice daily in a slow release formulation (MST tablets). The daily dose of morphine may vary from 20 mg to more than 400 mg. Large doses should not cause concern if pain relief is good and side-effects tolerable. Epidural and intrathecal administration is popular in some centres and implanted delivery systems can be used. These methods should only be used if the oral route fails for some reason.

Non-analgesic drugs   Other drugs can be used to supplement the analgesic medication. These are called adjuvant drugs or co-analgesics and include anticonvulsants, antidepressants, steroids and muscle relaxants.

Neural blockade

Nerve blockade may appear attractive in cancer but the potential benefits have to be weighed against the risks which are usually quite considerable. It is very difficult to target just the sensory components of a nerve so that motor and autonomic pathways may be at risk causing weakness or incontinence.

Examples of nerve blocks
- peripheral somatic nerve block e.g. intercostal for pain from rib metastases
- central somatic block e.g. epidural or intrathecal neurolysis
- sympathetic ganglion block e.g. coeliac plexus block for pain from pancreatic or other upper abdominal tumour

Neurosurgery

Cordotomy can be performed as an open operation or percutaneously with a special electrode and should be considered for unilateral pain that is not responding to oral analgesia.

Hospice care

Total emotional and physical care of the dying patient is essential and can be provided by special terminal care teams in hospital or in the community, and by special hospitals, usually called hospices.

Further reading

Alexander J I, Hill R G. *Postoperative Pain Control*. Oxford: Blackwell, 1987.
Bond M R. *Pain. Its nature, analysis and treatment*. Edinburgh: Churchill Livingstone, 1984.
Fields H L. *Pain*. New York: McGraw-Hill, 1987.

Melzack R, Wall P D. *The Challenge of Pain*. Middlesex: Penguin Books, 1982.
Sternbach R A, ed. *The Psychology of Pain* 2nd edn. New York: Raven Press, 1986.
Swerdlow M, ed. *The Therapy of Pain* 2nd edn. Lancaster: MTP Press, 1986.
Twycross R G, Lack S A. *Symptom Control in Far Advanced Cancer: Pain Relief*. London: Pitman, 1983.
Wall P D, Melzack R, eds. *Textbook of Pain* 2nd edn. Edinburgh: Churchill Livingstone, 1989.

19

Intensive care
D.R.G. Browne

- What is intensive care?
- Organization
    staffing
- Admissions policy
- Initial management of the critically-ill patient
- Assessment of respiratory failure
    general
    specific tests
- Mechanical ventilation
    initial management of a patient on a ventilator
    observations and monitoring of the ventilated patient
    patient problems on a ventilator
    ventilator problems
    modes of ventilation
    weaning patients from ventilatory support
- General management of the ventilated patient
    circulatory status
    renal function
    gastrointestinal function
- Nutrition
    total parenteral nutrition
    enteral nutrition
- Analgesia and sedation
- Control of infection
- Ethics and scoring systems

What is intensive care?

Intensive care is the term used to describe the management of the patient who requires special expertise that is not normally available on the general wards. The patient will require admission to a special unit that can provide that care. These units are defined as follows:

A general intensive care unit (ICU) is an area to which the patient is admitted for the treatment of organ failure that may require technical support including mechanical ventilation of the lungs and/or invasive monitoring.

A high dependency unit (HDU) is a unit which provides care which is intermediate between that available on the ward and the intensive therapy provided in the ICU.

Specialized areas also exist which include coronary care, paediatric, neonatal, postoperative recovery, renal and neurosurgical units. In a number of hospitals patients in some of these categories may have to be admitted to the general ICU if such specialized units are not available.

The Department of Health and Social Security (1970) has recommended that 1–2 per cent of the total number of acute beds in a hospital should be designated for general intensive care. This number is *in addition* to the number allocated to specialized units. The Intensive Care Society (1984) has recommended that such a unit should consist of 4–10 beds and should be situated close to the accident and emergency department; operating theatre and recovery room, X-ray, CT scanning and NMR facilities, and the general wards. A recent working party set up by the Association of Anaesthetists (1988) has recommended that each Health District should be provided with such general ICU facilities provided that the unit contains a minimum of 4 beds and has at least 200 admissions per year.

Organization

Staffing

The key feature of a successful ICU is enthusiastic and co-operative team work. *The ICU team* must include intensive-care-trained medical, nursing, and technical staff, physiotherapists, radiographers, dietitians, pharmacists, ward clerks and full-time secretarial support.

Nursing staff

The number of ICU-trained nursing staff required to run a general intensive care unit is determined by factors which include: the average bed occupancy in the unit; the 'dependency categories' of the patient admitted; the hours worked by the nursing staff; and the availability of other staff. The 'dependency category' of the individual patient is determined by the severity of the illness and includes the number of failing systems requiring technical support.

Medical staff

The special qualities required of the ICU consultant clinician have been defined (Safar & Grenvik 1971) as follows:
- decision, action-orientated attitudes and skills of the *anaesthesiologist* and *surgeon*
- knowledge, thoughtfulness and judgement of the *internist*
- inquisitive, data-seeking mind of *the scientist*
- diplomacy of a *UN ambassador*

The parent discipline of the individual ICU clinician is relatively unimportant provided that the individual has received adequate training and experience in intensive care. In the UK the majority of consultants in charge of general intensive care units are anaesthetists. This is probably because anaesthesia is a discipline which provides special expertise in airway care, oxygenation, tracheal intubation, ventilation, resuscitation skills, monitoring, and management of acute physiological changes, all of which are fundamental to the care of the critically ill.

A member of the junior medical staff should be resident on the ICU at all times. This resident doctor should have received adequate training and be proficient in the management of the airway, intubation techniques, basic ventilation procedures, invasive monitoring and other resuscitative procedures involving management of the patient in shock.

Admissions policy

Patients admitted to the ICU either require aggressive therapy for a life-threatening condition that is potentially reversible or require organ support until such time as a definitive diagnosis is made. Patients requiring ventilatory support may have to be given priority for admission to the unit if there are not enough staff and equipped intensive care beds to cope with the demand. In general terms patients admitted to ICU suffer from failure of the respiratory and/or the circulatory systems. In addition the patient may be suffering from sepsis, haematological disorders, neurological problems, gut dysfunction and liver or renal failure. The prospects of survival may decrease in inverse proportion to the number of failing organs. The ICU is not an area to which patients with a hopeless prognosis should be admitted, nor should such intensive therapy be used to prolong the process of dying.

Initial management of the critically-ill patient

Adequate oxygen delivery and appropriate uptake by the tissue cells are vital for survival of an organism and depend upon both adequate *respiratory* function and adequate *cardiovascular* function. Respiratory failure may be defined as a state resulting from the inability of the respiratory system to maintain adequate gaseous exchange with the subject breathing room air at sea level; while shock is the inability of the circulatory system to meet the needs of the tissues for oxygen, nutrients, and removal of toxic metabolites.

The interrelationship of these two systems may be summarized by listing the factors upon which oxygen delivery ultimately depends
- pulmonary gaseous exchange
- haemoglobin oxygen concentration (Hb) and saturation (SO_2)
- haemoglobin oxygen affinity
- cardiac output (CO)
- oxygen consumption ($\dot{V}O_2$)

Oxygen delivery may be improved by one or more of the following measures:

- administration of known concentrations of *oxygen* by Ventimask or by mechanical ventilation
- administration of *colloids* to improve circulating volume
- administration of *blood* to maintain haemoglobin of 10 g/dl
- administration of *inotropes* (dopamine, dobutamine) to improve cardiac function if the patient remains hypotensive in spite of a normal circulating volume
- administration of *vasodilators* such as glyceryl trinitrate (GTN) to reduce the workload of the heart if there is an increased systemic vascular resistance (SVR) that has not responded to volume repletion
- administration of *vasoconstrictors* such as noradrenaline to elevate the blood pressure if the SVR is reduced as a result of vasodilatation in septic-shock states

The remainder of this section will be concerned with the more detailed assessment and management of the patient in respiratory failure.

Assessment of respiratory failure

If the patient is in acute respiratory failure then immediate re-establishment of the airway, adequate alveolar ventilation and oxygenation must take priority over any further assessment.

General
This requires the following information:
- history
- general assessment of
    - cyanosis
    - distress
    - level of consciousness
    - ability to talk
    - patency of the airways
    - pattern of breathing (apnoea, stridor, wheezing, disco-ordination of breathing pattern, tachypnoea, use of accessory muscles)
    - presence of fatigue and exhaustion
    - ability to cough and take deep breaths
    - sputum retention
- clinical examination
- chest X-ray
- ECG

Specific tests

Arterial blood-gas (ABG) analysis on known concentrations of oxygen

Table 19.1 lists partial pressures of the arterial blood-gases (Pao$_2$ and Paco$_2$) to be found in a normal individual breathing a range of inspired oxygen concentrations at sea level (barometric pressure 760 mmHg, 103 kPa).

Table 19.1 The significance of blood-gas analysis

Inspired O_2 concentration (F_iO_2)	21% (Air) (0.21)	50% (0.5)	100% (1.0)
P_iO_2	159 mmHg (20.9 kPa)	380 mmHg (50 kPa)	760 mmHg (103 kPa)
PaO_2	100 mmHg (13 kPa)	250 mmHg (32 kPa)	637 mmHg (85 kPa)
SaO_2	100%	100%	100%
$PaCO_2$	40 mmHg (5.3 kPa)	40 mmHg (5.3 kPa)	40 mmHg (5.3 kPa)

Notes for Table 19.1
While the haemoglobin saturation (SaO_2) and the $PaCO_2$ *remain the same* as the inspired *oxygen concentration* is *increased*, the PaO_2 *should increase accordingly*.

An *'oxygen cascade'* exists between the partial pressure in the inspired gas (P_iO_2) and the resulting partial pressure in the arterial blood (PaO_2). This is due to
- dilution of the inspired gas with water vapour and carbon dioxide already present in the lungs
- ventilation/perfusion ($\dot{V}/\dot{Q}$) inequalities throughout the zones of the lung related to gravity. These will be exaggerated in pathological conditions such as
  - increased intrapulmonary shunting where some alveoli are perfused but not ventilated e.g. collapsed or consolidated alveoli
  - increased physiological dead space where some alveoli are ventilated but not perfused e.g. hypotension or pulmonary-arterial embolism.

In terms of arterial blood-gas analysis respiratory failure is said to be present if when breathing room air (F_iO_2 0.21) at sea level:
PaO_2 is less than 60 mmHg (8 kPa) and
$PaCO_2$ is more than 49 mmHg (6.5 kPa) or less than 35 mmHg (4.5 kPa).

Respiratory mechanics

Peak expiratory flow rates (PEFR)
Vital capacity (VC) — sitting/supine
Respiratory rate (minute volume)
Tidal volume (V_T) (minute volume)

These tests may reflect:
- the ability of the patient to cough and clear his airways
- the response of the patient to bronchodilator therapy
- the ability of the patient to maintain adequate ventilatory function in the supine position i.e. while lying flat to sleep at night
- deterioration over time on trend analysis as a patient becomes fatigued during a period of breathing on his own.

PEFR is a useful way to monitor the response of a patient to bronchodilator therapy but may not be practicable in a patient with respiratory failure who requires more intensive therapy.

VC measures the maximum expiration after a maximum inspiration. The normal value is 70 ml/kg i.e. 5 litres in a 70 kg man. *If the VC is less than 1 litre then the patient may require some form of ventilatory support particularly when lying supine at night*. This test is most useful in patients with respiratory failure resulting from *neuromuscular or myopathic disease states*, and trends may be particularly helpful in determining the ability of the patient to breathe on his own over a period of time. It has limitations in that it requires patient co-operation in order to perform this manoeuvre, it requires experienced personnel to assess the results, and an isolated measurement may not reflect the true ability of the patient to breathe adequately on his own over a period of time.

The respiratory rate or frequency (f) is a simple, non-invasive observation which is part of routine monitoring by the nursing staff. A rapid respiratory rate may reflect the underlying disease process and the ability of the patient to cope with breathing on his own.

Tachypnoea can become exhausting and may lead to a deterioration in oxygen delivery. Rapid, shallow breaths may maintain a 'normal' minute volume but at the price of small tidal volumes which may not provide adequate alveolar ventilation. *The respiratory rate is a significant measurement which must always be taken into account when assessing the patient and the arterial blood-gas analysis.*

Summary of assessment of the patient in respiratory failure

- Sputum retention or retained secretions, associated with an inability to cough, feature prominently in many types of respiratory failure.
- Although the patient may appear to have 'normal' blood gases (Pao_2 of 10–13 kPa) when breathing added oxygen, these are far from normal when breathing 50 per cent oxygen (Table 19.1).
- Blood-gas analysis must be assessed in relationship to
  - a known F_io_2 breathed continuously for 10 minutes prior to blood sample being taken
  - response to treatment (oxygen, ventilation, bronchodilators)
- Normal or low levels of $Paco_2$ may be present in the early stages of respiratory failure but if failure is allowed to progress then the $Paco_2$ may rise as the patient becomes decompensated and exhausted.
- Tachypnoea, increased work of breathing and disco-ordinate patterns of breathing should alert the clinician to provide some form of ventilatory support, including mechanical ventilation, as a matter of urgency.
- Some of the causes of respiratory failure are summarized in Table 19.2.

Mechanical ventilation

The patient may be ventilated by mask or through a tracheal tube passed through the nose or the mouth, or via a tracheostomy. A self-inflating bag with a face mask may be used in the initial stages of resuscitation prior to intubation. Special devices are now available to provide ventilatory support via a mask in patients where it is inappropriate to intubate (Carroll & Branthwaite). In general terms however, mechanical ventilation via a low-pressure cuffed endotracheal tube (ETT) which will also provide access for removal of secretions is the initial method of choice. The patient may need to be anaesthetized for the insertion of this ETT and muscle relaxants may be used to paralyse the vocal chords to aid its passage into the trachea.

Table 19.2 Causes of respiratory failure

Neurological problems
    respiratory centre deranged
    e.g. brain injury, drugs

Spinal cord lesions
    cervical cord damage (including diaphragm function)
    poliomyelitis
    polyneuritis
    tetanus

Neuromuscular junction problems
    neuromuscular blocking agents
    myasthenia gravis

Sleep apnoea

Respiratory muscle problems
    malnutrition
    sepsis
    myopathy

Chest wall problems
    flail chest
    kyphoscoliosis
    scleroderma

Upper airways obstruction
    infection — croup/epiglottis
    trauma
    tumour

Airway resistance increased
    asthma
    bronchitis and emphysema
    secretions

Pulmonary problems
    retained secretions
    infection
    pulmonary oedema
    inhalation of toxic fumes
    septic shock
    near drowning

Cardiovascular problems
    reduced circulating volume
    hypovoloaemic shock
    cardiac pump failure
    pulmonary-artery embolism

Metabolic problems
    metabolic acidosis
    catabolic states

Fatigue
If the patient is breathing with a respiratory rate of more than 35 breaths/min, or the Pa_{O_2} is less than 9.5 kPa breathing 50 per cent oxygen, or the Pa_{CO_2} is rising and the patient is unable to cough or is becoming exhausted, then the patient requires some form of mechanical ventilation irrespective of the underlying diagnosis.

Initial management of a patient on a ventilator

As soon as the patient has been intubated and attached to the machine, *the position of the ETT must be secured and checked to ensure it is correctly situated in the trachea.* Both sides of the chest must move equally on inflation and there must be no evidence of air being inflated into the stomach (p. 72). End-tidal CO_2 monitoring may also be used to confirm the presence of the ETT in the chest. A chest radiograph will confirm the position of the tip in the trachea. It is important that the correct site of this tube is checked every time the position of the patient is changed.

Observations and monitoring of the ventilated patient

General observations

- mental status, comfort and adequacy of pain relief
- anxiety — tranquillizers may be appropriate
- patient's colour — flushed (monitor temperature) or cyanosed (monitor with oximeter)
- chest movement must be equal on both sides with every breath

Monitoring the ventilator (every 30 min–1 h)

- switch on the ventilator!
- set the required inspired-oxygen concentration to be delivered
- monitor the concentration of the inspired oxygen
- set the tidal volume (V_T) at 10 ml/kg and monitor both inspired and expired volumes (beware leaks)
- set the respiratory rate at 12–14 breaths/min
- monitor inflation pressures (P_i) (normal range 15–20 cmH$_2$O)
- set high and low limits of the inflation-pressure alarm
- check humidifier
- check water traps present in the ventilator tubing

Monitoring the patient (every 15–30 min)

- pulse, blood pressure, central venous and/or pulmonary-artery pressures
- oxygen saturation (oximeter)
- end-tidal carbon dioxide (capnograph)
- spontaneous respiratory rate, tidal volume, minute volume
- temperature — hourly (central and peripheral)
- urinary output — hourly
- fluid balance
- secretions aspirated from chest — colour, quantity, thickness

Investigations (daily or more often if required)

- arterial blood gases on known F_iO_2
- urea, creatinine and electrolytes (serum and urine)
- Hb, platelets and bleeding clotting factors
- serum protein and albumin
- others as required e.g. blood cultures, phosphate concentrations
- chest radiograph

It is important to anticipate any problems which might arise while the patient is attached to a positive pressure ventilator. These are summarized below. *Such problems may occur at any time irrespective of whether the patient is being ventilated in the operating theatre, the intensive care unit, an ambulance, a helicopter, or during resuscitation.*

Patient problems on a ventilator
- inability to speak
  - remember such patients may **hear** what is being said
- cardiovascular effects
  - abolition of thoracic pump which hampers venous return and may lead to a reduction in BP
  - cardiac output may be reduced, especially in hypovolaemic states, and may lead to a reduction in BP
  - embarrassment of pulmonary circulation which leads to right heart failure
- pulmonary effects
  - rupture of alveoli in subjects at risk e.g. chronic obstructive airways disease (COPD)
  - right endobronchial intubation (collapse of left lung)
  - uneven ventilation, especially if high inspiratory flow rates are used
  - infection
- metabolic effects
  - hyperventilation may produce a fall in $Paco_2$, and a rise in pH with
    — fall in cardiac output and reduced perfusion of various organs
    — difficulty in weaning patients with obstructive airway disease
  - hypoventilation may produce a rise in $Paco_2$, a fall in pH and a fall in Pao_2 with
    — atelectasis
    — arrhythmias
- possible long-term effects
  - oxygen toxicity if 100 per cent O_2 has been required for prolonged periods
  - tracheal stenosis (rare with low-pressure cuffed tracheal tubes)
  - tracheal dilatation (if increasing volumes of air used to inflate cuff)

Ventilator problems
- obstruction
  - diagnosis— increase in inspiratory pressure on ventilator dial
    — decrease in expired tidal volume
  - causes • kink in corrugated tubing
    - kink in catheter mount
    - patient biting on ETT
    - mucous and debris inside ETT
    - cuff herniation, indentation or protrusion
    - foreign body in bronchus
    - endobronchial intubation
    - bronchospasm
    - pleural effusion
    - pneumothorax

- Leak
    - diagnosis— decrease in inspiratory pressure on ventilator dial
    - — decrease in expired tidal volume
    - causes • tubing attachments to ventilator
        - tubing attachments to humidifier
        - leaking expiratory valve
        - pilot balloon leaks from cuff on ETT
        - cuff leaks
        - ETT in oesophagus!

All these problems must be diagnosed urgently and treated appropriately. *Manual ventilation of the lungs using an inflating bag with added oxygen* may be required while the problems are being sorted out.

Modes of ventilation

The goals of ventilatory management are concerned with adequate gaseous exchange, adequate oxygen delivery and minimization of the oxygen cost of breathing. There are a number of different methods of ventilatory support which may be used to achieve these objectives (Table 19.3).

Table 19.3 Modes of ventilation

- controlled mechanical ventilation (CMV)
    - wave-form patterns
    - differential lung ventilation

- intermittent mandatory ventilation (IMV)

- positive end-expiratory pressure (PEEP)

- continuous positive airway pressure (CPAP)
    - mask
    - tracheal tube

- intermittent positive-pressure ventilation by nasal mask

- high-frequency jet ventilation (HFJV)

- extracorporeal membrane oxygenation (ECMO)

- low-frequency positive-pressure ventilation with extracorporeal CO_2 removal (LFPPV/ECCO$_2$R)

- negative-pressure ventilation
    - tank
    - cuirass

Controlled mechanical ventilation (CMV)

Fully-controlled mechanical ventilation by intermittent positive pressure (IPPV) is the commonest type of ventilation used during anaesthesia, when muscle paralysis is required. This mode of ventilation is frequently used in the initial stages of critical illness while the patient is being stabilized and later during transport of the patient for further investigative procedures. The disadvantages may include: reduction in venous return, reduction in cardiac output, reduction in organ blood flow, ventilation-perfusion inequalities, oliguria with salt and water retention and barotrauma. In order to overcome some of these problems two different techniques may be used in the ICU.

- *Wave-form patterns* may be altered by changing the inspiratory wave form and the inspiratory/expiratory time ratio may be altered for each breath. It may thus be useful to add a pause at the end of the inspiratory phase, with the lung fully inflated, to allow for better distribution of ventilation to lung compartments with different airway resistances. Delivery of the bulk of the tidal volume in the early part of the inspiratory phase, followed by a slow decline in flow, may allow more time for gas to enter the alveoli. In the presence of bronchospasm it may be helpful to prolong the expiratory-time phase in order to allow adequate time for expiration to take place.
- *Differential lung ventilation* involves the insertion of a double-lumen endobronchial tube so that each lung may be ventilated independently. This technique is commonly used in anaesthesia for patients undergoing thoracic surgery. In the ICU two separate ventilators may be required in order to ventilate each lung separately in order to allow for the different time constants of each to be accommodated. It may be particularly useful in the presence of unilateral lung disease.

Intermittent mandatory ventilation (IMV)

Intermittent mandatory ventilation allows the patient to breathe spontaneously in between mandatory tidal volumes delivered by the ventilator at a preset rate. A ventilator with such facilities provides the patient with a range of ventilatory methods extending from fully-controlled mechanical ventilation to spontaneous breathing without any ventilation from the machine at all. The level of mechanical ventilatory support required is judged by the clinical condition of the patient and the investigations already outlined. The advantages of this method are listed in Table 19.4.

Table 19.4 Advantages of IMV

- ventilatory support is matched to suit individual requirement
- reduced adverse effects of mechanical ventilation on respiratory, circulatory and renal function
- reduced need for sedatives and relaxants
- improved access for assessment of clinical status
- gradual transition from high mean airway pressures with ventilation to normal mean airway pressures with spontaneous breathing
- earlier start to the weaning process
- maintains respiratory muscle function
- avoids 'fighting' the ventilator
- more acceptable to the patient psychologically

Positive end-expiratory pressure (PEEP) and continuous positive airway pressure (CPAP)

Positive end-expiratory pressure and continuous positive airway pressure both *aim to elevate the airway pressure during expiration* in order to increase the functional residual capacity and improve arterial oxygenation. This technique is particularly useful in patients with tracheal tubes *in situ* as it compensates for the bypassing of glottic function imposed by the presence of the tube (Quan *et al.*, 1981). PEEP is the term conventionally used when the patient is being mechanically ventilated, while CPAP is used for the spontaneously breathing mode. Continuous positive expiratory airway pressure can be used in either mode with IMV.

Increasing use is being made of the CPAP mask as a form of ventilatory support which may avert the need for intubation. This technique is now used as a form of physiotherapy.

The *disadvantages* of PEEP/CPAP may include increase in physiological deadspace, barotrauma, redistribution of blood flow to poorly ventilated areas, alterations in regional blood flow, reduction in renal output, reduction in cardiac ventricular preload, and equalization of the cardiac right and left ventricular-filling pressures with shift of the interventricular septum (Jardin, 1981).

Positive-pressure ventilation by nasal mask

This technique applies positive-pressure ventilation via a tightly-fitting unobstructed nasal mask. This obviates the need for an endotracheal tube. *Full ventilatory support is given via this method.* It therefore differs from CPAP which only applies positive expiratory pressure at the end of each spontaneous breath.

This type of nasal ventilation is particularly useful for patients with chronic respiratory failure who get fatigued with the effort of breathing. An increasing number of patients are being taught to use this method in their own homes.

High-frequency jet ventilation (HFJV)

This includes a group of ventilatory techniques which use small tidal volumes (1–5 ml/kg) and rapid respiratory rates (1–15 Hz). The main advantage of these techniques is a reduction in peak airway pressures compared with fully-controlled mechanical ventilation. HFJV may be particularly useful in the presence of a bronchopleural fistula.

Extracorporeal membrane oxygenation (ECMO)

ECMO involves controlled mechanical ventilation with extracorporeal support using arteriovenous membrane oxygenation. This elaborate technique has been used in patients with severe and intractable respiratory failure in order to 'buy time' for the lung to repair itself. The results from such techniques have been disappointing.

Low-frequency positive-pressure ventilation with extracorporeal CO_2 removal (LFPPV/ECCO$_2$R)

This is a totally different concept from ECMO and involves 'resting the lung' (Gattinoni, 1986). The rationale behind this technique involves preventing further damage to the lungs by reducing their motion. Controlled intermittent positive-pressure ventilation is applied at the rate of 3–5 sighs/min, oxygenation (1–2 litres/min) is produced using an apnoeic technique via the trachea, and carbon dioxide is removed by means of an extracorporeal circulation.

The goals of this technique are

- *to overcome tidal-volume maldistribution* due to non-homogeneous lung compliance
- *to avoid high pressure/volume ventilation* with its related complications
- *to provide a better environment* for lung healing

Subatmospheric or 'negative' pressure ventilation

This type of ventilation enhances the normal pattern of breathing and is therefore more normal physiologically. It was originally developed during the poliomyelitis epidemics in the 1950s but these 'tank' ventilators were found to be unsuitable in patients with bulbar palsy and swallowing difficulties which result in tracheal aspiration of secretions in the presence of an unprotected airway. *These tank ventilators* are large and cumbersome but they continue to have a role to play with patients who require uncomplicated nocturnal ventilation. The *cuirass* jacket type of ventilator provides mobility and domiciliary care for patients who require continuous ventilatory support for periods of time during both the day and night and who do not require bronchial toilet or airway protection.

Weaning patients from ventilator support

Weaning patients from ventilatory support must be considered as soon as the underlying problems necessitating ventilation have begun to be resolved. Factors affecting the ability of the patient to wean successfully are summarized in Table 19.5.

Table 19.5 Factors affecting ability to wean

Failure of one or more systems:
• respiratory
• cardiac/circulatory
• neurological
• metabolic
Fluid and electrolyte imbalance
Feeding problems
Fever and infection
Fatigue of respiratory muscles

Most of these factors have been mentioned earlier and they must be identified and corrected accordingly. Successful treatment of infection and fever is particularly important because increased ventilatory requirements with high oxygen consumption have been reported in pyrexic patients. Ventilatory support may be needed to reduce the increased work load of breathing in such catabolic patients. If any of these factors are present then fatigue will occur when the rate of energy consumption of the muscles is greater than the energy supplied to them by the blood.

Careful monitoring of the patient is a fundamental part of the weaning process and the essential components are listed in Table 19.6. Particular attention must be paid to deterioration in any of these variables within a weaning period.

Table 19.6   Monitoring of patients being weaned from ventilators

- clinical status
- pulse and blood pressure
- temperature
- arterial blood gases on known F_iO_2
- respiratory rate
- pattern of breathing
- vital capacity
- tidal volume
- minute volume
- CO_2 production ⎫
- O_2 consumption ⎬ if facilities are available
- O_2 cost of breathing ⎭

Methods of weaning

The weaning process should be started with the patient in the sitting position and with all secretions aspirated from the chest. Weaning should begin early in the day and the appropriate system used to suit the needs of the patient (Browne, 1988).

In general terms the majority of patients on the ICU are weaned using IMV with PEEP/CPAP as required. Using this technique the rate of the ventilator can be turned up or down according to the requirements of the patient without having to change circuits. Refinements in modern ventilator design have now overcome the problems of increased respiratory workloads which were originally associated with patients breathing spontaneously through machines. The weaning process is monitored using the respiratory rate and blood gases as guidelines, while the ventilator rate is reduced progressively to zero with the patient breathing satisfactorily on his own.

The weaning process may be made more comfortable for the patient by using a tracheal tube passed through the nose rather than the mouth. The nasal route obviates the problem of the patient biting the tube and obstructing the airway. A tracheostomy tube may be easier to manage in the long term and has the advantage that the patient may be able to eat and drink normally once the larynx is competent even though he may still require ventilatory support. A further advantage of a tracheostomy is that special tracheostomy tubes have been designed which may allow the patient to talk when disconnected from the ventilator.

Extubation following successful weaning

Although the patient may be fully weaned from the ventilator, certain criteria must be met before that patient may be extubated. The tracheal tube may be removed only when it is no longer required for airway maintenance, airway protection, or bronchial toilet and physiotherapy. In some circumstances a mini-tracheostomy tube may provide useful alternative access for bronchial toilet to aspirate secretions from the chest.

General management of the ventilated patient

Circulatory status

As indicated at the beginning of the section on initial management, appropriate support of the circulatory system is as important as the management of respiratory failure. Methods for improving oxygen transport were listed in that section. Central-venous-pressure monitoring is an important guide for fluid-challenge therapy and inotropic support may be required if the patient does not respond. Cardiac dysrhythmias must be corrected by ensuring that the electrolyte balance is correct (with particular reference to the serum potassium) and then using the appropriate drugs, electrical pacing, or cardioversion as required.

Renal function

Patients requiring ventilatory support and who are critically ill will require catheterization of the bladder to monitor the urinary output on an hourly basis. This should be maintained at 1 ml/kg per h using appropriate fluid challenges in the first instance. Diuretics should never be used to treat a low urinary output in the presence of hypovolaemia. Renal function must be monitored by measuring the serum creatinine and urea on a daily basis. The creatinine is an important measurement with which to diagnose impending renal failure as the presence of an elevated urea may be due to a number of other factors such as catabolic states. Patients with impending renal failure should be managed with the advice of renal physicians.

Gastrointestinal function

Gut failure is increasingly recognized as an important element in the critically-ill patient. A nasogastric tube should be passed into the stomach and aspirated at regular intervals. 'Adynamic ileus' is a common response to stress, and normal gastric and colonic function may not return for many days. Stress ulcers may also occur and prophylactic measures should be taken in all patients. Such measures may include the administration of drugs such as ranitidine or omeprazine which inhibit the production of acid gastric contents. Some authorities consider the administration of topical gut antibiotics may be useful in protecting against liberation of toxins, infection and multiple organ failure.

Nutrition

Feeding by the normal *enteral* route should be used whenever possible but in the critically-ill patient requiring ventilatory support, gut failure may also be present. *Intravenous total parenteral nutrition* (TPN) should then be used as malnutrition may have profound effects on subsequent patient management. The effects of malnutrition on respiratory function are outlined in Table 19.7. The diaphragm loses mass in proportion to loss of body weight and this may be associated with fatigue and subsequent ventilatory failure. Nitrogen and potassium are lost from the body as part of the systemic response to stress and as a result the muscles themselves are thought to become myopathic in critically-ill patients. Any such muscle weakness may inhibit the weaning process from mechanical ventilatory support.

Table 19.7 The effects of malnutrition

- severe respiratory muscle weakness
- ineffective cough leading to alveolar collapse
- decreased production of surfactant leading to alveolar collapse
- decreased production of elastic fibres in lung parenchyma
- impaired immunocompetence leading to infection
- decreased ventilatory response to hypoxia or hypercarbia
- increased work of breathing

After Rochester D F and Aora N S (1982).

Total parenteral nutrition (TPN)

TPN involves the aseptic insertion of a designated central venous catheter (preferably 'tunnelled' subcutaneously to avoid infection), through which the appropriate nutrients may be administered until gut function returns. Comprehensive accounts of optimal regimens for parenteral nutrition have been given by Willatts (1984) so only broad outlines will be given.

Parenteral nutrition should aim to supply water, nitrogen, carbohydrates, fat, electrolytes, trace elements and vitamins. In some circumstances a mixture may be prepared by the pharmacy using a 3-litre bag, the contents of which can then be given to the patient over 24 hours. In the critically-ill patient however, fluid balance may be a problem in that fluids may have to be restricted. A more flexible system is therefore required.

It is important to provide sufficient energy to allow the utilization of amino acids for protein synthesis. This may range from 200 kcal/g nitrogen to 125 kcal/g nitrogen in the hypercatabolic patient following trauma or sepsis. This energy may be provided from carbohydrate in the form of glucose and fat in the form of intralipid solutions.

Glucose administration should not exceed more than 4 mg/kg per min. This is to avoid excessive production of carbon dioxide which occurs in the presence of high glucose loads. Glucose should be administered on a continuous basis throughout the 24 hours and blood sugar should be monitored at hourly intervals. Insulin may be required to maintain the blood glucose within the normal range.

Intralipid is the compound used for the administration of fat in the UK. It is preferable to give intralipid during the early part of the night to avoid any interference with blood analysis which may result from lipaemic serum. Intralipid has the advantage that it provides a high-energy source and can be given via peripheral veins if necessary. Both glucose and fat may be equally effective in their nitrogen-sparing effects, so both energy sources can be used in equal quantities.

Amino-acid solutions provide the source of nitrogen and there is a wide variety of manufactured products on the market with little to choose between them. These solutions should contain a mixture of the essential and non-essential amino acids (L form) in balanced proportions avoiding excess glycine. The nitrogen content available from the various products may range from 9 g/litre to 14 g/litre and 18 g/litre. Amino-acid solutions should always be administered simultaneously with glucose. Intralipid may be added to the combination as appropriate.

Many of the amino-acid solutions contain electrolytes such as sodium, potassium, calcium, magnesium and chloride. Serum electrolytes should be monitored closely and supplements administered as required. Particular attention should be paid to phosphate levels as hypophosphataemia has been associated with respiratory difficulties.

Various solutions are available which contain mixtures of water-soluble vitamins (e.g. Parentrovite), fat-soluble vitamins (e.g. Vit lipid), and minerals with trace elements (e.g. Addamel). Each of these preparations together with folic acid should be added daily to the feeding regimen.

Water, albumin and blood products should be given, if required, as part of the planned fluid-balance protocol for the day.

Complications of parenteral feeding may include sepsis, thrombosis, electrolyte disturbances, glucose intolerance, respiratory distress, metabolic acidosis and impairment of liver function.

Guide for basic TPN regimens

Many critically-ill patients may need to have fluid restriction so i.v. feeding should begin with 500 ml 20 per cent dextrose and 500 ml of an amino-acid solution (9 or 14 g/litre nitrogen) given concurrently over 24-hour periods. 500 ml Intralipid 10 or 20 per cent may then be added at a later stage overnight. As more space for feeding becomes available the volume of 20 per cent dextrose and amino-acid-containing solution may be increased to 1 litre of each. As the patient's condition improves the amino-acid-containing solution may be changed to one containing 18 g/litre nitrogen. If fluid restriction remains an important part of patient management then smaller volumes of more concentrated solutions may be given over 24 hours e.g. 500 ml 50 per cent dextrose, and 500 ml amino-acid solution (18 g/litre nitrogen).

Vitamins, minerals, essential elements, and folic acid *must supplement all feeding regimens*.

Routine monitoring must include daily weight, serum electrolytes, creatinine, urea, Hb; twice weekly serum calcium, phosphate, protein, albumin, liver-function tests and weekly serum magnesium and zinc levels.

Enteral feeding

This is the provision of nutritional support via the normally functioning gastrointestinal tract and should be used whenever possible to avoid the complications of TPN. Enteral feeds can be given by mouth, by nasogastric, nasoduodenal or nasojejunal infusions or by a feeding gastrotomy or jejunostomy. The commonest method for the ICU patient is the nasogastric tube. Enteral feeding should be introduced gradually if the patient has required nutritional support by the parenteral route and the TPN regimen should be reduced appropriately as the enteral feeding is increased.

A wide variety of sterile, canned, commercial preparations are available which can be prescribed according to the particular needs of each individual patient. The enteral feed can be administered via a narrow-bore nasogastric tube or via a large-bore Ryles tube if gastric emptying is uncertain. A feeding pump may be useful to control the drip rate if the feed is infused over a 12–24 hour period. Special enteral preparations are available for specific requirements and include: concentrated feeds for fluid-restricted patients; low-glucose high-fat feeds for patients weaning from ventilatory support who may not tolerate the glucose content of the normal feed; and high-nitrogen-containing feeds for patients who have been catabolic and require protein to improve muscle function.

Analgesia and sedation

The provision of adequate pain relief is fundamental to the management of all patients undergoing intensive care. The clinician must be particularly alert to this problem as the patient with a cuffed tracheal tube on a ventilator cannot verbalize his discomfort and it may be inappropriate for him to communicate by other means. The diagnosis of the source of the pain is important and surgical advice must be sought if necessary. Local analgesic nerve blocks or epidural opiates may be useful adjuncts to the more routine methods of i.v. opiate infusions supplemented by bolus doses for painful therapeutic manoeuvres. Pethidine, morphine, diamorphine, fentanyl, codeine phosphate and indomethacin are the most frequently used analgesic agents at present (Chapter 18).

Sedation is a term which includes relief of anxiety as well as sleep in the intensive care situation. There is no satisfactory single agent which works well with every patient all of the time. Anxiolytic agents include the benzodiazepines such as lorazepam, midazolam and diazepam. The need for sedation may range from anaesthesia for therapeutic manoeuvres or surgery, to night sedation with the patient being mobilized and alert during the day. Agents include thiopentone, etomidate or propofol for induction of anaesthesia; propofol, ketamine, midazolam or chlormethiazole for continuous infusions; and temazepam, chlormethiazole or chloral for night sedation. Alcohol may also have a useful role to play.

In practice a combination of analgesics, sedatives and anxiolytic agents are used in a variety of different ways to improve the well being and comfort of the patient. The level of sedation must be constantly assessed and great caution must be used with continuous infusions of such drugs as midazolam and fentanyl because their effects may be particularly prolonged in the presence of sepsis or liver or renal failure.

Control of infection

A patient in the ICU is particularly prone to infection for a number of reasons:
- depression of the immunological system as a result of the ongoing illness
- the presence of intravascular cannulae, three-way taps and transducers, urinary catheters and tracheal tubes
- infection from items of equipment if adequate precautions have not been taken (e.g. nebulizers, humidifiers) or cross infection from items such as stethoscopes
- pulmonary aspiration of organisms from the pharynx or regurgitated from the gastrointestinal tract around a leaking tracheal-tube cuff. This problem may be exaggerated in patients treated with antacids or H_2 receptor antagonists.
- super infection by resistant organisms as a result of antibiotic treatment
- malnutrition
- pulmonary oedema

Handwashing with hibiscrub or iodine is mandatory for every single individual who attends or visits each patient. This must be done both before and after seeing the patient in order to avoid cross infection between patients. All invasive procedures should be carried out under strictly sterile conditions. *Disposable gloves* should be worn for all procedures concerning any form of *contact with body fluids*. Advice should be sought from the microbiology and control of infection departments on a daily or more frequent basis, with reference to further protective manoeuvres, the appropriate investigations required, and specific antibiotic therapy as and when needed. The physiotherapist also plays a key role in the prophylaxis and management of pulmonary infections.

Ethics and scoring systems

The aim of intensive care is to provide the patient with the appropriate support until such time as he is fit to leave the unit. In the presence of inadequate resources to meet the demands for such therapy, clinicians are being asked to look for methods which will define those patients who will benefit most from such sophisticated and expensive technology.

Various 'severity of disease' scoring systems have been developed to look at this problem but it is difficult to make judgements on such predictions for a number of reasons. These reasons include individual variation in the response of the patient to the disease process, the advent of new methods of treatment, and the ultimate quality of life of the patient discharged from the ICU to the general ward, and then hopefully from the hospital to the community.

The scoring system which is currently being assessed on a national basis in the UK is known as the APACHE II severity of disease classification system (Knaus, 1985). This system scores 12 physiological measurements (such as temperature, mean arterial blood pressure, heart rate, electrolytes etc.) according to their degree of deviation from the normal range. Additional scores are given for the depth of coma, the age of the patient, the presence of defined chronic disease and whether any emergency surgery was performed immediately before admission to intensive care. The sum of the score is an expression of the degree of physiological derangement. *The higher the score, the worse the outlook.* The term APACHE was coined from the initial letters of the phrase **A**cute **P**hysiological **A**nd **C**hronic **H**ealth **E**valuation.

The aims of the APACHE scoring system are:
- to provide a prognostic indicator of outcome for groups of patients with a clearly defined diagnosis
- to compare different policies and treatment regimens
- to compare efficiency of intensive care in different hospitals over a period of time
- to provide a means of clinical audit
- to rationalize an expensive commodity

Recent studies have shown that when clinical judgement is used in combination with the Apache II scoring system, a specific computer programme analysis can provide an accurate prediction of death (Chang, 1989).

In general terms, however, it may have to be the *quality of life* as well as *the overall outcome* which will be the determining factor in whether the application of this technology is justifiable for future patients suffering from similar disease states. This area is a minefield of ethical and moral dilemmas which are constantly changing in the face of scientific advances and financial constraints. The emphasis in patient management in the future may have to be **care** rather than **cure**. This may range from the ability to enable the patient to make a full recovery, returning to work or the community, to providing facilities to enable the patient to leave this world peacefully.

Further reading

Rochester D F, Arora N S. Respiratory muscle failure. *Medical Clinics of North America* 1983; **67**: 573–97.

Browne D R G. Weaning patients from ventilators (Part 2). *Hospital Update* 1988: 1898–906.

Chang R W S, Lee B, Jacobs S. Accuracy of decisions to withdraw therapy in critically ill patients: clinical judgement versus a computer model. *Critical Care Medicine* 1989; **17:11**: 1091–7.

Gattinoni L, Pesenti A, Mascheroni D, *et al.* Low frequency positive pressure ventilation with extracorporeal CO_2 removal in severe acute respiratory failure. JAMA 1986; **256:7**: 881–6.

Knaus W A, Draper E A, *et al.* Apache II: a severity of disease classification system. *Critical Care Medicine* 1985; **13**: 818–29.

Safar, P, Grenvik A. Organisation and physical education in critical care medicine. *Anesthesiology* 1977; **47**: 82–95.

Willatts S M. Design of an optimal parenteral nutrition regime. *British Journal of Parenteral Therapy* 1984; **5**: 117–23.

Index